Psychosomatic Disorders in Childhood

also by Melitta Sperling

The Major Neuroses and Behavior Disorders in Children

Psychosomatic Disorders in Childhood

Melitta Sperling, M.D.
edited and with contributions by
OTTO E. SPERLING, M.D.

JASON ARONSON
NEW YORK • LONDON

LC: 76-22870

ISBN: 0-87668-274-3

Library of Congress Cataloging in Publication Data

Sperling, Melitta.
    Psychosomatic disorders in childhood.

    Bibliography
    Includes index.
    1. Pediatrics—Psychosomatic aspects. I. Sperling,
Otto E. II. Title.
RJ47.5.S63   618.9'2008

Contents

Contents

Classical Psychoanalysis and Its Applications

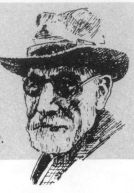

A SERIES OF BOOKS
EDITED BY ROBERT LANGS, M.D.

Robert Langs
THE TECHNIQUE OF
   PSYCHOANALYTIC
   PSYCHOTHERAPY, VOLS. I AND II

THE THERAPEUTIC INTERACTION,
   TWO-VOLUME SET

THE BIPERSONAL FIELD

THE THERAPEUTIC INTERACTION:
   A SYNTHESIS

Judith Kestenberg
CHILDREN AND PARENTS:
   PSYCHOANALYTIC STUDIES IN
   DEVELOPMENT

Melitta Sperling
THE MAJOR NEUROSES AND
   BEHAVIOR DISORDERS IN
   CHILDREN

Peter L. Giovacchini
PSYCHOANALYSIS OF CHARACTER
   DISORDERS

PSYCHOTHERAPY OF PRIMITIVE
   MENTAL STATES

Otto Kernberg
BORDERLINE CONDITIONS AND
   PATHOLOGICAL NARCISSISM

OBJECT-RELATIONS THEORY AND
   CLINICAL PSYCHOANALYSIS

William A. Console
Richard D. Simons
Mark Rubinstein
THE FIRST ENCOUNTER

Humberto Nagera
FEMALE SEXUALITY AND THE
   OEDIPUS COMPLEX

OBSESSIONAL NEUROSES:
   DEVELOPMENTAL
   PSYCHOPATHOLOGY

Willi Hoffer
THE EARLY DEVELOPMENT AND
   EDUCATION OF THE CHILD

William Meissner
THE PARANOID PROCESS

Mardi Horowitz
STRESS RESPONSE SYNDROMES

HYSTERICAL PERSONALITY

Victor Rosen
STYLE, CHARACTER AND LANGUAGE

Charles Sarnoff
LATENCY

Heinz Lichtenstein
THE DILEMMA OF HUMAN IDENTITY

Simon Grolnick,
Leonard Barkin, Editors
in collaboration with
Werner Muensterberger,
BETWEEN FANTASY AND REALITY:
   TRANSITIONAL OBJECTS AND
   PHENOMENA

ARONSON

Series Introduction

It is an honor and a pleasure to have for this series a second volume from Melitta Sperling, here most ably assisted by her husband, Otto, himself a prominent psychoanalyst, who upon her death assumed editorial responsibility for the present work. The wide acclaim accorded her first volume, *The Major Neuroses and Behavior Disorders in Children*, attests to the depth and clinical usefulness of her uniquely perceptive investigations. In the present work are presented Dr. Sperling's pioneering studies of psychosomatic and pregenitally founded disorders, studies every mental health professional, concerned on any level with these often puzzling and difficult-to-treat syndromes, will welcome. In this, her final effort as a psychoanalytic researcher and practitioner, her remarkable qualities, both professional and individual, are more than evident. She will long be remembered as a classical psychoanalyst whose investigation and treatment of a wide range of emotional disorders opened new avenues of understanding where confusion had prevailed.

Robert Langs, M.D.

Preface

Melitta Sperling was successful in the treatment of cases which previously had been in psychoanalysis but without results. When asked how somebody could learn her technique short of supervision, she would point to the case histories which she had published. "Theories may come and go, but the case history is the fundamental truth." It is true that reading is very important; the psychoanalyst can treat only relatively few cases. Reading gives him the opportunity to borrow from the experiences of others. However, what is often not explicit in a case history is the influence of the therapist's personality.

One of the outstanding character traits of Melitta Sperling was her courage. Often when the experts had given up, she would take over and rescue the patient from the operating table or from the psychiatric hospital. If I compare her technique with my own, the following comes to mind. When I treated ulcerative colitis with psychoanalysis in Vienna in the 1930's, I waited until the patient was discharged from the hospital, where he had been treated with Peru balsam enemas. In the symptom-free interval, I would treat him in my office, aiming at a prevention of a relapse. He was still, however, under supervision and treatment by his internist. When the symptoms returned, he went right back to the hospital. How different was the technique that Melitta Sperling used.

She regarded psychoanalysis as a powerful instrument that could have an immediate effect on the acutely ill patient. Therefore she would not wait for a symptom-free interval. Sometimes a child would be brought to her office wrapped in a blanket with high fever and bloody diarrhea. In order to prevent a splitting of the transference, she would insist that the psychoanalyst be the primary physician, while the internist or other specialists serve only as occasional consultants. Only too often, when a psychiatrist prescribes medication, the patient regards the drug as the therapeutic agent and what he says as merely an expression of his bedside manner. A patient of Melitta Sperling had to put all his hopes of recovery not in play, not in drugs, not in the "magic couch," but in the insights which he could arrive at in the psychoanalysis. She was suspicious of tepid positive transference, which is only an adjustment of the patient to the psychoanalytic situation without real cooperation. With a benevolent perserverance, she would pursue resistances even if it took years. The child had to know that he was responsible for his apparently physical symptoms, that he could replace them with others or stop them altogether.

Therapeutic successes as reported in the nonanalytic literature are not convincing. Often the prominent symptom is replaced by another which is not as spectacular and which had not been recognized by the author as a replacement. In contrast, in many cases reported in this book there is not only a follow-up of many years but also a consideration of silent symptom substitutes like accidents, impoverishment of the personality, or failure in school or job or social life.

November 1975   Otto E. Sperling, M.D.

Introduction

In this volume I deal with my experiences in the psychoanalytic treatment and investigation of psychosomatically sick children. In the ten years of pediatric practice preceding my psychoanalytic training, I had made the observation that emotional factors and the mother's handling of her sick child seemed to play an important role in the child's illness and in the speed of recovery. I also realized that the fact that my prescriptions were more effective with some children was due to the positive relationship I had established with their mothers.

In 1940, with the help and support of the late Dr. B. Kramer, Chief of the Pediatrics Department of the Brooklyn Jewish Hopsital, I established the Children's Psychiatric Clinic there. At that time it was not a common thing for a psychoanalyst to psychoanalytically treat physically sick children in a hospital setting. This association with the pediatric department of a general hospital afforded me the opportunity to select my patients from various other departments such as allergy, dermatology, gastroenterology, and neurology and to conduct treatment and research on a great variety of psychosomatic syndromes, some of which had been neither investigated nor treated psychoanalytically in children before. This association also made it possible for me to study children with severe illness (bronchial asthma, ulcerative colitis, etc.) in the hospital ward during the acute phases of the illness. Some of these experiences are reported and discussed in this book. Here I should like to state briefly that there can also be advantages to working psychoanalytically within a general hospital. There, physicians who feel threatened in their abilities to treat these patients can be convinced of the effectiveness of the psychoanalytic approach. These physicians can see the patient and follow up the course of treatment in regularly scheduled clinical conferences. One has to be careful, though, not to expose the patient by giving the medical and other personnel a chance to misuse personal information about him. For this reason, intimate disclosures of the patient and notes of the analyst should not be entered into the official charts but into a separate file kept by and only accessible to the analyst.

I was also consulted by pediatricians, social workers, and mothers about problems with infants and children of preverbal age. This kind of practice is usually not within the domain of psychoanalysts or psychiatrists since one essential prerequisite for such treatment is a patient's ability to communicate with the analyst. New methods and modifications of existing ones had to be found to make such treatment not only possible but also successful.

Two discoveries deserve special mention here, both from the standpoint of child development theory and from the standpoint of the technique for treating the psychosomatically sick— especially young children. One discovery is the psychosomatic type of object relationship. The other is the introduction of simultaneous treatment of mother and child with its various modifications, such as (1) treatment of the mother preceding that of the child, (2) concomitant treatment of mother and child, (3) intermittent treatment of mother and child, (4) indirect treatment of the child through treatment of the mother, and (5) treatment of the mother after conclusion of the child's treatment. The clinical material of this volume abundantly illustrates the dynamics of the mother-child relationship in operation.

The psychosomatic type of object relationship is one of the pathological vicissitudes of the child's symbiotic relationship with his mother. In this type of relationship, the mother, because of her own neurotic needs, encourages bodily illness and dependence of the child by the special care she gives to the child when he is sick. She rejects any overt expression of "crazy" neurotic behavior and any expression of "bad" aggression or sexuality. To be sick and dependent means to be "good." Aggressive and other objectionable (to the mother) and forbidden (sexual) impulses have to be repressed and are discharged through bodily channels in the various psychosomatic symptoms. In reality, the child's illness does make him more submissive. Still the struggle with mother goes on, but only in the symptoms, using identification and aggression (turned against the self) as the main mechanisms. Besides innate constitutional factors, the mother's preoccupation with certain organs and organ functions result in an early acquired disposition in the child to respond with a disturbance of these specific organs and functions in a traumatic situation. That is to say, not only the choice of psychosomatic illness but also the specific symptomatology depend to a large degree on the quality of the mother-child relationship, as I shall try to show in the various chapters of this book.

The simultaneous treatment of mother and child proved a method which not only made it possible to treat these patients successfully but which also permitted observation both of the mutual effects of the mother-child dynamics and of changes in these during the treatment. I should add that, in my method of simultaneous treatment, both mother and child are treated by the same analyst, but in separate sessions. Some child analysts who apply simultaneous treatment, particularly in England, have mother and child treated by two different analysts who do not communicate directly, but rather through a supervisor. I have come to believe that such an approach unnecessarily complicates the treatment. Mother and child are a unit and should be treated as a unit. In addition, the team approach does not permit the analyst to experience and observe in operation the unconscious rapport between the mother and her child nor to perceive the changes which occur during treatment. It would seem to me that this misapplication of the method of simultaneous treatment is due, in part, to the fact that the role of the mother-child relationship, in both the genesis and maintenance of the child's illness, is not sufficiently understood nor accepted.

Although seeming to accept a unifying mind-body concept, most child analysts divide the psychosomatically sick child between themselves and medical specialists. But once such a division is made, it becomes difficult to convince the child that certain bodily symptoms are controllable and should be controlled by the patient. Particularly with hospitalized children, the team approach and anaclitic therapy are the most frequently used. However, these approaches may render psychoanalytic treatment inapplicable later, because the child, who at first has been indulged and considered incapable of tolerating frustration, comes to consider analytic treatment as an imposition which he resents rather than desires. Preparatory or concomitant treatment of the mother and some educational work with the hospital personnel are necessary steps for a successful outcome. Most important is to speed up the discharge from the hospital and to prepare the patient for clinical or office treatment because the hospital setting does not lend itself well to this type of psychoanalytically oriented treatment. The techniques of treatment and, in particular, the management of the transferences and resistances from the child, the family, and the various physicians, are illustrated and discussed on the basis of the case material in this book.

PART 1

TECHNICAL AND THEORETICAL CONSIDERATIONS

1

The Concept of Psychosomatic Disease

by Otto E. Sperling, M.D.

Most people, if exposed to danger, show two groups of reactions. On the one hand, they experience anxiety and an impulse to run; on the other, they are aware of changes in body functioning—either perspiration or trembling or acceleration of the pulse and heart pounding or diarrhea or any combination of these symptoms. The degree of these reactions is very different in different people. When the danger has passed, psychological equilibrium is established and the physical symptoms disappear. When experimentally produced, such reactions in different body systems are the subject of psychosomatic research, but they are not psychosomatic diseases.

In some people the reaction to danger is only physical. These people deny or repress any psychological sense of anxiety and complain only about the phenomena in their body, which they regard as physical disease. In these cases, in a psychoanalysis, the repression of anxiety or other emotions can be lifted and the person can learn to deal with the danger in an appropriate way. These also are not psychosomatic diseases.

If a person has a paralysis of the arm and careful examination by the neurologist can reveal that the symptom is not based on a disease of the central nervous system or any peripheral nerve, or any other organ, we say the paralysis is functional or psychogenic, and not organic. We know that anything psychological is going on in the brain, but brain research cannot explain it. Psychoanalysis can explain the paralysis: a fantasy is translated into body language. The arm might be genitalized (Ferenczi, 1926). It might represent the penis and be being used for the expression of unconscious conflict. The diagnosis would be conversion hysteria. If this disease had existed for a long time and had led to an immobilzation of the joints and an atrophy of the musculature of the arm as a consequence of its not being used, such secondary complications would be organic and should be treated by the proper specialist. They would not be a psychosomatic disease.

The opposite process can also take place. The success of open heart surgery can be frustrated or annulled by a fully unexpected, severe psychological reaction, even psychosis. Any operation can symbolize a castration and thus mobilize a psychoneurosis. The unwillingness of the patient to undertake rehabilitative measures during convalencence may require the services of a psychotherapist. It was always known that psychological factors had an important influence on the cause of tuberculosis. I remember, for instance, a case of a severe exacerbation of tuberculosis which occurred in a woman after she had seduced the husband of her sister. She denied remorse, but an unconscious feeling of guilt had apparently reduced her resistance to the disease. Psychological factors can probably, in some cases, also reduce the resistance against colds (K. Menninger, 1934; Saul, 1938). Sugar has been found in the urine of football players after exciting games and in students after hard examination, and hyperglycemia occurs in aviators and soldiers exposed to danger. Suggestion under hypnosis has altered the blood sugar level (Dunbar, 1938a). The course of diabetes mellitus can be influenced by depression, by anxiety, and by unconscious conflicts (Weiss and English, 1949). In these situations, psychoanalysis can help, but it cannot substitute for diet and insulin treatment.

Psychosomatic diseases are different. These are organic diseases which produce visible changes in x-rays and at autopsy, often with changes in the chemistry. They have been the domain of the internist or other specialists, and have been treated with bed rest, drugs, diets, and change of climate. In conversion hysteria, Freud (1905a) had conceded that there is a somatic compliance "offered by some normal or pathological process in or connected with one of the bodily organs." The location of the hysterical symptom might have been motivated by a previous organic disease, or by some inferiority of this organ. But this is only of theoretical importance. The organ is not really sick; it is only a *locus minoris resistentiae.* In the practice of psychoanalysis, it is more important that this organ is fit for the projection of a fantasy. The insistence on somatic compliance is a resistance. The patient is made to feel that he is fully responsible for his disease, that he has created it, maintains it, and that he is the only one who, with the help of the psychoanalyst, can undo it. Whether it be conversion hysteria or psychosomatic disease, the patient must accept the responsibility for the disease.

My experiences with war neurosis (1950) have taught me that the ability to blame somebody else for the disease can worsen very substantially the prognosis of any disease. The fracture of a leg, if it occurs as a sports accident, would be cured in four months. But if it happens in a war, the patient may never stop limping. After a fracture it is necessary to mobilize the affected joint and to strengthen the musculature: a process which can be very painful. If somebody else is responsible for the fracture, the patient is not able to mobilize enough energy and endurance for this task. The same applies to psychosomatic disease. If this is an ailment which has befallen the sufferer like any other disease, and if it is the responsibility of the psychoanalyst to cure him, the patient is not able to mobilize enough energy to overcome his resistances and to make the necessary effort in the treatment.

The psychosomatic diseases dealt with in this volume are organic diseases which have proven accessible to psychoanalysis and psychotherapy, and which, when treated in this way, show better results than with any other treatment. It was already known during the Middle Ages that the pilgrimage to certain shrines could cure diseases which had resisted the efforts of medical doctors. Among physicians, George Ernst Stahl was the first one who believed that the knowledge and understanding of how the soul functions is more useful than the knowledge of chemistry and physics. In a dissertation published in 1702, under the title *De Medicina Medicinae Necessaria,* he pointed out "the stupendous, sudden and quick effect of the so-called passions and affects on the body." Toward the end of the nineteenth century, as hypnosis was used more and more in the treatment of hysteria, it was found out that it also could stop an asthmatic attack and mucous colitis. Most convincing was the fact that psychosomatic symptoms could be induced by hypnosis—for example: urticaria, wheezing, vomiting, migraine, and a variety of skin reactions (Seitz 1953). Among psychoanalysts, Smith Ely Jelliffe was the first to use psychoanalysis for the treatment of psychosomatic diseases. In 1916, he wrote with Elida Evans, "Psoriasis as an Hysterical Conversion". He also treated migraine and epilepsy with psychoanalysis. In Vienna it was Felix Deutsch (1923) who first extended the use of psychoanalysis for the treatment of the effort syndrome. For many years he was a most important contributor to psychosomatic medicine. Still, when Groddeck (1923) demonstrated that he treated organic disease like conversion hysteria, he shocked the psychoanalysts. He was the first to maintain that menstrual cramps are psychogenic. In spite of the valuable contributions by such pioneers as Dunbar, Alexander, and Binger, not many psychoanalysts are willing to take on a psychosomatic case for treatment, and psychosomatic cases are not acceptable for supervision. The reason might be that in some cases, when cortisone treatment has brought psychosomatic diseases to a sudden stop, psychosis has followed. The alternation of psychosomatic disease and psychosis has been observed by a number of researchers (Brody, 1952; Kerman, 1946; Lidz et al., 1952). This danger has been overestimated. In the many years of Melitta Sperling's experience, and my own, the end result of psychosis has never occurred. In the case of Barbara (chapter 25), a mild psychotic episode occurred which could be dealt with in the psychoanalysis (M. Sperling, 1955c). Another reason for analytic reticence may have been the false assumption that in psychosomatic cases a division of labor is necessary. The internist must treat the somatic symptom and the psychoanalyst, the neurosis. The team approach, however, is not very useful in the treatment of psychosomatic cases. Melitta Sperling found that in order to prevent the splitting of the transference it is necessary to wean the patient away from specialists and family physicians. She found also that when drugs are prescribed in psychotherapy or in psychoanalysis the associations dry up. The patient then expects to be cured by the drugs. It is necessary that the patient put all hopes for a cure on the psychoanalysis. Otherwise, there is not enough energy available to overcome the resistances. She did not accept the authority of internists or surgeons and convinced the patient that the disease was his own responsibility, even if the symptoms were of an organic nature. She realized that cuddling the patient creates later obstacles; she would adhere to strict neutrality—giving no gifts, no feeding, no special sympathy.

If the psychoanalyst adheres to these principals the treatment of psychosomatic diseases is not much different from the treatment of conversion hysteria. As a matter of fact, conversion hysteria has practically disappeared. In cases where conversion hysteria would have occurred in Freud's day, we see today psychosis or psychosomatic disease. In the First World War, cases of war neurosis had the symptoms of convulsions, fainting, stiffness and trembling, as in Parkinson's Disease, paralysis of the legs, etc. After the Yom Kippur War in Israel, when I talked with Israeli psychiatrists and inquired about war neurosis, the answer was, "We have no war neurosis. Our soldiers are all enthusiastic fighters." When I inquired about ulcers of the stomach they conceded that the incidence was high. "Some soldiers did not tolerate the Army food." These ulcers of the stomach were the equivalent of the hysterical convulsions during the First World War.

The determination as to whether a symptom is organic or functional has been criticized by Halliday (1943). "A little consideration shows that the words organic and functional are merely examples of technical slang which express in convenient form the following: In certain illnesses...a structural technique or approach (e.g. anatomical, histological) provides a positive finding.... In other illnesses the application of the structural approach yields a negative finding, whereas the application of other techniques of approach provides a positive finding. . . . Many writers . . . seem to have imagined that by using these words a fundamental etiological basis for the division of illness has been achieved." In my opinion this differentiation is indeed very important as long as we keep in mind that in some cases organic diseases can be cured by psychological means. Halliday cited as an argument for his criticism the experience that some warts could be removed by suggestion (by painting the wart with color). Another example was the experience that the bleeding after a tooth extraction, in a case of hemophilia, could be stopped by hypnosis. This does not mean that hemophilia or verrucae are psychosomatic diseases. It only means that the arterioles which lead to the wart and to the hemophiliac's tooth, which are controlled by the autonomous nervous system, can be influenced by the hypnotist to go into a spasm. (Idiopathic Raynaud's Disease is in fact such a spasm occurring in the artery of a finger.)

I do not wish to enumerate here all the possible variations of the influence of the mind on a physical disease and all the possible influences of a physical disease or deformity on the mind. But to maintain that every disease is psychosomatic is misleading. It is better to keep in mind that symptoms fall into two categories; some are predominantly organic and others predominantly functional. Diseases fall into three categories: some are essentially *somatic*; some, like conversion hysteria, are essentially based on *functional* symptoms; and psychosomatic diseases show *organic* symptoms which are produced and maintained by psychological processes, often on the basis of somatic disposition.

A transition from conversion hysteria to psychosomatic disease is also possible. At a time when psychoanalysts did not think that psychosomatic symptoms were their business, Federn (1934) observed that the end result of analyzed cases of conversion hysteria was disappointing; they often ended up as a psychosomatic disease.

Alexander (1943) and Fenichel (1945) maintained that psychosomatic diseases are caused by unconscious *attitudes* but only in hysteria does real conversion occur—i.e. representation of a fantasy in the afflicted organ. Melitta Sperling (1973) could go beyond the findings of Alexander and others. By the use of the proper psychoanalytic technique for a long enough time she could show that not only in hysteria but also in psychosomatic disease, fantasy is represented in the symptom. "In hysteria ....conversion is dealing with the unresolved oedipal conflicts," while in psychosomatic disease conversion is of a pre-oedipal nature.

The use of the words *organic* and *psychogenic* should not be interpreted by the reader to mean that I believe that body and soul are different substances. In reality, I convinced myself early in life that the psyche is a function of the brain. When somebody is hit on the head and falls unconscious, there is no psychic life, no sensations, no feelings, no dreams, no fantasies, no memory. Only in awakening from unconsciousness might one dream.

The training of the psychoanalyst makes it necessary to confine oneself to the psychological aspect of psychosomatic disease; it is up to neurologists, physiologists, and psychophar-macologists to deal with the physical aspects of psychosomatic disease. For example, Richmond et al. (1962) and Bridger and Reiser (1959) have found that the autonomous nervous system in some psychosomatic diseases functions in a similar fashion to that in the neonate and infant. Patients with rheumatoid arthritis often show marked generalized peripheral and cutaneous vasomotor lability. Mason (1963) found that in psychosomatic diseases, there were significant alterations in multiendocrine profiles. Mason et al. (1960) delineated separate circuits from the hippocampus to hypothalamic nuclei in the brain, which are involved in the stimulation of various adrenal hormones. Mirsky (1958) found in duodenal ulcer a hypersecretion of pepsinogen into the blood which is genetically determined. Finally, immune mechanisms and the proteogenic immunological functions of reticuloendothelial structures have been implicated in some psychosomatic diseases (Moos and Solomon, 1965; Solomon and Moos, 1965). Still, our understanding of the pathological physiology of these diseases is incomplete. As interesting as these finding are, they have no therapeutic significance. The psychoanalytic situation, on the other hand, offers the opportunity to see the causative connection between traumatic experience and the symptom in rich and colorful detail. A caution is in order here. This need to establish a causative connection between experience and symptom can also misfire. For example, a patient with general paresis can be convinced that his loss of memory is a punishment for masturbation in his adolescence.

In recent years, several attempts have been made to formulate a general metapsychology of psychosomatic disorders. Giovacchini (1959) has concentrated his observations on the ego state. Schur (1955) has emphasized ego regression. It is true that the ego's capacity to perceive and evaluate dangers is impaired in some cases. For example, a girl on the brink of death, suffering from anoerxia nervosa, might exercise to lose weight; and an adolescent with ulcerative colitis might be fully unaware of the possibility of death. But the theory of regression to early infancy or to traumatic experiences in the perinatal and earliest neonatal epoch could not be substantiated in my studies. Nor could I find the idea of traumatic experiences *in utero* (Sontag, 1944) very convincing.

In my experience, ego regression is not the central problem. Most psychosomatic patients display age-adequate ego function; for example, reality testing, synthetic function, memory and intelligence. Regression is important, but not to the extreme of infancy. Even more important in my experience is object relationship in all its aspects, not just from the point of view of separation (Schmale, 1958) or object loss (Engel, 1962).

2

Problems in the Analysis of Children with Psychosomatic Disorders

In this chapter I should like to point out some of the major difficulties I encountered in analytic work with children suffering from psychosomatic disorders. These children are regarded as organically sick by their environment particularly if their ailments are unaccompanied by neurotic manifestations. In fact, the more severe the physical symptoms, the less apparent is the underlying neurosis. Such children usually have a history of long standing illnesses and continued unsatisfactory contact with doctors. One child I treated had been in a hospital for a whole year. Many of them had been hospitalized at one time or another. The tendency of parents to regard the condition as primarily physical is fostered by the medical profession, which is itself only slowly becoming aware of the role of psychological factors in the etiology and tenacity of certain illnesses heretofore regarded as basically organic.

The reluctance to accept psychoanalytic treatment encountered in parents where children present overt psychoneurotic behavior manifestations will, therefore, be infinitely greater in psychosomatic cases.

I came to understand that this attitude on the part of parents is due not exclusively to ignorance or lack of insight, but that the mother prefers the child to be sick rather than have her own motivations exposed and that actually this preference expresses the unconscious wish of the mother that the child should die.

As a matter of fact, in work with such a mother, the degree of insight exhibited is amazing. In many cases the mothers told me that they had always known the child's problem to be an emotional one, but that this interpretation was never apparent to anyone, especially the doctors.

I should like to illustrate my findings with a case.

Freddie (4)

Freddie was referred to me at the age of four by the hospital, where he had been severely sick for several months with ulcerative colitis. He had had his first attack at the age of eighteen months. He was hospitalized twice at that age and had a severe recurrence at three and a half. In this case for the mother to accept psychiatric treatment actually meant to admit her guilt. On many occasions her husband had accused her of having made the child sick. In giving me the history she remarked, "Boys in my family don't live long." Two brothers died at a young age while all five sisters are still alive. In this interview she told me that her older son had died as an infant in a strange accident. Mother and child were sleeping in a summer bungalow where a stove overturned. Both were found asphyxiated. The child was dead, the mother was revived. Her husband then seemed to blame her for the child's death. She herself felt that if she had shared the bungalow with her sister (she had wanted to, but her husband did not permit it) this accident might never have happened.

In connection with the short-lived boys in her family, she casually remarked, "Freddie is taking his time." She was very proud that she had successfully trained him when he was very young. When only fourteen months of age, Freddie became disturbed when a drop of food soiled his bib. Since she herself was a meticulously clean person, she could not understand why her child had to have "such a messy disease." Just when she had cleaned the bathroom, Freddie would have to run and, unable to hold his stool, would dirty the freshly washed floor. Similarly, when she had finished dressing him in clean clothes, he would have to run and again dirty himself. The mother couldn't stand that.

When his condition improved, he was able to attend kindergarten. He maintained control over his bowels, whereas at home he would have to run to the bathroom constantly. Several weeks later, Freddie got the grippe and had to stay home. When he recovered, the mother called me on the telephone, because, as she explained, "she couldn't face me." She was determined not to continue Freddie's treatment nor would she send him back to kindergarten. Maybe at some later date she would bring him back. This was the mother's reaction to the threat of interference with her unconscious wish to destroy Freddie.

Characteristic of the mother's attitude toward Freddie is the following: when Freddie was four and a half years old, he once teasingly exposed his penis to his sister, five years his senior. The mother became so infuriated that she threatened to cut off his penis, holding before him the big kitchen knife. Next day she was angry and surprised that Freddie clung to his father and wouldn't let him go to work.

A year later, I saw Freddie in the hospital, acutely ill (106° temperature and severe bloody diarrhea). The pediatrician strongly recommended that psychoanalytic treatment be resumed. I agreed to treat both child and mother at the clinic, but the mother could not accept the offer. I learned later that he was in another hospital with a severe attack of ulcerative colitis.

Obviously, the child in such a case cannot be saved, unless, as I stress in chapter 7, one succeeds in changing the mother's attitude.

Diet

In all psychosomatic cases, diets play a paramount role. I came to understand what a powerful instrument the diet becomes in the hands of the mother. In many cases the diet is made the focus of tyranny over the child. Unfortunately, the medical profession often helps to provide these mothers with rationalizations and scientific alibis for their sadism.

It is interesting to observe the reaction of the child in such a situation. Even though the child may understand the necessity for a special diet, he will be hostile and uncooperative and accuse his mother of cruelty because he feels the unconscious need of the mother to punish him by depriving him of the foods he likes.

A modification in the unconscious attitude of such a mother brings about a startling change in the behavior of the child.

Children who have fits of temper over food, reject food, or express their rage in physical symptoms will accept severe diet restrictions when they recognize the sincerity of the motive. I was particularly impressed with the frank admission of the mother in the case of a five-year-old boy who, since infancy, had suffered from mucous colitis with severe diarrhea. He had always been subjected to rigid diets. Every transgression was punished by severe beatings. With some interpretation to the mother, she was able to lift the restrictions and stop the beatings, after which the child's colitis symptoms disappeared. The mother one day said to me, "Now that I let him eat whatever he wants and I don't beat him up, he has no diarrhea, but he doesn't behave better at all. He is even more fresh and unmanageable than he was!" It was necessary to help the mother tolerate the child's released aggression during this transition period. Restricting him too violently would force him to again convert his sadism into physical symptoms.

Food taboos often become associated in the child's mind with sexual taboos. There is the unconscious expectation that the transgression of such taboos will be followed by castration (illness). It is important in eliminating or changing a diet to work this fear of transgression out with the child and the mother; it is advisable that the physician who imposed the restriction should himself lift it (take back the castration threat).

In the case of seven-year-old Robert, suffering from severe ulcerative colitis, I had gotten the mother to take the child out of the hospital when he was still severely ill. She promised to cooperate by disregarding the diet and allowing him to eat whatever he wanted. Frequently when she had some difficulties in adhering to it, she would threaten to send him back to the hospital.

Maternal Attitudes

This attitude of the mother leads me to a discussion of the child's anxiety lest he be sent away from home. Since most of these children had at some point in their illnesses been hospitalized, the danger is a realistic one. In Robert's case, the suspense was so intolerable that he ended it one day by unconsciously arranging for an accident. He fell out of the bed and hurt his leg and head. He was taken to the clinic that day by his mother. He told me about the accident in a highly excited state and showed fear that his mother would leave him at the hospital. After I had reassured him that he would go home, he told me he had had a nightmare that night. He found himself driving an ambulance and then crashing and ending up in the hospital. He understood the interpretation that this was his way of solving an intolerable situation of suspense. By falling out of the bed and hurting himself, he wanted in a characteristically masochistic fashion to bring about his hospitalization instead of suffering suspense like Damocles with the sword hanging over his head. As if the child were actually thinking, "Well, if my mother wanted to give me away and I have to go back to the hospital, I will at least bring it on myself."

Sometimes the severity of the symptom is in direct proportion to the need of the child to test mother's patience or love. Psychodynamically this is analagous to the need of an insecure child with behavior disorder to test the mother's acceptance of him by means of bad behavior. Here the child formulates its feeling in this way: "She has to love me even if I'm bad; you don't have to be a mother to love a good child." In the case of psychosomatic disorders the idea is, "She has to keep me with her even if I am very sick and a lot of trouble. If she sends me to a hospital then she doesn't love me. I'll die [kill myself] but it'll be her fault."

I am thinking, here, particularly of an eight-and-a-half-year-old girl suffering from ulcerative colitis. In her fourth and last attack, she was taxing her mother's strength and patience to the utmost by the severity of her symptom. In this way she was really testing the mother to find out if she would keep her home or send her back to the hospital. Preceding that attack of ulcerative colitis, the mother had said, "I won't send you back to a hospital anymore, no matter what happens." This was exactly what the child was trying to find out. The masochistic provocation on the child's part can be stopped by psychoanalytic interpretation. As for the mother, she must be guided in the same way as one would be in treatment of a neurosis with behavior symptoms. The threat of hospitalization, conceived of by the child as a threat of abandonment by the mother, is a real one in such cases and corresponds to the unconscious wish of the mother to rid herself of the child.

An equally important factor is the anxiety of the mother which in an over-compensated form represents the unconscious death wish. The fear that the child might die in such cases is justified in reality because ulcerative colitis represents an actual danger to life. In cases of bronchial asthma, the subjective experience of dying is an extremely painful one for the child and very disturbing to the mother. The lessening of the mother's anxiety is in itself a therapeutic factor, as if indicating to the child, "I don't have to die, she really doesn't want me to." When the mother's anxiety is lessened, she will be able to carry out the analyst's suggestions and bring the child for treatment even if it should be acutely ill. The psychoanalytic treatment may go on for years, but the analytic interpretation of an acute attack equals surgical procedure in promptness of effect and can be considered emergency treatment. A child whom I treated for ulcerative colitis was brought to my office, wrapped in blankets and running a temperature of 104. In this case, for instance, the physical condition was completely changed after the session, and the child got up the next morning feeling perfectly well.

In these cases the analyst obviously assumes far greater responsibility than that involved in the treatment of all other types of psychoneurosis. The results, however, justify it and demonstrate the value of the psychoanalytic method in the treatment of psychosomatic disorders.

3

The Role of the Mother
in Psychosomatic Disorders
in Children

This chapter examines somatic reactions produced in children in response to an insoluble conflict with the mother. The significance of parental attitudes in the personality development of the child is well known from psychoanalysis; however, there is comparatively little known about the parent-child relationship in the specific area of psychosomatic disorders.

After treating twenty children with various psychosomatic disorders, together with their mothers, I found a certain quality existing in the relationship between the mother and these children which, in my opinion, served as a dynamic force precipitating as well as perpetuating the child's illness.

The mother, in every one of these cases, had an unconscious need to keep the child in a helpless and dependent state to a degree which I have encountered only in the mothers of psychotic children. Mother and child represented a psychologic unit in which the child reacted to the unconscious need of the mother with correspondingly unconscious obedience; it was as though the child were given a command to get sick, which meant in reality, to stay dependent and helpless.

The somatic reaction of the child, in these cases, comes with amazing speed. The most severe symptoms may develop so rapidly that the untrained observer, unable to find the connections, usually falls back on rationalization. Equally severe symptoms may suddenly be resolved without therapy, and for no apparent reason. It is as if one were to observe two parallel curves—the mother and child curve—where a specific change (elevation or decline) in the mother curve produces a specific reactive change in the child curve.

Since the method used for my study and the therapy was analytic, fragments from the analyses of both children and mothers whom I have treated either in succession or simultaneously will be presented. I shall limit myself to two cases, children of varying ages and with varying symptoms.

John (6)

John's mother presented the symptoms of chronic depression with somatic equivalents.

She had severe difficulty in the handling of her two children. Her symptoms, which appeared in an acute episode after the birth of her first child, returned in a permanent form with the birth of John. She had not wanted another child so soon, but when she became pregnant accidentally two years after her first child's birth, she hoped at least that she would have a girl. In fact, she was prepared with a girl's name which she gave to John and changed only in the second year of her analysis.

She found it difficult to care for John in his first year because she suffered from fatigue and severe migraine. John was a feeding problem and the older child whined and clung to her; both children constantly suffered from colds. At about two years of age, following a tonsillectomy, John developed spells in which he behaved as if he were dazed and faint. She was advised to "slap him out" of these states and to pour cold water over him. She soon recognized, however, how badly John reacted to this treatment and discontinued it. By this time, John had developed attacks of bronchial asthma and had also become a behavior problem.

The analysis of the mother (of which only significant parts relating to John can be presented here) revealed that to her the child unconsciously represented her younger brother, born when she was two and a half years old. She had exhibited radical changes in behavior in reaction to the birth of this brother. Her mother observed that she had changed from a healthy baby to a moody, sick child. She had carried over to John this unresolved relationship with her brother. Analysis helped her to become conscious of her death wishes toward John, which she acted out in inconsistent and often sadistic behavior. It also helped her to recognize that she was using his illness and difficult behavior to rationalize her rejection of him and that unconsciously she needed to have him sick and dependent upon her.

At the start of the mother's analysis John was six years of age and under medical care. The psychosomatic nature of his asthma and allergies was neither recognized nor accepted by either the father or the attending allergist. The mother's preoccupation in analysis centered about the physical symptoms of John and herself. The parents invariably found valid and concrete explanations for John's asthmatic attacks—weather, food, exposure, and so forth. John had an attendance record of only fifty days for an entire school year prior to treatment of the mother. He was also under severe dietary restrictions which he himself feared to violate. The mother, who had gained some understanding of his problem through her analysis, began to introduce previously forbidden foods into his diet and, through her reassuring attitude, helped him to accept these new foods without allergic reactions. Within a few weeks, he had abandoned his restrictive diet completely, though he continued to suffer frequent and severe asthmatic attacks.

Toward the end of the first year of the mother's analysis, the relationship between them improved to the extent that John began to talk about himself to his mother. This was a new experience for both mother and child. John had always shied away from his mother, who would habitually grab and shake him or hold him so tightly as if to "squeeze the breath" out of him. Now John would sometimes say, "You know when I get asthma? When you yell at me and punish me and beat me up." The mother had observed that when she reprimanded him severely for urinating on the toilet seat or when he came home occasionally from school with a bowel movement in his pants, he would develop an asthmatic attack. She observed also that he would become very cranky and have asthmatic attacks when she withdrew into her bed with migraine.

It·was in this phase of the analysis that the mother began to accept the significance both of the emotional factor and of her own role in John's illness. She had always been concerned about John's physical condition, prohibiting him from running around and putting him to bed to prevent an asthmatic attack whenever she noticed signs of wheezing. This method never worked; whenever he would start to wheeze, the attack always followed. Some examples may illustrate how the mother handled John during this phase and the results of her approach. One afternoon, the mother, who had noticed John wheezing heavily in play with another boy after his visits to the movies, began to talk to him about a boat he had made. After a while, John said, "I am wheezing."

Mother: Why are you wheezing? You went to the movies and you enjoyed yourself.
John: I was running around with my friend.
Mother: That should not make you wheeze.
John: But I ran a lot.
Mother: That's no reason.

John looked at his mother as he had on many occasions to see whether she actually meant what she said, whether it was all right for him not to have an attack. There was no sign of wheezing at all after this conversation.

It seems of interest to report an incident illustrative of a reaction diametrically different from the one cited above—in which the mother's sensitivity to the child's reactions obviated an asthmatic attack. The mother had prepared John's bath, cautioning him not to play but to wash himself quickly since she was in a hurry to leave for an appointment. Upon returning to the bathroom, she found John stretched out in the tub with his penis erect, playing with the soap. She got very angry, grabbed him, gave him a forceful scrubbing, and then pulled him out of the tub. Immediately after this, John had a severe attack of asthma, necessitating treatment and forcing the mother to remain at home. In the analytic session the next morning the mother brought out feelings concerning the size of the penises of her two boys. She thought that her older son had a rather small penis while John's appeared to her unusually large for his age. She realized that her anger with him on the previous night had been disproportionate and related it to the sight of his penis. That night the mother had dreamed that John lay on the railroad tracks, crushed by a train. Though becoming aware both of her impulse to harm him (particulary by choking) and of some of her motives for this was initially disturbing to her, it markedly changed her attitude to John and consequently his attitude to her.

The following episode, also occurring at this time, before John himself entered analysis, shows how the understanding of her unconscious motivations enabled the mother to help him. One day he came home from school wheezing terribly. He could hardly walk upstairs and immediately asked for the ephedrine gun.

His mother casually suggested that she take his coat off and quickly took out some electric trains in which John became interested. John began to play, completely forgot about the gun, ate his supper, and slept through the night. In the morning, he dressed himself—this being a most unusual thing for him because such a wheezing attack would always render him sick the next day and he would frequently remain in bed for a prolonged period. On leaving for school, the mother said to him, "Come home well today." When he came home that afternoon, he smiled to her and said, "Here I am as you wanted me."

John had always been a behavior problem at home and in school. His difficulties in adjusting to a group and to the school situation in general, in addition to his inability to learn, became even more pronounced after his physical symptoms began to subside. For this reason and because both parents used his behavior to rationalize their rejection of him, I decided to take John into treatment. In the analysis, John was very provocative and destructive at first, testing me to see if I would react in the same way as his mother and teacher, that is, by becoming angry and sending him away. In school, he was sent out of the room; at home, his mother retreated to her bed with a headache when he angered her. John was very distrustful of women, often making cryptic remarks, such as : "My mother is a murderer and all her friends are too. You know what they do—they hunt corpses—boys' corpses." It was significant that he brought this out at the time when his mother's analysis revealed her extreme resentment of John and me. The transference situation lent itself very well to the mother's reliving of the phase in her life when, through the birth of her younger brother (my taking John into treatment), she had lost her mother to the baby (her analyst to John).

The true reason for John's inability to function as a boy physically and intellectually was his mother's inability to accept him as a boy. In painstaking analysis, the mother had to be shown again and again that she did not accept John as a boy. To her unconscious, he had to be dead or a girl, that is, either sick or a good boy who was dull and could not learn. She felt that her mother had rejected her because she was a girl and consequently had considered her inferior and dull. Her brother had gone to college while she had not finished her studies, taking only a business school education and then going to work.

One day when John showed his mother a picture he had made in my playroom, she said to him, "I didn't think you had it in you." This was after two years of analysis. Unconsciously, she wanted John to be incapable of performing and in this way had practically tabooed John's intellectual functioning. It was also very difficult for her to tolerate aggressive behavior on his part and, on such occasions, she would ask him, "Why can't you be a good boy?" to which John would reply, "But then I can't do anything I like." (Despite this protest, he would comply with his mother's wishes.) With the rationalization that John did not know what to do with his free time and that he had no friends in his neighborhood with whom to play, the mother had taught him to knit. John would take his knitting to school with him and while the other children did work, he sat by, knitting like a little girl. In a session with me, when he brought his knitting along and sat with knees bent girlishly under him, counting the stitches, he carried on a discussion with me, telling me that I was very old-fashioned to think that knitting was not a proper activity for boys, that his mother had told him that boys and girls do the same things and that this was the modern spirit. Only after the mother, in her analysis, had overcome this basic rejection of John was he able to assert himself as a boy and to overcome his intellectual inhibition. He himself asked for remedial tutoring and was eager to make up for lost time. He is actually a boy of superior intelligence, rating an IQ of 128.

It would seem of interest to report an episode which occurred during John's treatment and which reflects the attitude of the father regarding John's condition. John had always been allergic to animal hair and therefore could not have a pet, nor was he allowed to come close to any animal. Whenever John visited his aunt who had a dog, he would come home with a severe wheezing attack. The parents could see this only as a reaction to animal hair, although John was not permitted to come close to the dog. Whenever the parents took John visiting, they were always very tense, kept after him constantly, reprimanding and nagging, with the result that John behaved notoriously badly in other people's homes. Particularly with her husband's relatives, the mother was greatly concerned lest John expose her unfavorably. After John had been in analysis with me for several months, I had worked out with him and his mother a plan whereby he could have a dog to show his parents that he was not really allergic toward dogs but rather toward his parents' handling of him. It was a great event in his life when his wish was fulfilled. But I had not reckoned with the father, who had been very cooperative on the surface but had apparently been unable to accept the psychologic implications of John's allergies. The day after John received the dog, the father—usually very easygoing with John—chose a minor instance to punish him severely, hitting and threatening him. This was rather unusual behavior for the father. The mother, who seemed to sense the underlying unconscious motivation in her husband's behavior, became extremely angry at him and protected John against him. When I spoke to the father on the next day, he himself was so startled at his sudden outburst of temper that for the first time he proved amenable to my interpretation that in this way he had sought to offset our plans to prove to him the emotional basis of John's allergies. By severely upsetting and frightening the child on precisely the day after he had gotten the dog, he could be almost sure to provoke an attack. John, however, held his own and, after a year of owning a dog without any allergic reactions, succeeded in convincing his father.

Ann (4)

When Ann started psychoanalytic treatment, she was four years of age. She had been referred to me when she was three, because of severe and persistent vomiting, anorexia, and abdominal cramps with periodic episodes of diarrhea for which no organic cause could be found. It was only when the child developed a very intense phobic attachment to the mother, refusing to allow her out of sight, that the mother acted upon the referral to psychiatry. In the psychoanalytic treatment of the mother, I learned that prior to Ann's birth her mother had had an obsessional concern regarding her husband, who suffered from mild diabetes. Her attitude toward her husband changed markedly upon the discovery of his diabetes, as did her entire behavior; she could not work, developed a sleep disturbance, and found it impossible to concentrate on anything except her husband's diabetes. As soon as Ann was born, she completely lost her anxious preoccupation with her husband's ailment and devoted herself exclusively to the child. Soon after the child's birth, she thought that the child was not taking enough food; she changed the formula and increased the number of feedings, with the result that at seven weeks, Ann developed anorexia, vomiting, and diarrhea for which she had to be hospitalized. After a short stay in the hospital, the child was discharged and put on a diet and new formula. Her symptoms continued and she was hospitalized again at eleven months. At the age of four, she still had not been given any solid foods but was on a formula elaborately prepared and fed to her by her mother with a spoon. The mother maintained that only she knew how to prepare Ann's food and how to feed her. Up to the time of her treatment, the child had never had a feeding unaccompanied by vomiting.

Analysis of the mother revealed that Ann's intense need to hold on to her mother was a reflection of the mother's inability to let Ann out of her sight even for a moment. She was in a constant dread concerning Ann. She did not permit her to taste candy or solid food for fear that the child would choke on it instantly. Even at such times when the child was in a real need of glucose due to a run-down condition caused by her continuous vomiting, the mother could not carry out the doctor's suggestion to allow Ann to suck on a lollipop.

The mother, the youngest of five children, had been a particularly demanding and possessive child. She always had to have her own way and would threaten suicide if her mother did not comply immediately. She remembered with satisfaction an incident which happened when she was about eight years old. One day she asked her mother for some money; her mother refused her. The grandmother, who lived with the family and who took my patient's threats to kill herself seriously, stood up on a chair to reach for her purse in order to give her the requested money. The grandmother fell, broke her hip, and was laid up in the hospital for several months. Ann's mother felt no regret but instead was pleased that she had gotten what she wanted.

To her mother's illness and death, Ann's mother reacted in a way which amazed her and which she could understand only after analysis.

She had been so concerned about her mother that when the doctor came to treat the mother, he had to attend to my patient first. All during her mother's illness, she had a rapid pulse and could neither eat not sleep. On the day of her mother's death, however, she heaved a sigh of relief, ate a complete meal, and had her first sound sleep for weeks. She had never realized how dependent she had been upon her mother and that this dependency had expressed itself in her possessive and domineering behavior. In retrospect, she could understand that she had been unable to tolerate a situation filled with such suspense as her mother's illness, a situation over which she exercised no control. She accepted her mother's death as something which *she* wanted to happen to end the intolerable suspence. This reaction could be understood as a defense against an impending depression and as a mechanism which enabled her to maintain her fantasy of omnipotence.

After her mother's death—she was about twenty years of age at the time—she went to live with a married sister to whom she tried to transfer her need for control. She then married a man whom she could dominate, and when, in her first year of marriage, her husband developed a mild diabetic condition, she became extremely disturbed. Her husband's illness represented a severe threat to her omnipotence; and her extreme insecurity, helplessness, and dependence threatened to break through. She had carried over to her husband the relationship she had maintained with her mother and was reacting to his illness as she had to her mother's. As soon as Ann was born, she transferred this relationship from her husband to the child, transforming her role from a passive into an active one.

Only after the mother had gained some understanding of her need for complete control over Ann was she able to relinquish her hold on the child to some extent. The child reacted to this not only by giving up her phobic clinging but, to the mother's amazement and frustration, Ann showed a very strong desire for independence. When Ann first began her play analysis, she had to have her mother with her in the playroom and continually asked her permission for everything we did. But she apparently understood my casually interjected interpretations regarding her insecurity in relation to her mother, because on her fourth visit she decided to come in by herself. And when leaving my office, she told her mother, "I don't want you to come in with me into the playroom anymore. I have a much better time without you." This was a big step forward, not only in Ann's life but also in her mother's, because throughout the year past Ann had refused to remain with anyone except her mother for any length of time, not even with her father or her nursemaid whom she had had since she was one year old and whom she liked a great deal. The mother had thought—and as we understood, unconsciously wished—that Ann would never let go of her. At the same time, the degree of her disturbance about Ann's clinging behavior was so extreme that it can hardly be described.

It seems to me of great interest to report an episode which occurred after about six months of treatment, at a time when Ann's condition had so improved that she had given up her clinging to her mother and was playing outdoors with other children. She had also been asking for some solid foods—bread, fish, meat—which she would eat when her father or grandmother were in the house but not at her regular mealtimes when her mother fed her. She had also completely stopped vomiting. Suddenly, there was a relapse into phobic clinging and refusal of any solid food. In the session with her mother, it was revealed that Ann's relapse had set in on the day after the mother's visit to her gynecologist for a checkup. During her pregnancy with Ann, the mother had undergone a gynecologic operation, and there was some question as to whether she should or could have another child. She had seen this doctor once before, more than a year ago, and the day after that, as she distinctly remembered, the phobic behavior of Ann had started. On her way to the doctor this time, she had thought about this and wondered whether the same would happen again. The mother was able to recognize that she had been unwilling to let go of Ann (her fantasy of omnipotence) and that the fleeting thought she had had about a recurrence of Ann's symptoms had expressed her unconscious wish for it. The morning after this session, the mother said to Ann in a casual way, "I am going shopping now and Mary [nursemaid] will take you out this morning." Ann, who on the preceding days had clung to her mother, cried bitterly, vomited, and complained of bellyache whenever she attempted to leave her, accepted this suggestion very readily. The mother realized that actually she had clung to Ann and had not wanted to leave her and now that she was determined to let go of her, Ann accepted this without disturbance.

In her play sessions with me, Ann, who at first showed marked anxiety whenever the topic of food came up, was prepared for the acceptance of solid foods. She avidly played a game in which she fed steak to her doll-children for all their meals and nothing happened to them. It was difficult, however, for the mother to surrender her monopoly of the food control over Ann even though she permitted the child more freedom now in other areas. When Ann began to bombard her mother with questions as to when she would have "regular food," the mother felt guilty but could not accede with ease to the child's request. She understood that this meant setting Ann free, allowing her normal independence. Ann, in turn, was testing her mother constantly during this period. Often she would come to her to tell her that she had cramps and would carefully watch her mother's reaction. When her mother did not look up from her book, Ann said, "How can you read when I have a bellyache?" The mother responded, "Because there is no need to worry about your bellyache. Just go and play with your toys and it will disappear." After a while, Ann came running back to her mother, full of smiles, to tell her that the bellyache had disappeared. Once Ann was sucking hard candy at home, something which she did in every one of our play sessions but which she had not yet done at home. She suddenly made a noise, as if she were choking, and she watched her mother's face very closely. When the mother remained calm ("It does take a lot out of me," the mother would tell me) Ann said, "Don't you hear? I am choking!" The mother replied, "You're a big girl now and you know how to suck a candy." Ann continued to test her mother for some time before she was convinced that this change in her mother's attitude was a real one.

From the psychoanalytic study of twenty mother-child pairs, certain features seem to emerge as characteristic for these mothers of children suffering from various psychosomatic disorders:

1. The carry-over of an unresolved emotional conflict from childhood and the acting out of this conflict with the child (The child may represent an unconsciously hated sibling or parent)
2. Projection of part of the mother's own person onto the child
3. A need for control over the child, so intense that in some of these cases the child is regarded and treated as if he were a part of the mother's own body (a phenomenon described as appersonation by Otto E. Sperling)

The use of projection and the need for control, in which the child's individuality is completely disregarded, leads to a certain impairment of reality testing with reference to the child. Because this specific relationship is limited to one of the children in the family, the behavior of the mother may not appear to be particularly disturbed, especially since her reactions can easily be rationalized in the case of a sick child. Only through the observations made in psychoanalytic study can one recognize the degree of disturbance in the mother's behavior toward the child. The mother's attitudes can be transferred in an equally irrational and exaggerated way onto other relationships, e.g., from child to husband. I should like to cite an example of this: After Mrs. S. had understood (through analysis) that her only daughter had represented to her a hated sister and after she had been able to resolve this relationship with the child, she transferred it to her husband. When the husband developed a psychogenic tremor, Mrs. S. reacted to him in an irrational and exaggerated fashion similar to that which she had displayed previously with her eleven-year-old daughter who had suffered from a tic disorder. She would stay up nights, for instance, to observe whether her husband had the tremor in his sleep. Ann's mother behaved similarly; in her case, the sequence of consequences was reversed. She first had this relationship with her husband and then transferred it to her child.

In summarizing the attitudes of the mothers and the reaction of their children in cases presented here, we note the following:

To his mother, John represented not only her hated brother but also a penis symbol—her penis. She used to grab him playfully and put him on her lap, pressing him tightly to her pubic region. As a little girl, she had done this with a dog whom she would hold pressed against her body so that its penis stuck out, as if it was hers. This second role which John played in his mother's unconscious cannot be dealt with more extensively in this brief synopsis. However, it may be said that she projected onto John the conflict around her own sexual role—whether to be a woman or to imagine herself a man. John, in turn, complied unconsciously with his mother's wishes and at the same time rebelled against them in his symptoms and behavior.

The analysis of Ann's mother brought out her great need to be indispensable to Ann. In the child's helplessness and dependency, the mother managed to cover up her own unconscious dependency and insecurity. Through Ann, she re-enacted her own childhood, playing the roles both of the child and of the mother. She had arranged an inseparable union between herself and the child in which both were equipped with magical control over the life and death of one another. This feeling manifested itself also in the conscious attitudes of the mother. She felt that because Ann could not be without her even for a day, she (the mother) was not allowed to fall sick. With obvious satisfaction, she indicated that she had never been ill since Ann's birth because no one else could minister to the child. When Ann was hospitalized as an infant, the mother had to be called in to feed her because Ann would not take the formula from the nurses. The mother had fed Ann with a spoon practically from birth on, so that Ann did not even know of bottle-feeding. Ann responded to the mother's need for control over her by remaining dependent (sick) and at the same time controlled the mother through her physical symptoms and phobia.

In the case of fifteen-year-old Helen (see chapter 12), similar mechanisms were at work. Helen represented to the mother a part of herself, the mother treating her as she herself would have wanted to be treated and also expecting her to behave as she thought she herself would have responded. She did not allow Helen to express her individuality. Helen's illness was the outcome of an unsuccessful attempt to break away from her mother. Unable to resolve her conflict whether to hold on or to let go of her mother, she became sick and so remained dependent though rebelling against this in her very symptoms.

The pathogenic conflict of the child in such cases arises from the specific relationship to the mother. Some of these mothers behave as if the physiologic act of having given birth to the child (separation) had not been accepted as a fact in the unconscious.

Moreover they do not tolerate frank neurotic or rebellious behavior of the child and suppress it, often with great cruelty. In the case of a seven-year-old girl with ulcerative colitis, the mother had the idea that she could not let the child grow up to be like one of her husband's family, if it destroyed both the child and herself. It almost did destroy the child. When the child developed bloody diarrhea, the mother became extremely anxious and overindulgent, only to relapse into her former behavior as soon as the child improved (see chapter 7).

The solution of this conflict with the mother is achieved somatically by the child. The mother from whom the child cannot separate himself emotionally nor in reality is given up in the somatic symptom or symptoms (asthma, anorexia, vomiting, diarrhea, etc.). Meanwhile in reality, through the illness, the dependency upon the mother is not only maintained but overemphasized. In addition, the child derives a secondary gain from illness and the satisfaction of arousing profound guilt feeling in the mother.

This specific relationship of mutual dependence and "magical" control existing between mother and child is an important predisposing factor in the development of a psychosomatic disorder in a child. I have limited myself in this chapter to demonstration of this one factor—the child's relationship with the mother—in the genesis of a psychosomatic disorder because, in my cases, the mother was *the* important person and her neurosis decisive for the reactions of the child. The choice of symptoms, the somatic compliance, and other factors operating in such conditions are dealt with elsewhere in this section.

Psychosomatic Medicine and Pediatrics

While observational studies are valuable confirmation of the significance of the mother-child relationship for the well being of the child, they show mostly the phenomenological aspects, namely, the observable deviate behavior or impaired physical functioning of the child. However, a knowledge of the psychological factors that produce these abnormalities and of the dynamics operating in their production is needed for a comprehensive understanding.

A study of the mothers of psychosomatically sick infants and young children conducted concurrently with the treatment of the young patients was my objective when, during the investigation of a variety of psychosomatic disorders in children, I treated both mother and child psychoanalytically. Not only was it possible through this method of investigation to observe in operation the fundamental workings of the mother-child relationship, but it was also possible to see how the modification of the unconscious needs of the mother manifested itself in a change in the somatic responses of the child. It was found that in young children even severe psychosomatic disorders were still reversible, if it was possible to improve the relationship existing between mother and child.

This chapter will present a survey of clinical entities in children which have been studied by myself and other psychoanalysts, psychiatrists, and pediatricians.

Feeding and Eating Disturbances in Children

These are the earliest and most frequent psychosomatic disorders in children. The significance of the mother-child relationship and the effect of the personality of the mother on the child's reactions have been recognized and emphasized especially by psychoanalytic investigators. Spitz (1951) considers that the mother's personality may be a "disease-provoking agent," referring to such an abnormal influence as a "psychologic toxin" causing "psychotoxic diseases of infancy." These earliest somatic casualties which are the first indications of a profoundly disturbed mother-child relationship are treated only rarely by the child analyst or child psychiatrist. I shall therefore present briefly one of my cases.

Infant

The mother of a five-month-old infant was referred to me by a pediatrician who had recognized that the mother's psychological disorder was the cause of the child's symptoms. The situation was as follows: the mother had given birth to a healthy, well-developed eight-pound boy whom she had to breast feed in the hospital. Even then she experienced much anxiety. She worried that she might not have enough milk and urged the doctor to prescribe a formula to have on hand at home in case breast feeding should not be sufficient. At home she began to add the formula after each feeding. She would wake the child when he fell asleep after breast feeding and force the bottle upon him. Because the child began to vomit after each feeding, the mother consulted a pediatrician who told her to stop the additional feedings. However, she did not accept this advice. As time went on, the child refused to take the breast, continued to vomit, and developed colic. She consulted another pediatrician who advised her to starve the child for some time until he could take food again. At this the mother became panicky, abandoned any schedule, and was obsessed by only one desire—to get food into the child. The child was losing weight rapidly, and at this point the mother consulted the pediatrician who referred her to me. I learned from the mother that she had not wanted this child, and particularly not a boy. She had wanted to get rid of the pregnancy which had been an accident, but her husband would not agree. She feared that something would happen during birth, or that the child would be born dead. Another child, a daughter twelve years old at the time, had never presented any difficulties to the mother.

Psychoanalytic investigation revealed that she had unconsciously identified her son with her younger brother who had died in infancy when my patient was five years old. She had always felt guilty over the death of this brother without having been conscious of her death wishes against him. She had by force of repetition-compulsion re-enacted with her own child this unresolved conflict with her brother. The resolution of this conflict in the course of her analysis helped her to accept the little boy as her son rather than to regard him as a substitute of the hated little brother and restored her ability to feed and care for her child properly.

In cases where a deep-rooted, unresolved, infantile conflict is the basis for the mother's inability to function as a mother, advice and manipulation of conscious attitudes do not help because the mother, while intellectually understanding and accepting help, is unable to apply it (M. Sperling, 1950d).

The progressive development of a severe feeding disturbance arising from a distorted mother-child relationship, and the therapeutic approach which takes into consideration both partners of this relationship may be illustrated by the following case (see also chapter 3).

Ann (4)

A four-year-old girl, Ann, was referred to me for treatment because of feeding difficulty, abdominal cramps, diarrhea, and phobic behavior. The feeding difficulty had started very early and the mother had tried formula after formula and consulted pediatrician after pediatrician. At seven weeks and again at eleven months of age, Ann had to be hospitalized with colic, diarrhea, and severe anorexia. The mother had to be called to the hospital to administer food because Ann would not take food from the nurses. At four years of age she was still fed on a formula consisting of liquid and semisolid food. Her mother would not allow anyone to prepare the food nor to feed the child.

Every feeding was a major disturbing event. The child would gag and vomit during each feeding and have cramps; the mother would become extremely anxious, expecting a catastrophe at any moment. Ann was not allowed to have any solid food because her mother was afraid that she would choke. But it was not the feeding difficulty nor Ann's psychosomatic complaint which had prompted the mother to accept referral to psychiatric treatment. Though she had completely "devoted her life" to the care of her child, she could not tolerate Ann's phobic clinging to her. On such occasions, she was cruel with Ann, threatening to leave her. This, of course, only increased Ann's phobic clinging. In her analysis, the mother realized that she resented Ann's clinging to her because this meant a shift in control. With the food she was controlling her. It was of interest to observe in their simultaneous treatment how sensitive the child was to her mother's gradual giving up of the "food control." Ann tested her mother on innumerable occasions until she was convinced that her mother would allow her to eat normally, which in this case also meant to grow up normally.

A theoretical evaluation of the various types of eating disturbances in children has been contributed by Anna Freud (1946). Sylvester (1945) has reported a case of anorexia in a four-year-old child in whom the dynamics underlying the anorexia were found to be similar to those in melancholia. I found that in the more severe cases of eating disturbances the mother's unconscious conflict about food (food as a magic control over life and death) was reinforcing the child's unconscious fantasies. This interplay of the unconscious of child and mother must be taken into consideration as a factor in treatment.

Psychogenic Diarrhea, Mucous Colitis, and Constipation

It would seem that these conditions in children have not attracted much psychiatric attention as yet, although I have found that they occur rather frequently and that they respond readily to psychotherapy. In the psychoanalytic treatment of children suffering from persistent or recurrent attacks of nonbloody diarrhea and abdominal cramps, certain common features in the personality structure and also certain common traumas in early childhood were found consistently. The association of psychogenic diarrhea with phobic behavior was found in a number of these cases and reported in two studies.

It was found that the onset of the diarrhea occurred almost typically between the ages of one and a half to two years. This age period, as we know from psychoanalysis, represents the height of the anal-sadistic phase in the psychosexual development of the child. The personality of the mothers of these children also showed certain features in common: especially marked were compulsive traits, ambivalent attitudes with a need for control over the child, and over-emphasis upon anal functions. Because of the mothers' attitudes, toilet training had been a particularly traumatic experience for these children. It was conducted unusually early and rigidly and led to abrupt repression of anal impulses or did not allow for adequate expression of such impulses. In those cases where the child had colic from infancy, there was a marked exacerbation of the symptoms around the age of two. In cases where toilet training had been accomplished early, shortlived relapses into soiling occurred around the age of two before the condition of chronic or intermittent diarrhea had established itself fully.

Understanding of these factors would enable pediatricians to watch for early signs and encourage them to abandon the routine approach to the treatment of diarrhea. The indiscriminate dispensing of diets, enemas, suppositories, injections, and sedatives in these cases is harmful for the child and, in many instances, only serves to provide the parents with a rationale for their own neurotic needs. In the case of a five-year-old boy with mucous colitis, it was found that the mother had used the rigid diet prescribed by the pediatricians as a disguise for her sadistic and punitive impulses towards the boy. During the phase when the dietary and other severe restrictions had been lifted and the child's aggression, released from the somatic symptoms, had become manifest in his behavior, the mother one day said to me, "Now that I let him eat whatever he wants and don't beat him up he has no diarrhea, but he doesn't behave better at all" (chapter 2).

In the psychoanalytic treatment of a twelve-year-old boy with mucous colitis and phobias (chapter 10), it was found that the diarrhea represented the somatic equivalent of an emotional conflict, namely, whether to hold on to or to separate from his mother. The diarrhea, by an unconscious equation of mother and feces, represented the symbolic giving up of the mother, while in the phobic clinging he was holding on to her in reality.

These findings were confirmed in the psychoanalytic treatment of other children; for example, the case of a six-and-a-half-year-old girl who suffered from psychogenic diarrhea, abdominal cramps and who also exhibited phobic behavior (chapter 9). The necessity to consider the unconscious needs of the mother, which appear as a resistance in the treatment of the child, came out clearly in this case. Sudden withdrawal of the child from treatment could be prevented through an understanding of the behavior of the mother as an acting out of unconscious needs and through interpretation of these needs to the mother.

Withdrawal from treatment in such a case often appears justified to the mother, since the aggravation of the child's condition proves to her the ineffectiveness of psychotherapy. Actually in such a case the child's aggravated condition is due to the increased unconscious resistance of the mother towards the child's treatment. In this case, the child was allowed to complete treatment successfully.

Investigating the role of emotional factors in idiopathic celiac disease, Prugh (1951a) found no single etiologic factor operative. His observations regarding the personality of the mother and the time of onset of symptoms in the children suggest some similarity between factors prevailing in celiac disease and psychogenic diarrhea.

In her study of a case of constipation in a two-year-old child, Sterba (1949) brings out the interesting connection between food and elimination in the child's mind. Finch (1952), in discussing a case of constipation in a four-and-a-half-year-old child, portrays "the battle for the stools" raging between the child and his family. He also draws attention to the fact that the original routine of giving enemas, for the giving of which the child had to be restrained forcibly, had been instituted upon medical advice. Obviously this is an area in which pediatricians need much education.

Bronchial Asthma and Allergic Conditions

The studies of French, Alexander et al. (1941), on psychogenic factors in bronchial asthma, in which eleven cases of children were included, revealed that the basic conflict in asthma is one between the urge to cling and the temptation to separate. These studies also brought out important findings about precipitating factors, defense mechanisms, and certain common features of the character structure of the asthma patient.

Gerard (1946) has studied five children with bronchial asthma psychoanalytically and corroborated the previous findings. She found that although the sensitivity to allergens in these children was not changed by psychoanalytic treatment, asthma attacks did not occur in these children when they were exposed to allergens thereafter. Gerard states that the specific emotional condition of the child is at least of equal importance to the allergic sensitivity in the production of asthma. She also stressed the ambivalent attitudes of the mothers, which alternate between rejection and overprotection, and found that the sex of the child was frequently the reason for rejection of the child by the mother. Clinical observations have corroborated these findings (Swanton, 1947; Miller and Baruch, 1948).

I have approached the study of bronchial asthma through concurrent and/or intermittent treatment of mother and child, and would like to illustrate this with the treatment of a boy who was suffering from allergic manifestations and bronchial asthma. By the psychoanalytic treatment of mother and son, I could obtain deeper insight into the specific dynamics of the mother-child relationship operating in bronchial asthma (see chapter 3).

John

The allergic manifestations and bronchial asthma of this boy, John, were treated for one year indirectly, that is, through his mother, who was undergoing psychoanalysis with me. John himself became my patient when he was seven years old, after his asthma had already been greatly improved but not yet cured. His behavior and learning difficulties had become very obvious by this time.

During the phase of indirect treatment, John's reaction to the change of the mother's feelings and attitude towards him was very interesting. Prior to her analysis, when he would wheeze or show any signs of an incipient attack, his mother would put him to bed immediately and keep him there for days. After she had gained insight into her unconscious need to have him sick and dependent on her and had realized that to let him be well meant to her to let him be a boy, she treated his wheezing in a different fashion. Each time he drew her attention to this symptom, instead of sending him to bed, she would reassure him and would tell him that the fact that he was wheezing did not mean that he would have to have an asthma attack and stay in bed. John apparently was very sensitive, or should we say "allergic," to his mother's "unconscious." He had previously responded to her unconscious demands as though he were ordered to get sick. Now he was cautiously and consistently testing his mother to find out whether she had actually decided to let him be well—that is, to let him be a boy. The lifting of the severe dietary regime imposed upon John because of his allergies had been handled in the same way. The mother gradually introduced item after item of the previously forbidden foods until John was on a full diet within a few weeks.

Migraine and Psychogenic Headache

Friedman and Katz (1950) report on a series of children, who were referred from the Headache Clinic of a general hospital for psychiatric help, drawing attention to the fact that such conditions do occur frequently in children. They found a correlation between the episodes of headaches and emotional conflict in these cases.

In a study (chapter 18) which included nine children in whom migraine and persistent or recurrent headache had been a prominent symptom, I found that the onset of the headache could be traced back to a situation in which intense rage impulses had to be repressed suddenly. It was found that the original traumatic situation in which the child had to repress repeatedly such rage impulses often related to the birth of a sibling and to the child's repressed hostility and envy of this rival. The headache in these cases could be interpreted as the somatic expression of the unconscious impulse to kill the hated object instantly through an attack upon the head. The child could not allow himself to be conscious of such an impulse because he might not be able to resist its urgency and actually kill the object in a fit of rage. The connection between psychogenic headache and petit mal and epilepsy will be pointed out in the next section.

Petit Mal and Epilepsy

In 1932 Bartemeier, in a paper entitled "Some Observations of Convulsive Disorders in Children," opened a wide area for research and therapy in epilepsy and petit mal. Since then, however, very little work in this field has been done. Innovations in the treatment of epilepsy and petit mal have been primarily pharmacological and dietary with electroencephalography as a diagnostic tool.

Krug, Hayward, and Crumpacker (1952) report the residential treatment of a nine-year-old girl with petit mal and enuresis. They stress as important factors in this case the emotional deprivation in the early life of the girl and her feeling of being "unloved and of being unlovable." The hostility and the aggressive behavior of the girl are interpreted as defense against being hurt. This girl had very hostile feelings toward her mother, whose interference prevented her from accepting her femininity. Treatment lessened the intensity and frequency of petit mal attacks. The EEG remained unchanged. The report considers the petit mal attacks as precipitated by certain emotionally charged situations in a child with a "physiologically altered nervous system." This interpretation is based on an acknowledgment of an epileptic constitution. We know, however, from the work of Freud (1950d), Kardiner (1932), and others that epileptic reactions can be elicited from any human being under given circumstances.

Encouraged by the insights and therapeutic results obtained in psychoanalytic work with children suffering from migraine and/or other forms of headache I undertook to study and to treat psychoanalytically children with petit mal and epilepsy. Seven children have been studied; in all cases the diagnosis had been established by careful and repeated neurologic examinations. Some of these children had been treated for years with antiepileptic drugs such as dilantin and glutamic acid in high doses without effect and were beginning to show signs of deterioration and definite features of the epileptic personality.

I found that the basic unconscious conflict in all these cases was one between extreme passivity and extreme aggressivity. While I do not consider this conflict in itself specific for petit mal or epilepsy, I regard the attitude of the patients towards this conflict, in which either outcome is associated with death, as a specific dynamic factor in this condition (see chapter 20).

Boy (7½)

A seven-and-a-half-year-old boy (see chapter 20), had developed petit mal at the age of four and a half. A characteristic feature of his developmental history was the fact that his mother did not allow any outward manifestation of aggression. Play thearapy, his associations and his dream material revealed that his first attack had occurred when he was crossing the street with his mother and became frightened of being run over by an oncoming truck. It was found in analysis that this fear was the expression of his unconscious wish to fall and to be run over, an indication of his strong suicidal impulses. When in the course of the treatment the child acquired confidence in his ability to handle self-destructive impulses, his murderous impulses directed against his brother and mother became apparent. Together with the emergence of these object- and self-destructive impulses occurred a marked change in the child's behavior and symptoms. In lieu of the petit mal he developed attacks of headache. When he was helped, through further treatment, to tolerate consciously his impulses without fear of acting them out in reality, the attacks of headache ceased.

On the basis of my findings I would interpret the petit mal as an unconscious functional elimination of those parts of the mind which serve the perception of certain noxious stimuli from within and from without. Perception of these stimuli would lead to an explosive reaction endangering the life of the patient and that of people in the environment.

I consider this defense mechanism which the child adopts in dealing with dangerous impulses and with a threatening and very frustrating reality as specific for petit mal and epilspsy. It is also my impression that there is a definite interrelation between psychogenic headache and petit mal and epilepsy in these cases. The change from the symptom of petit mal to the symptom of headache in the course of treatment I attribute mainly to a decrease in the suicidal impulses and to an increased tolerance of such impulses consciously.

Environmental factors in the etiology and maintenance of petit mal and especially the interrelated dynamics of the maternal attitudes and the child's responses are of utmost importance. It is hoped that further studies will corroborate these findings and that a full recognition of the importance and possibility of changing such attitudes through psychotherapy will prove an essential factor in the prevention of petit mal and epilepsy (chapter 18).

Obesity

Hilda Bruch (1945) found that to the obese child physical size represents safety, power, and strength and that the child's fear of becoming "skinny and weak" is a factor in his resistance to weight reduction. She considers the eagerness of physicians to treat these children with hormone injections harmful because such treatment creates the impression of physiological deficiency. She states the commonly made prediction of sexual maldevelopment is incorrect and gives rise to anxiety in the child and to guilt feelings in the mother because so many of these mothers had wanted their sons to be daughters. Treatment which aims at reduction of food intake meets with resistance. Success depends largely upon the ability and willingness of the mother to let the child grow up and the child's willingness to do so.

Ulcerative Colitis

Chapter 7 describes the treatment of two children in some detail. This paper, published in 1946, in which experience gained in the treatment of four more children was used in the formulation of the psychodynamics, opened a new approach to the treatment of ulcerative colitis. A report by Finch (1952) and the observations of Prugh (1951b) on a series of children with ulcerative colitis seem to corroborate some of my findings. Despite these reports on successfully treated patients, resistance to the use of psychoanalytic techniques in the treatment of ulcerative colitis is still widespread. Child psychiatrists or psychiatrically trained pediatricians who treat ulcerative colitis seem to prefer various forms of supportive psychotherapy on a conscious level. The general practitioner is certainly not expected to be equipped for, nor skilled in, major surgery, but the surgeon should be able and willing to do such surgery when necessary. As regards psychoanalysis, this argument applies equally to the treatment of children suffering from ulcerative colitis.

In a publication by Hulse and Rapoport entitled "What Can Pediatrics Expect from Psychoanalysis" (1952), the authors, after a general discussion of some psychoanalytic principles with which they feel pediatricians ought to be acquainted, proceed to give their own technique in dealing with psychosomatic cases in a pediatric ward. "No attempt to probe or interpret is made. The therapeutic approach is limited to giving the child a realistic perspective. For example, if a child with ulcerative colitis balks at a transfusion, it is pointed out to him why it is necessary. At the same time he is assured that as soon as he begins to take more food and his physical condition improves such procedures will be eliminated. The therapist, in short, attempts to be the good realistic parent."

This "common sense approach" also brings to mind the case of a seven-year-old boy in an acute delusional state whom I saw as a consultant in the pediatric ward. He had been hospitalized because of an upper respiratory infection; during his stay in the hospital he had spoken of his fears and especially of a "turtle phobia" he had. The resident pediatrician decided to use "the common sense approach" and to cure the boy of his phobia by showing him a turtle with the intention of thereby proving to him that there was nothing to be afraid of. The result was an acute panic with delusions. The boy saw turtles everywhere, in his bed, on the floor, on the walls; he could not be calmed down.

The turtle phobia of this boy, who was later treated by me in the Child Psychiatric Clinic of the same hospital, could be understood and resolved in psychoanalytic psychotherapy. It was found that a turtle represented to him a highly emotionally charged symbol. As is characteristic of the unconscious, it operates with the mechanisms of condensation, displacement, and projection, and can in this way often express in one symbol the total conflict of the patient. This boy, who was a latent schizophrenic, expressed his intense sibling rivalry and murderous impulses in relation to the turtle which in projection became an extremely frightening object to him which he avoided phobically. Why the turtle was made the symbol could be understood only through analysis of certain experiences actually relating to a turtle which my patient once owned and which his brother had let fall out of the window. To explain why and how this lent itself to be used by the boy in this way would lead us too far astray here. However, one significant element should be mentioned, namely, that the mother, who was a very immature person, would keep only one of the boys home at a time while the other was placed away from home. It was therefore necessary to eliminate the rival in order to be with the mother. Only through an understanding of the historic and dynamic development of the presenting symptom was it possible to arrive at the final interpretation which made the symptom unneccessary.

To return to the discussion of ulcerative colitis, it is obviously unwise and not in keeping with the dynamic of this disease to limit oneself during the acute phases to assuring the child that as soon as he begins to take more food he will not need transfusions. This is what parents, doctors, and nurses tell the child anyway and is of the same value as attempting to induce a patient who is in a severe depression to eat by telling him that if he ate he would not need to be fed artificially. I am thinking of a nine-year-old girl with ulcerative colitis whom I saw for the first time when she was acutely ill in the hospital. Surgery had been advised, but she was so ill that the surgeon feared that she might expire on the operating table. I had been called as consultant against the vehement advice of the attending physician, apparently in order to allay the conscience of the mother who had refused to accept psychotherapy for the child when it had been suggested to her a year before.

In the first meeting with the child I told her that I knew how she felt and what she was doing, namely, that she felt like destroying herself and was actually doing so. I also told her that this was not the only solution and that I could assist her in finding a better one. From the way she responded I recognized that she felt that I understood. After I reassured her that I could and would help her and that I would speak to her mother about taking her out of the hostpial, we made an agreement: I explained that in order to help me to help her she would have to stop this suicidal undertaking and start eating. I explained to her that her mother felt justified in keeping her in the hospital because she was not eating and because she needed frequent transfusions. The change in the child's condition after I left her was nothing short of miraculous. Amazing in such cases is the speed with which the most severe clinical symptoms can develop and subside.

I had had some information about this child through a preliminary interview with her mother. On the basis of this information I was able to understand that the patient was intensely jealous of her younger sister, whom the mother overtly preferred. It also was obvious in the very first interview with the mother that she was extremely reluctant to yield the child to the psychiatrist, owing to her unrecognized fear of being exposed and interfered with in her relationship with the child. The fact that she had, for a whole year, refused to accept the advice of a reputable pediatrician to see me, though the child had been sick on and off with ulcerative colitis, was suggestive of such an attitude. It was also evident—this again is typical of mothers of children with ulcerative colitis—that she wanted to rid herself of the child. She was in a good position to rationalize this wish because no one could keep such a sick child at home (chapter 2). It was obvious from the start that the resistance of this mother would be very strong; this proved true throughout the treatment.

This case once more emphasizes the fact that it is essential to include the mother in the treatment, or to reckon at least with the mother's resistances and to be prepared to meet them, if one wants to treat successfully a case of ulcerative colitis in a child. Disregard of this factor and disregard of the dynamics of ulcerative colitis account, in my opinion, for the poor therapeutic results in most cases.

Recognition of some of these factors places the pediatrician in a key position regarding the treatment and prevention of psychosomatic illness. Obviously the most economic way to deal with this problem is by prevention, and the analogy with immunology readily offers itself. Once we know what is causing the disturbance, how and when it started, the road is clear for action. We have seen that psychosomatic disorders have their source in the early mother-child relationship. Therefore, the work of prevention must begin there. Or better still, the work should begin with the mother before the child is born. There are certain behavior patterns and symptoms which some women exhibit before and during pregnancy which demonstrate conspicuously that these women must, and inevitably will, establish a type of relationship with the child which will be conducive to the development of a psychosomatic response in the child. Prenatal mental hygiene clinics, where expectant mothers are screened and treated according to definite indications, would seem therefore to be an important step in this direction (M. Sperling, 1952).

Psychosomatic Disorders
in Adolescents

Puberty and adolescence are crucial phases in the life of young people, during which their ability to renounce the attachment to the original love objects and to form new relationships with persons of the same and of the opposite sex is being tested. The influx of sexual energy at this period of life disturbs, to a considerable extent, the precarious balance which the child has been able to establish during latency. It is well known that many neurotic and character disorders have their onset at this particular period of life. It is less well known that a variety of psychosomatic disorders also begin during this period. This is probably due to the fact that youngsters who appear organically sick are usually not referred for psychiactric treatment. An additional reason may be the fact that a reverse reciprocity exists between psychological and somatic manifestations in a psychosomatic disorder, that is, the more apparent the somatic manifestations are, the less apparent is the underlying neurotic structure. During the phase of active somatic illness, the individual does not appear neurotically sick, and there is little incentive for the parents or their advisers to have such a child treated psychiatrically.

The disposition to react with a psychosomatic disorder to a particular life situation is acquired early in life. The conflicts motivating such an individual are conflicts of the pre-oedipal phases, and the fixation points and regression in psychosomatic illness go back to the oral and anal phases of development. This disposition is rooted in a specific mother-child relationship, of which the outstanding feature on the part of the mother is her need to keep her child in lifelong dependence for the satisfaction of vital emotional and bodily needs. The complementary specific feature in the child is an unconscious compliance with these needs of the mother, that is, to be sick and dependent (see chapter 3). The specific somatic symptoms of the child, in these cases, are structured similarly to neurotic symptoms in which both the forbidden wish and the punishment are executed at the same time. In the psychosomatic symptom, both the compliance with the unconscious wish of the mother and the rebellion against it are expressed simultaneously. Although most investigators in the field of psychosomatic medicine consider rejection of the child (by the mother) as the significant feature of the mother's personality, I could, with the help of a specific research method which I used for the study of such cases, namely, the simultaneous psychoanalytic treatment of mother and child, arrive at a different conclusion.

In the simultaneous psychoanalytic treatment of mother and child, in which the interaction between the unconscious wishes of the mother and the responses of the child can be observed and treated analytically, I found that the mother rejects the child only when he is well and attempting to assert his independence, but that she rewards him when he is sick; that is, when he submits to her wishes (M. Sperling, 1955c). Low tolerance of frustration and emotional immaturity have been described as characteristic features of the psychosomatic patient. These features, however, are not specific for these patients; they are also characteristic for psychopaths, addicts, impulse-ridden characters, perverts, and other pregenitally fixated individuals. The specific characteristic feature of the personality of the psychosomatic patient, namely, that feature which differentiates him from the above-mentioned categories, is the specific structure of his superego. This, in turn, is the outcome of the specific mother-child relationship operating in these cases. During certain phases of the treatment, the behavior of psychosomatic patients may temporarily become that of impulse-ridden characters (M. Sperling, 1959d).

I am emphasizing this point because I want to indicate that the decisive factor is not so much the difference in the ego, particularly its strength or weakness, which accounts for the psychosomatic reaction, as it is the different structure of the superego of such patients. The aforementioned changes in the behavior of a psychosomatic patient occurring during treatment can be understood as resulting from changes in his superego. That means that his superego has become more permissive and less punitive and not that the ego has become weaker in the treatment process.

This report, prepared by Dr. Roy Lilleskov under supervision of Dr. Henry I. Schneer, is given to illustrate what may appear to be, but is not, a psychosomatic disorder.

Boy (12)

A twelve-year-old Jewish boy, a seventh grader in junior high school, was referred to the Kings County Hospital Child Guidance Clinic by the Kings County Hospital Pediatric Department after a ten-day diagnostic hospitalization failed to disclose organic pathology. His symptoms were overweight and colitis. His mother was not precise, but she felt that soiling was the problem. She said, "He had celiac disease when he was a baby. The doctor said if he lost weight the soiling would go away too." She continued, however, to refer to colitis. She expressed concern that he had no friends because of the smell. Almost daily, he has a bowel movement in his trousers.

From the report of a psychiatric interview with the boy, he was observed to be markedly obese, friendly, but constantly making self-reassuring comments and seeking approval. Whether complaining or not, his smile presented the same quality of bland acceptance. His soiling and eating were discussed in the same passive manner. He blames his trouble on being lazy but "can't do anything about it."

He recalled his life by school grades, for example: "In the first grade my mother went to work. . . . In the fifth grade I broke my leg. That is the year we had four teachers. I hate that. Getting used to new ones."

Of his soiling, he had this to say: "I get cramps and I have to go. I can't wait. It happens any time. No special reason. It's because of the colitis. There is nothing I can do about it."

He would like to be thinner but not "skinny" like one child they call "the stick." He overeats and cannot stop: "not because I'm hungry, I just want to eat."

His family consisted of an obese mother, forty-three, and his father, forty-six, described as a "giant," six feet tall, three hundred pounds" who was able to load three hundred-and-fifty-pound packages of fish at the market. The father was considered to be impulsive, impatient, and generous, and he would strike the children when annoyed. During her marriage the mother had a surgical repair for a pendulous abdomen. She also has been diabetic for the past five years. She described with much guilt how she would become enraged over the patient's soiling. For her diabetes, the patient would inject herself in the morning, and the older son would perform this service in the evening. The older son, seventeen, is tall and slim, not as bright as the patient, and "spoiled" owing to childhood allergies. The patient feels that he is always picked on by the brother. There is a twenty-two-year-old married daughter of whom little is known. A maternal grandmother, incontinent of urine and feces, lived with the family during the patient's second and third years of life.

Concerning the patient's development, he walked and talked at ten months. The mother attributed feeding difficulties to "severe food allergies" of her children. When the patient was thirteen months old, he had a severe diarrhea during which he lost weight. For months he continued to have three to four stools a day, loose and filled with mucous but not foul. Celiac disease was diagnosed. He was placed on a banana-and-rice diet, and, by the time he was two years old, he recovered his weight. Coincidentally, he was having a recurrent tonsillitis between the first and second years. When he was two years and four months old, he had a tonsillectomy. He weighted twenty-seven pounds then. When he was three years old he weighed seventy-seven pounds. The voracious eating since the tonsillectomy has now culminated in a weight of two hundred and ten pounds in a boy five feet, three inches tall.

For several years the mother was concerned with the small size of his genitalia. He was given androgen injections. Last year, however, a leading endocrinologist said that there was no sign of an endocrine problem and that hormone therapy should cease. In regard to his sexual history, the mother took pride in the lack of modesty in the home. When the father is shaving, the mother may be in the bathtub while one of the children uses the toilet.

At school, the patient is considered "very intelligent." He is in an advanced class.

Psychological testing of the patient place him in the superior range of intelligence. The Rorschach, TAT, and figure drawings did not reveal any indication of a psychotic break.

I do not consider this case a true psychosomatic disorder. The mucous colitis of this patient, on closer investigation, reveals itself to be really a form of soiling. I do not consider obesity a psychosomatic disorder, and the structure of the superego of the obese patient confirms my view. In the case of this boy, too, the structure of the superego is that of an impulse-ridden character. The outstanding feature in his case is a lack of instinctual control. My diagnosis of this boy would be: a character disorder closely related to addiction. As you may know, in some cases of obesity, the treatment is actually like that of addiction, for the obese patient behaves toward food as an addict does toward a narcotic.

Here, again, I want to stress the fact that I consider the differences in the structure of the superego to be of primary etiological significance. I did not find the ego of these addict-type patients particularly deficient. In fact, in certain aspects these patients reveal particular abilities in manipulating reality and people. In the Rorschach test of this boy, there was no evidence of psychosis. The superego originates from the incorporation of parental prohibitions, interdictions, and commands. The family history of this boy reveals a very permissive, seductive environment and parents who were lacking in emotional control themselves. We would expect that, by identification with the parental figures, he would develop a superego of the kind which would permit the behavior described in the case history.

In psychosomatic patients, however, the superego is very harsh. The psychopath or delinquent permits himself to release his destructiveness and his aggression externally to the outside world and to the objects in reality. Therefore, they attract much attention. The literature on adolescence deals mainly with the problems of delinquency. The psychosomatically sick adolescent does not attract very much attention because he suffers, whereas the delinquent adolescent makes other suffer. The element of suffering is essential to justify the diagnosis of psychosomatic illness. It is not mental pain or manifest anxiety which the psychosomatic patient experiences. These are the very feelings which he tries to avoid at the price of bodily suffering. There is a great deal of suffering involved in psychosomatic illness which, in some cases, may even lead to what I have called "psychosomatic suicide."

A beautiful illustration of this is the following observation reported by the internist Cullinan (1938). A young girl, gravely ill with ulcerative colitis, was receiving the last rites. The priest told her of the suffering of her parents, how they grieved and cried. Shortly after the priest left her, the patient got off the bed and said that she thought her parents had suffered enough. This was the end of her ulcerative colitis attack—one which had not responded to medical treatment.

In this connection again, the differences between the personality structure in psychopathy and psychosomatic illness are of interest. The psychoanalytic concept that, unconsciously, every suicide represents a murder is a familiar one. Neither the psychosomatic nor the obsessive-compulsive nor the depressive patient is prone to commit murder. This can be understood on the basis of the structure of the superego, which does not permit the acting out of destructiveness in reality but which prompts them to turn this destructiveness inside and toward themselves. These destructive impulses, in the case of the psychosomatic patient, are then released through the bodily symptoms.

The concept of profiles in psychosomatic diseases, introduced by Dunbar (1947), is of interest. According to this concept, certain personality types are prone to develop certain psychosomatic disorders, such as the peptic-ulcer type described by F. Alexander (1943, 1950). The problem of specificity of symptoms should also be mentioned here. It has been found that the same patient can develop different psychosomatic symptoms at different times and also that persons of different personality types can develop the same psychosomatic syndromes. This would seem to contradict the concept of specificity of symptoms. The phenomenon of change of psychosomatic symptoms in the course of treatment has been described by Engel, and by myself (1957). Just as, in a psychoneurosis, the symptoms may change when the underlying unconscious fantasies have been analyzed but the basic conflict has not yet been resolved, so the same can occur in a psychosomatic disease. Concerning the fact that different personalities can develop the same psychosomatic disease, careful analytic study of such cases revealed, rather, the significant basic similarities in these patients.

Psychosomatic Disorders in Adolescence

In describing some of the psychosomatic disorders most frequently encountered during adolescence, I shall use the conventional approach and classify these disorders according to organ systems. Most frequent are the disorders of the gastrointestinal system, comprising the mouth, the intestines, and the anus. The mouth is the organ for intake and, in the infant, the primary organ for contact with the outside world. The first object relationships are established through the mouth, so to speak. In the unconscious, food and mother remain associated all through life. The mouth is also an important organ for the development of reality testing and differentiation between the inside and outside worlds. Ernst Simmel (1932, 1933), a well-known German psychoanalyst of the old guard, suggested that there may be a libidinal organization preceding the oral phase which he called the gastrointestinal libido organization. In this way he was stressing the significance of the whole gastrointestinal system in the early instinctual development and not just that of the mouth, which is considered to be the most important and earliest erotogenic zone. I think it may be of interest to learn how Simmel arrived at this concept: Simmel was the man who founded what can be considered the first psychosomatic hospital in Germany during World War I. In this hospital he treated his patients with the psychoanalytic technique, and it was as a result of his experiences with these patients that he formed this idea.

The respiratory system is another organ system to be afflicted frequently with psychosomatic disorders. The psychologic mechanisms operating in certain psychosomatic diseases of the respiratory system are similar to those which we find in the disorders of the gastrointestinal system. The physiological processes of inhaling and exhaling can be used symbolically by the unconscious to express conflict of separation and fantasies of taking in or letting go.

Disorders of the circulatory system are not too frequent in adolescents.

The skin, owing to the fact that it represents the boundary of the body from the outside, becomes the seat of a number of psychosomatic disorders which, from a psychoanalytic point of view, can be understood as expressions of conflicts between the inside and the outside.

One of the most frequent disorders of the gastrointestinal tract found in puberty and adolescence is anorexia nervosa. It can be a very serious condition. There are patients who have to be hospitalized and fed artificially. This behavior toward food is similar to that of patients suffering from depression. We actually find, in the psychoanalytic treatment of patients with anorexia nervosa, a very close dynamic interrelationship between anorexia and depression. In some instances anorexia has been described as an equivalent of depression, the refusal to eat being an outstanding symptom in severe depression. Anorexia nervosa occurs more frequently in girls but is also found in adolescent boys. From a dynamic point of view, one should think in such a case of an unconscious feminine identification as an important dynamic factor. Very often anorexia is associated with nausea and vomiting. Unresolved sexual problems and unconscious pregnancy fantasies and wishes also are significant dynamic factors.

In anorexia nervosa there is a severe inhibition of the oral instincts to the extent that the patient stops eating and may have to be fed artificially. The exact opposite is true for obesity. In these cases, overeating and excessive gratification of oral instincts in reality are common. It is for this reason that I do not consider obesity as a psychosomatic disorder. I consider obesity as an impulse disorder and would place it in the category with drug addiction and alcoholism. The decisive difference between this type of patient and the psychosomatic patient is precisely that the impulse-ridden character gratifies his impulses in reality with a disregard of the consequences of his action for himself and others, whereas the psychosomatic patient, consciously unaware of his impulses, can gratify them only partially and in a distorted way via the somatic symptoms. In the psychosomatic symptom, as in the neurotic symptom, the need for punishment is gratified by the pain and suffering associated with the illness. As one patient suffering from chronic ileitis put it, "This [the ileitis] makes me a martyr and not a maniac." In his case, and this is so in every case, the illness brought essential gains. It was the key to the heart of his wife. Had he shown his true feelings in his overt behavior, it certainly would have brought him not sympathy but disapproval from his wife and others.

The alternative in these cases, however, is not either to be sick (i.e., a martyr) or to act out destructive impulses in reality (i.e., a maniac) as this patient presented it. It is possible for these patients in psychoanalytic treatment to achieve the adequate instinctual control necessary for healthy functioning.

Ulcerative and mucous colitis are psychosomatic disorders of the lower gastrointestinal system, frequently occurring during adolescence. Abdominal cramps and diarrhea are characteristic features in both conditions. Ulcerative colitis is the more serious illness and is associated in most cases with fever, anorexia, and bloody diarrhea. The onset is generally sudden. The course of this illness is characterized by spontaneous remissions and exacerbations and often leads to chronic invalidism and even death if not treated. For detailed studies on this subject I refer to chapter 7. I can only summarize here some of my findings.

In its severe form, ulcerative colitis is the somatic equivalent of a melancholic depression. The fixation and regression are primarily to the oral-sadistic level. In its milder forms it can be understood to represent the somatic equivalent of certain perversions or severe character disorders. In these cases the fixation and regression are primarily to the anal level of psychosexual development. The specific quality of object relationship in ulcerative colitis and its etiologic and dynamic significance have been demonstrated and emphasized in my studies of this illness. I should mention here that gastric and duodenal ulcers occur in older adolescents and that the same unconscious conflicts have been found to be at work in these conditions as in young adults.

Another condition seen not too infrequently, particularly in adolescent boys, is hemorrhoids. Of course this does not mean that every case of hemorrhoids in an adolescent is a psychosomatic disorder, but there are some instances in which this condition is a true psychosomatic disorder, that is, the somatic expression of an unconscious conflict. I am thinking of one case, that of a 17-year-old boy who developed acute and severe hemorrhoids during his analysis. Since the boy was suffering badly, his father had arranged with the proctologist for surgical removal of the hemorrhoids. I was able to get a postponement of the operation so that we had a chance to understand, in the analysis, what had happened. After resolving the conflict and becoming conscious of his fantasies, the hemorrhoids cleared up as dramatically as they had appeared. The proctologist was so baffled by this that he wanted to know what medication we had used so successfully. He could not understand that merely talking could have such an effect upon hemorrhoids.

I shall now mention some of the disorders of the respiratory system, such as hay fever, rhinitis, nervous coughing, sneezing, etc., referred to as "allergies of the upper respiratory system" occurring in adolescents. In this connection it may be of interest to learn that the psychoanalytic treatment of certain allergic conditions, while freeing the patient from his allergic reactions, does not change the (constitutional) allergic condition. After treatment such patients may be found to be sensitive to the allergens, for example, in skin tests, but when exposed to these allergens they show no clinical manifestations. This phenomenon demonstrates the significance of the emotional factor which, in these cases, apparently is a specific factor to trigger off the allergic clinical reactions. I have observed this phenomenon in cases of hay fever, bronchial asthma, and food allergy in adolescents.

Of the disorders of the circulatory system, angioneurotic edema and migraine headache occur not too infrequently during adolescence. I had an opportunity to treat also an adolescent girl with hypertension. On follow-up seven years later, it was found that her hypertension did not recur even in situations of stress.

Of the disorders of the skin to be found in adolescents, dermatitis and eczema are the most frequent. In my material there was a preponderance of girls in whom the dermatitis was associated with a particularly severe itch and uncontrollable scratching. Because of some of the dynamics unfolded in the psychoanalytic treatment of these girls, I am inclined to think that girls may be more prone to develop dermatitis. Although psychological factors undoubtedly play a role in acne, I would not consider acne to be a psychosomatic disorder. It would, rather, seem that acne is secondarily used in certain conflicts of adolescence and may be aggravated and maintained by this.

PART 2

ULCERATIVE COLITIS

6

Ulcerative Colitis
in Children: Current Views
and Therapies

Ulcerative colitis is a disease of the lower gastrointestinal system. Clinically it manifests itself in attacks of abdominal cramps and bloody diarrhea, commonly associated with fever, nausea, and weight loss. The onset is generally sudden but can also be insidious. The course of the illness is characterized by sponteneous remissions and exacerbations, often leading to chronic illness and surgical intervention. In some cases it may even prove fatal. To the pediatrician and the internist, chronic ulcerative colitis has been and remains an enigma, as a survey of the recent medical literature on ulcerative colitis in children confirms. The etiology of this disease is unknown and accordingly the treatment at best is aimed at symptomatic relief. There is no known medical treatment which can control the course or severity of the disease.

The purely medical approach to the treatment of this disease has proven so unsatisfactory that surgery has become a rather frequent procedure. In fact, very recently Lynn (1965), a pediatric surgeon of the Mayo Clinic, earnestly suggested that in every case of ulcerative colitis in a child, total colectomy and permanent ileostomy should be performed not later than six months after the onset of the first symptoms of ulcerative colitis. Lynn states that, "The entire medical treatment of ulcerative colitis in children should be viewed as preoperative. A child who suffers from bouts of ulcerative colitis over a prolonged period, even though they are brief and well tolerated, must be considered a candidate for surgery."

Actually, the course of this illness in children is more severe than in adults and the response to medical treatment is less satisfactory. The earlier the onset of the ulcerative colitis, the more severe will be its course.

A recent follow-up study on eighty-four children with onset of ulcerative colitis in the presteroid era revealed a high mortality rate, 33 percent, and a high incidence of major surgery, also 33 percent. Another 33 percent were alive without surgery but with chronic recurrent ulcerative colitis. Of the latter, 10 percent had carcinoma of the rectal colon and 18 percent had strictures or complications such as obstruction (Korelitz and Gribetz, 1962). The introduction of steroid therapy during the past decade has resulted in more dramatic remissions and raised the hope of more effective treatment of ulcerative colitis in children. However, these dramatic effects when they occurred were limited to reducing severe attacks, especially first attacks; their influence on the later course of the illness has been less satisfactory. This therapy has undesirable side effects, especially when given over a long period of time, and contributes to complications. A follow-up study of thirty-seven children aged two and a half to eleven and a half years, treated with steroids during the first three years of the disease, later revealed an even higher incidence of chronic complications compared with the results in the presteroid era, and a higher frequency of retarded growth and development, possibly accentuated by direct hormonal influence (Korelitz and Gribetz, 1962; Korelitz, 1964). The authors of this study concluded that this treatment has not reduced the incidence of surgery, that its effect is nonspecific and anti-inflammatory and it may be useful in severe cases preliminary to surgical intervention. Lynn (1965) expressed concern that steroid therapy might mask signs and symptoms of a disintegrating colon or complicate the picture in bowel perforation. In his view, "Steroids should not be used without the concurrence of the surgeon who will become responsible in the event of failure of this regimen." This is a rather sad but realistic view of present-day medical treatment of ulcerative colitis in children.

Let us now take a look and compare this situation with what psychiatry and especially psychoanalysis have contributed to the dynamic understanding of this disease and its treatment. Understanding of some of the emotional factors operating in ulcerative colitis has come from the psychiatric investigation of adult patients, beginning with the pilot study of Murray in 1930. In 1946 I published my first account of successful psychoanalytic treatment of children suffering from ulcerative colitis. This was the first psychoanalytic study of children with this disease and opened up a new approach to the treatment of ulcerative colitis in children (see chapter 7). Subsequent reports by other investigators (Finch and Hess, 1962; Mohr et al., 1958; Prugh, 1950, 1951) on a series of children with ulcerative colitis corroborated some of my findings concerning some common features observed in these children and their families. The findings of these authors although obtained in most cases by observational and interview methods and not in psychoanalytic treatment, are helpful for an understanding of the personality disturbances of these children. An observation by Finch and Hess (1962) is of particular interest. They state, "All of these children were torn between the need to express hostility and the need for a close dependent relationship with the mother which resulted in conformity and compliance." While this finding in itself is not specific and can be observed in a variety of neurotic disorders in children, for instance, phobias, it deserves attention because it indicates the presence of a conflict between aggression and dependency. These authors dealt with one aspect of this conflict, namely, the repression of aggression resulting in conformity and compliance, but they did not explore further the vicissitudes of these repressed aggressive impulses and their role in the illness proper, that is, in ulcerative colitis. I would like to outline some dynamic formulations concerning the nature and etiology of ulcerative colitis in children which I developed from psychoanalytic work with ulcerative colitis children and their mothers over a period of twenty-five years.

Ulcerative colitis is not a disease of adulthood as is commonly assumed. It originates in childhood, although it may remain latent and the clinical manifestations may appear only later in life (Portis, 1949). This finding is in full accord with our knowledge of the causes of mental illness, derived from psychoanalytic theory and practice. Early experiences and unresolved conflicts of childhood predispose and condition certain behavior later in life. The nature of these experiences and the age at which they occur are factors in determining the severity and form of the reaction which may be precipitated by a specific emotional situation later in life. The disposition to react with bodily symptoms to emotional trauma is acquired very early in life. In fact, in infants and very young children, bodily pathways are the only outlets for distress arising from any source.

It has been found that certain life situations are conducive to the onset of ulcerative colitis in adults (separation, real or feared object loss, and similar traumatic situations). In children certain developmental phases constitute such vulnerable life situations. In the young child, the age between one and a half and three years is such a time. Other such times are the beginning of latency and start of school and later the start of puberty and adolescence. Actually, the onset of ulcerative colitis in young children usually occurs between one and a half and two and a half to three years of age (M. Sperling, 1959c). This is a time when the child not only has to give up soiling and pleasure in his excretions and has to acquire sphincter control, but also has to undergo an important psychological transformation. From a passively dependent infant of the oral phase, the child develops into the aggressive and even destructive toddler of the anal phase who now has the necessary physical equipment for the execution of some strivings for self-assertion and independence from his mother. During this age, certain attitudes of the parents, especially of the mother, may interfere with a satisfactory development of the anal-erotic and anal-sadistic drives and provide the basis not only for a bowel disturbance but also for a disturbance in the child's ability to handle and to express adequately aggression and sexuality later in life. The pregenital roots for the development of character disorders go back to these phases. The fixation to the anal-erotic and anal-sadistic phases of development and the regression to these fixations under traumatic circumstances in later life are of particular importance in ulcerative colitis.

In some cases, the anal-erotic needs of the mother which are usually covered up by reaction formations may lead to a relationship with her child which I have referred to as "toilet symbiosis" (1959c). Mother and child often spend many hours of the day and night together in the toilet. In one case, the child, eight-year-old Lisa, who had suffered from ulcerative colitis since the age of one and a half years, would get abdominal cramps during mealtimes and would often interrupt eating to run to the toilet. The mother frequently had the meal brought into the bathroom and would feed the child there. This mother, whom I had the opportunity of studying in a lengthy analysis, was an intensely anally fixated woman who spent many hours every day with her own anal procedures in the toilet. She was afraid to be in the toilet when there was no one at home. When her child improved and was ready to attend school, this became a problem for the mother, because she needed to have someone in the house in the morning when she had to spend time in the toilet. This specific phobia was only one manifestation of a generalized chronic and crippling phobic state from which this mother suffered and which she had been able to cover up by rationalizations and manipulations and by the help of the "sick child" (M. Sperling, 1967a). In spite of the obvious signs of disgust from the mother, or even the child, manifested during cleaning procedures (these children soil themselves frequently and thoroughly and refer to the soiling as "accidents"), we found that these are instinctually gratifying experiences for both and are difficult to renounce.

For treatment of more severe cases of ulcerative colitis, especially in young children, I introduced the method of simultaneous treatment of mother and child. This technique was necessary for therapeutic reasons, but at the same time it proved to be an invaluable research tool which permitted me to gain a deeper understanding of the interrelated dynamics of the mother-child relationship operating in these cases (1959d). The most significant contribution which came from this work was the discovery of a specific relationship, the psychosomatic type, between mother and child, in which a premium is set by the mother on her child's illness and dependence upon her. This psychosomatic relationship originates early in life, but its pathological effects become apparent first during the anal phases of the development of the child when the ability to initiate actively a gradual separation from the mother develops because of the maturational processes of this age. During the preceding oral phases of development separation is a passive experience for the child and is initiated by the mother. This aspect of the dependent relationship is obvious and has been accepted generally, namely, the dependence of the child upon the mother for gratification of his needs. However, the other aspect, the dependency of the mother upon her child for the gratification of her own neurotic needs, is not obvious and therefore not generally accepted. Once this "psychosomatic" relationship is established, it interferes with the regular progression of the subsequent developmental phses. I would like to demonstrate the dynamics of such a mother-child relationship, its pathogenic effects, and its modifications in the treatment of a case of ulcerative colitis in a child not yet four years old.

Freddie (4)

Freddie was referred to me by the hospital in which he had been treated for severe ulcerative colitis for several months. Mother and child were each seen twice a week in separate sessions. I would like to give the developmental history in some detail because it is rather typical for cases of ulcerative colitis in children with early onset of this illness. Freddie's mother took pride in the fact that she had achieved sphincter control with him at the age of one year. At the age of one and a half he showed fears of touching and fear of dirt. He would display signs of anxiety if a speck of food fell on his bib. The onset of his diarrhea occurred at this age (when a child should be still permitted to soil himself). In this case, however, neither the mother nor Freddie had ever allowed themselves openly to acknowledge and to gratify their anal impulses. Identification with the compulsive mother caused unusually severe and early repression of anal impulses in this child, leading at the age of one and a half years to the formation of an oversevere prestage of the superego with compulsive features. Freddie could allow himself to soil only at the cost of illness. At the same time, this forced his mother to handle the fecal matter which she consciously abhorred but to which she was unconsciously attracted. The mother's conscious reaction to his illness is best highlighted by her remark to me, "I am such a clean woman and he has such a messy disease."

Freddie did not respond to any medication, and in addition to the diarrhea, he developed bleeding and a high fever. An infectious origin of the diarrhea was suspected and a tonsillectomy was performed. No improvement ensued, however. After several weeks in the hospital he was discharged unimproved, but was hospitalized again after a short stay at home because of an acute exacerbation. This time he was admitted to a hospital where there was particular interest in the psychosomatic approach to ulcerative colitis. All types of treatment and medications were given, but there was no response. After some time, when he had been taken off medications and the dietary restrictions were lifted, Freddie began to improve slightly. During this time he had a psychiatric workup and the parents were seen by a psychiatric social worker.

The description of the boy's behavior in the hospital confirmed the impression of an early, unduly severe reaction against anal impulses. He remained in the hospital for several months, and the only therapy consisted in letting him play with other children. He was discharged much improved. The parents, who had been given some understanding by the social workers were advised to let the child eat and play normally instead of overprotecting him as they had previously done. The child remained well until the age of three and a half years.

At this time during his oedipal phase when the child began to masturbate, the mother threatened his genital impulses just as abruptly as she had earlier suppressed his anal ones. Characteristic of the mother's attitude toward Freddie is the following: when Freddie once teasingly exposed his penis to his sister (five years his senior) the mother became so infuriated that she threatened to cut off his penis, holding before him a big kitchen knife. Following this, Freddie developed an acute phobia (he was clinging to his father and would not let him leave the house) and shortly thereafter an exacerbation of the ulcerative colitis. The child responded to his mother's interference with his developing sexuality by an acute repression of his sexual impulses, which found release and expression in a renewed exacerbation of the original symptom of bloody diarrhea.

Freddie was again admitted to the hospital. From there he was referred to me for ambulatory treatment, which the mother accepted after some hesitation. In the playroom he exhibited anxious, phobic, behavior. He was anxious about not being able to control his diarrhea and continuously ran from the playroom to the bathroom. He was afraid to touch things, especially clay, and when he did so, had to wash his hands immediately. On the one hand, the boy's sexuality was abruptly suppressed by the severe prohibition of masturbation, and at the same time, he was stimulated and seduced by both parents. The father, who had very strong latent homosexual tendencies, had an almost paranoid attitude toward his wife and suspected her of infidelity. Whenever he quarreled with her, he would take Freddie into bed with him, clearly indicating that he used Freddie as a substitute for his wife.

Symptoms such as bloody diarrhea serve to gratify infantile sexual impulses, whose normal outlet has been blocked by prohibition and repression; they also serve as a release of the aggression against the prohibiting parents, which the child dares not feel consciously and is unable to express directly. The multiple purpose and the overdetermined meaning of the symptoms explain why these conditions resist treatment so stubbornly. The symptoms serve important dynamic functions in the patient's unconscious life. He cannot give them up if he has no other more adequate way of dealing with his needs.

Freddie would characteristically spare his father and awaken his mother when he had to go to the bathroom at night. This only added to her resentment against him. The mother felt that her husband and son had "ganged up" on her. She told me that she was one of five sisters and two brothers. The brothers had died young, but all the sisters were alive. She had had a son before Freddie was born, who had died in an accident in infancy. Her attitude to Freddie is shown by her remark, "The boys in my family don't live long, Freddie is taking his time."

In psychotherapy, Freddie improved remarkably. In treatment, the child has to be allowed to relive in a modified form the developmental phases that he has missed in life and to work through the pregenital drives in symbolic play activity. Only after this has been done can normal ego development take place. The important thing is the acceptance by the child and the parents of the existence of his oral and anal impulses, not their direct gratification.

The fact that this boy developed a condition such as ulcerative colitis so early in life is attributable in a large measure to the unusually strong and early repression of oral and anal aggressive impulses in response to his mother's needs. She demanded complete submission and allowed no overt instinctual manifestations or gratifications. Freddie had earlier been a severe feeding problem, indicating that the mother-child relationship had been disturbed from the beginning. Freddie's mother, like the mother of Lisa (who also developed ulcerative colitis at one and a half years of age) was an intensely anally fixated woman for whom Freddie's illness provided a legitimate setting for the gratification of her own repressed anal impulses. Freddie's mother, like Lisa's mother, needed a sick child, because her older child had just started school and she knew that she would not have another baby. As in Lisa's case, there was an acute marital crisis and Freddie's mother too needed someone whom she could control and who would be completely (for his very life) dependent upon her. But Freddie's situation was even more difficult because his mother did not allow him to be a boy and did not permit any expressions of aggression. His aggression was turned entirely against himself. There has been no manifest display of aggression until play analysis was undertaken at the age of four. The consequent turning outward of the destructive impulses was accompanied by immediate and striking improvement both in the ulcerative colitis and in the child's total behavior. When Freddie began to assert himself by attending kindergarten and evidenced some overt aggressive behavior, his mother suddenly withdrew him from treatment. She could not tolerate any improvement in the child which threatened to interfere with his dependent relationship to her. In addition to the basic reasons which led to this specific relationship with Freddie, namely, her own unresolved relationship with her mother and brothers and her very strong repressed anality, she needed Freddie to be sick for other reasons as well. At that particular time his illness also served to keep the unsatisfactory marriage going (see chapter 2 and 1952b).

This case brings out the importance of taking into consideration such an attitude of the mother when one treats a child with ulcerative colitis. In Lisa's case, I worked first with Lisa's mother in preparatory analysis for one year before starting Lisa's treatment and then intermittently during the three and a half years of Lisa's analysis and thereafter for another three years. Winnicott (1966), reporting the unsatisfactory outcome of a case of ulcerative colitis, states, "Unfortunately I was unable to see early enough that the ill person in this case was the mother. It was the mother who had the essential split, and the child who had the colitis. But it was the child who was brought to me for treatment." Even those physicians who discount the importance of psychogenic factors in ulcerative colitis have recognized the powerful influence of the mother on the patient and consider the mother in certain cases of ulcerative colitis in children a greater problem than the child himself (Crohn, 1963).

A General Therapeutic Approach

I began my work with ulcerative colitis children on a pediatric ward of a general hospital. Every kind of medical treatment had been tried on these children without success. I worked under the watchful eyes of the pediatricians and other specialists and presented my cases regularly in clinical conferences to the medical staff. In some cases, I was called as the last resort when surgery was contemplated. The Chief of Service gave me complete freedom to treat my cases as I saw fit, and it was because of this arrangement that my work with these children was successful.

The findings of this and subsequent work with ulcerative colitis children and their mothers revealed that in the severe cases the underlying psychiatric disorder resembles that of a melancholic depression or the depressive phases of a manic-depressive psychosis. It seems to represent the somatic dramatization of the same conflict, with relatively little mental pain, that in depression is expressed psychologically. The psychological equivalents of the somatic manifestations in ulcerative colitis can range from melancholic depression and paranoid schizophrenia to pregenitally fixated character disorders and neuroses. The degree of severity of the manifest clinical, somatic pathology corresponds to the degree of severity of the latent psychopathology in the child's personality and in the interrelated family dynamics, but especially those of the mother-child relationship.

It indicates a total ignorance of the psychodynamics of ulcerative colitis to advocate, as a therapeutic approach in the acute phases of this illness, limiting oneself to assuring the child that as soon as he begins to take more food he will not need transfusions. This is what parents, doctors, and nurses tell the child in any event and is of the same value as if one were to attempt to induce a patient who is in a severe depression to eat by telling him that if he ate he would not need to be fed artificially. Yet this approach in which the child is treated by a team of physicians (pediatrician, internist, surgeon, and child psychiatrist) with the major emphasis upon medical treatment in the acute phases has been recommended by certain child psychiatrists (Hulse and Rapoport, 1952). McDermott and Finch (1967) consider the team approach as "the best approach" in the treatment of ulcerative colitis in children. Their gloomy statistics, however, "75 percent of the youngsters hospitalized since the formation of the physician team required surgery," does not support such a claim. The splitting of the patient between the specialists can be disastrous for the patient. It makes for a division between the somato- and psychopathology and makes it difficult if not impossible to correlate the somatic and psychological factors operating in ulcerative colitis. The poor results reported with this method would indicate that this is not "the best approach."

The attitude of the surgeon in the cases of children with severe ulcerative colitis is best described with the comment of a surgeon made to the mother of a nine-year-old boy with severe ulcerative colitis, when instead of accepting his suggestion for major surgery she accepted, as an alternative, referral to me. "How can you take your sick child to a psychiatrist when he needs surgery? What will she do (the psychiatrist)? Speak to his stomach?" Such an attitude throws the mother into severe conflict and will be used by some mothers as a rationalization against psychiatric treatment. This mother followed the advice of a consultant pediatrician and told me later, as many mothers have, that she had always known that her son had an emotional disturbance, but that the d octors did not think so. This boy did remarkably well in his treatment with comparatively little work with the mother, because she was willing to release her son from his dependent relationship with her. At the time of this writing, this boy is a young man, twenty-five years old, married, and has not had a recurrence of ulcerative colitis since the age of nine and a half years. He was in treatment with me for three years. In 1964, I published a twenty-year follow-up study of a child whom I treated successfully for severe ulcerative colitis when he was seven and a half years old.

I have follow-up studies from three to twenty-three years on patients whom I have treated for ulcerative colitis. From 1942 to the present I have treated twenty-one patients intensively and eleven for shorter periods of time. I have seen in consultation forty-five patients and I have supervised the treatment of nineteen cases, a total of ninety-six cases. All these patients had at least one hospitalization, but most of them had several. They all were severe cases of ulcerative colitis before they came for treatment, and none of them developed cancer. I think this is of particular interest in view of the frequency of polyposis and cancer in medically treated cases.

This chapter reflects my concern over the major role that surgery is taking in the treatment of ulcerative colitis in children. My treatment is aimed at making medical treatment and surgery unnecessary. I was successful in thirty out of the thirty-three cases I have treated. One of these three cases was Freddie who was withdrawn from treatment by his mother, and the others were two adolescent girls who were subjected to colectomy when they were hospitalized for reasons other than the ulcerative colitis itself. I want to illustrate this eagerness of surgeons to remove the colon of patients who have or had ulcerative colitis with a recent supervisory experience. The patient, a nine-year-old-boy with chronic ulcerative colitis who had been doing well in his treatment, suddenly developed acute abdominal pain and fever. The pediatrician diagnosed an acute abdomen due to the ulcerative colitis. The patient said that he did not think that this was ulcerative colitis because it did not feel like it and he knew how the pain in ulcerative colitis felt. The analyst also did not think that it was ulcerative colitis and arranged with the pediatrician to be present in the operating room. When the boy was opened up and acute appendicitis was found, a colectomy was prevented only because the parents, forewarned by the analyst, steadfastly refused to consent to the surgeon's request.

Concerning the therapeutic approach, I would like to outline some general guidlines. It is essential to understand that ulcerative colitis, that is, idiopathic ulcerative colitis for which no known external or internal etiological cause can be established medically, indicates the presence of a psychiatric disorder; that the symptoms of the ulcerative colitis are the somatic manifestations and expressions of the specific unconscious fantasies and conflicts; and that we treat not the symptom or the diseased organ(s) but the patient who produces and who needs and maintains these symptoms. The clinical manifestations and course of ulcerative colitis in a child reflect the severity of the underlying psychopathology not only of the patient, but also of his family, especially of the mother. I have always assumed complete responsibility for the treatment of my patients and if I accept a patient with ulcerative colitis, it is with the understanding that I manage the treatment and determine the necessity for intervention by other specialists, re-examinations, and whatever procedures may be indicated. From the very beginning, my aim in treatment is to help the patient understand that his somatic symptoms are meaningful and are his (preverbal) way of expressing and discharging feelings and conflicts of which he is not aware consciously. The growing understanding of the patient that he is not at the mercy of the somatic symptoms but that he is the one who produces them and also the one who can stop them is extremely important and helpful. The emphasis in treatment is to encourage the patient to wean himself from medications and medical treatment. This approach is diametrically different from the team appraoch. The team approach fosters the patient's dependence upon medications and medical treatment and puts the responsibility for control of the ulcerative colitis upon the treating physician who then extricates himself from this "dilemma" (McDermott and Finch, 1967) by turning the patient over to the surgeon.

In the treatment approach which I am using and advocating, all medical personnel previously involved in the treatment of the patient have to accept that their contact with the patient will be reduced to a minimum or eliminated entirely after the patient has been weaned from steroids or whatever medication he had been taking. The patient is sent, however, for periodic checkups. This places a great responsibility upon the analyst or child psychiatrist. The results, however, justify the procedure and demonstrate the value of this approach in the treatment of ulcerative colitis.

I would also like to give a few general suggestions about the handling of the mother. With children of prelatency age, it is best to work with the mother first, and in many cases, this may even be sufficient so that no direct work with the child may be necessary. Even severe symptoms may still be reversible if it is possible to change the relationship existing between mother and child. In such cases, the mother has to be helped to modify her unconscious needs and to achieve sufficient security so that she can relinquish this relationship with her child. With this technique, I was able to achieve a complete cure with a follow-up from five to fourteen years in five children aged three to five years. I have seen similar results in supervision of the treatment of young children with ulcerative colitis. With children of latency age, work with the mother preceding or concomitant with the treatment of the child is necessary. With children of puberty age and adolescents, I prefer to work directly with the child, unless, as in the most severe cases, the underlying psychiatric disorder is of a schizophrenic or borderline nature. In such a case, it is preferable to divide the treatment of mother and child between two therapists (one for the mother and another for the child) if treatment is concomitant; or if the treatment is to be carried out by the same therapist, it is preferable to treat the mother first. This is similar to the treatment in severe character disorders (Sperling, 1959d).

This chapter attempts to assess the current views and therapeutic approaches in the treatment of ulcerative colitis in children. The purely medical approach, the team approach (combined medical and psychiatric treatment), and the psychoanalytic approach have been discussed and the therapeutic results compared. The psychoanalytic approach which I have developed and used since 1942 takes into consideration the psychosomatic mother-child unit and the pregenital conversion nature of the somatic symptoms in ulcerative colitis. The approach of treating the somato- and psychopathology as different but inseparable expressions of the same unconscious conflicts, fantasies, and impulses has proved to be the most successful method in treating ulcerative colitis in children.

Psychoanalytic Study of Ulcerative Colitis

The importance of psychogenic factors in ulcerative colitis has been emphasized by several investigators. Cecil D. Murray first demonstrated that there exists a definite relationship between emotional disturbance and the onset of bloody diarrhea; also he expressed the opinion that this disease tended to occur in a definite type of personality, characterized by emotional immaturity that shows itself in lifelong dependence upon parents, and in sexual maladjustment. His impressions have been confirmed in a number of case reports by A. J. Sullivan and E. R. Cullinan and others. In a personality study of forty patients, E. Wittkower could show that ulcerative colitis is a disease of the mentally ill. Almost all the patients showed character disorders, clinical neurosis, or psychosis. In his opinion, similar precipitating events would not lead to this symptom in other individuals.

Although a great deal of psychoanalytic study has been made of gastrointestinal disturbances, especially by Alexander and his coworkers, there exists very little analytic literature on ulcerative colitis. A case history published by G. E. Daniels on the treatment of a patient with ulcerative colitis and depression confirms my observations.

Although emotional disturbance as a precipitating and constant factor in the etiology of ulcerative colitis has been stressed by all investigators, the cause and nature of this illness have remained unknown.

Robert (7)

Robert was first seen by me after he had been ill with ulcerative colitis for more than one year. He had developed colitis when he was about six years old, a few weeks after he had started school. When his mother attempted to place him in kindergarten at five years old, Robert had become terrified, refused to stay, and his mother had to have him withdrawn.

Robert, aged seven, had two sisters, twelve and fourteen years old. While the girls had presented no difficulties, he had been a difficult child from birth. He was, indeed, a problem to his mother even before he was born. She had to spend almost all of the first three months of this pregnancy in bed, and when she was six months pregnant her whole body became swollen. She had not wanted Robert nor, in fact, any children, but she had never done anything to get rid of them. Her husband, who at that time had lost his father, insisted on trying to have a boy to whom he could give his father's name.

Robert is described as having been a very irritable and stubborn baby. He was a very fearful child, much more demanding than his sisters had been, and he had frequent tantrums. The father was "always more demonstrative" with the boy than the mother, and left all the disciplining or punishment to her. Robert always became extremely moody whenever he was punished. His mother was very defensive about the role that she might be playing in the child's illness and repeatedly wanted to be reassured that she had not contributed to his illness by mismanagement.

I first saw Robert in a pediatric ward to which he had been admitted the fourth time since the onset of his illness more than a year previous. He had been treated with several courses of sulfonamides, high protein diets, low residue and gelatine diets, cod-liver oil, enemas, vitamins, and liver extracts; and finally he was taken off all milk and milk products. He would improve spontaneously and then have another attack of bloody diarrhea, cramps, and fever. He required frequent transfusions. An x-ray examination revealed loss of haustrations with ulcerations of the large bowel. Bacteriological studies of material taken directly from the colon were negative for pathogenic organisms.

At the time treatment began, he was acutely ill, weighed about thirty-nine pounds, and had bloody diarrhea, abdominal cramps, and temperature up to 106. He was described in the hospital as a moody, irritable, uncommunicative child, interested only in his diet and his stools. He never engaged spontaneously in conversation, and answered mostly in monosyllables. Whenever his mother visited him in the hospital, he demanded that she go immediately and buy him crackers or peanuts. If she refused, he would begin to cry, complain of cramps, and sit on the bedpan.

In my first contact with him, he regarded me very suspiciously and reserved judgment. When I told him that I could very well understand how he felt in the hospital helplessly exposed to the nurses and doctors who did not give him the things he wanted, his face lighted. I told him that I could help him to get the things he wanted, and that this would help him to get well much faster, and I gave him the feeling I understood how lonely he felt in his futile struggle against everybody. The first thing he wanted me to bring him was a horn. It gave him great satisfaction to use this horn to annoy the other children and the nurses in the ward. He readily accepted my suggestion that he express his anger in some acceptable way, such as tearing up paper. He asked for scissors to cut up cardboard. He told me a dream the second time I saw him: "The bed next to me was empty and the boy in it had disappeared." He told me he had been very angry with this boy who teased him. Robert quickly accepted me as a valuable accomplice in getting him concessions. He ate much better when a number of previously forbidden foods were added to his very rigid diet. After four weeks during which he was brought in a wheelchair to me in the clinic twice a week, his general condition had improved somewhat. He was still running a high temperature and had bloody stools. He became more and more insistent upon going home and sought my aid in persuading his mother, who was frightened at the mere mention of taking him home. After I talked to his mother to prepare her, Robert was dicharged from the hospital having first been given a blood transfusion. He weighed about forty-nine pounds, his temperature ranged to 103, and the bloody diarrhea continued. He was to be brought to the clinic twice a week, and his mother agreed to come whenever it was necessary to discuss the situation with her.

At home there was constant fighting about food between Robert and his mother, who threatened repeatedly to send him back to the hospital. It was difficult to persuade her that it was better to let him have the food that he desired, especially since his cravings were for pickled herring and smoked salmon for breakfast and all kinds of delicacies during the day. He complained that the things his mother cooked did not taste right, that whenever she turned on the gas there was a bad odor in the house. After three weeks he began to improve gradually. His weight increased, his temperature remained almost normal during the day, (rising during the night), and the frequency of his stools decreased. It was evident that despite her knowledge that food did not cause the diarrhea, Robert's mother used it as a threat to return the child to the hospital from her need to have him away from home. He was up for long stretches of time during the night with frequent bowel movements which roused him from bad dreams. In these dreams he would find himself at the hospital being given injections, being tortured by Japs, or killing Japs himself.

"I was lost on the street and I looked for a car. There was only an ambulance. I asked the man to drive. He didn't know where to drive to take me out of the place where I was lost. I drove and crashed."

This dream he related one day when he was brought to the clinic having fallen out of bed and hurt himself during the night; his mother had told him he would have to be hospitalized He came in crying— frightened that he would have to remain. I told him that, because he felt that he could not stand the suspense of impending hospitalization any longer, he had tried in his dream to put an end to the suspense. He was able to understand that his falling out of bed was the result of his unconscious decision to end an intolerable situation. My reassurance that I would keep him out of the hospital calmed him considerably.

In a discussion with his parents the same day, the father blamed the mother for making Robert sick, and she in turn blamed him for spoiling the child, complaining she could not "go on any longer," that she could not manage Robert with his father in the house, and that one of them had to leave. Her very ambivalent attitude toward Robert had to be resolved if his treatment was to be successful.

The boy improved steadily. He gained sixteen pounds during the first three months at home although he had had measles. His temperature returned to normal, with occasional elevation in the evening and during the night. Blood disappeared from his stools. He gained control of his bowel movements during the day but awoke frequently at night and had to run to the bathroom. His father's employer, who had donated blood for Robert in the hospital several times, arranged with me that I see Robert once a week in my office in addition to the two times that I saw him in the clinic.

In play analysis, Robert acted out his sadistic impulses towards his parents. With clay, for instance, he would make one figure and put it on top of another figure; then he would dismember the first figure, tearing off the head and extremities, then squashing the clay and throwing the whole thing away. This was his conception of parental intercouse. In this connection, it transpired that Robert had been sleeping in his parents' bed since he was an infant. The parents had intercourse freely in his presence assuming that he was asleep but without bothering to make sure. At about the age of two he became unmanageable, would break windows, throw things, and have frequent temper tantrums. On many occasions, especially during the night, he would soil himself. His nightmares, frequent awakenings at night, and running to the bathroom had a direct connection with observation of parental intercourse and represented his reactions to these experiences. In this manner, he managed to keep his parents awake, to separate them, and so to prevent intimacy between them. He would either take his mother's place with his father or, preferably keep his father busy emptying the bedpan.

"I dreamed I was a pig. A man chopped off his neck. They wanted to eat it but the pig was still walking with his neck chopped off.

"I was sleeping in my bed and all of a sudden I woke up and I saw a big rat coming towards me. I got very afraid and started to run away. I jumped out of the window and I climbed up a tree. The big rat with a big mouth and long ears and popping eyes started to climb after me and wanted to eat me up."

This was a nightmare from which he awoke with fear and diarrhea. On the basis of previous similar material, we connected it with his own impulse to devour whenever he was very angry. To the question with whom was he so angry that he was afraid of his own oral aggression, he laughed and said, "I won't say it." Asked to say what he was thinking, he replied, "This time it is my father and not my mother." At this time he was sleeping with his father. We had discussed with him and with his mother a change in sleeping arrangements. Robert was to sleep alone, but he was resistent at that time to give up sleeping with his father. It was apparent that Robert was working out the Oedipus

Complex on an oral sadistic level. His mother's observation that the child had begun to masturbate, which he had not done before, could therefore be considered as progress in his development.

The change in his behavior during this phase of treatment was very striking. While a few weeks before he had been afraid to touch playthings, he was now breaking or tearing whatever he played with. With clay he would frequently make animals which bit him. He would then squash or break them to pieces. At home this aggressive behavior was creating difficulties. He became extremely demanding, had temper tantrums, was destructive, and threw knives, especially at his older sister (a mother substitute). While analysis enabled him to give expression to his aggressive impulses, thereby making his physical symptoms unnecessary, Robert now repeated his earlier behavior when only by means of temper tantrums could he get his way. Although his mother punished him by beatings and deprivations, he would provoke her to outbursts of violent temper—satisfying to him because it proved to him that he was stronger than she. Besides, he could induce his father to indulge him and derive much gratification from playing one parent against the other.

Since his ability to tolerate tension was still very limited, he was almost in a constant temper tantrum. In his illness, a reaction to a traumatic situation (starting in school, separation from mother, hospitalization), he had regressed to the level of oral sadistic fixation, partly relieving his feelings of complete helplessness and extreme fury by oral sadistic incorporation of the frustrating object, and anal elimination of this incorporated object—but at the price of his own physical destruction.

Since this phase of the analysis represented repetition of early infantile behavior, it was essential to guide mother and child through this period of retraining in a more successful way than had originally been done. His uncontrolled behavior demonstrated that he had really never received adequate training from his parents, who were emotionally immature and had great difficulty controlling their emotions. While the mother usually became very angry, the father tended to be more detached with an impulsive need to run away when the situation became difficult or to indulge himself and Robert in a very childish way. The father, to whom I had suggested psychiatric treatment, could not accept this idea, and the mother, who was working with me, was not too helpful, because of her own limitations and ambivalence. The task of adptation was left to the child.

One day Robert and his mother arrived at the clinic, both very excited. In a fit of temper he had broken dishes at home, thrown a knife at his sister, and threatened to break everything in the house. All that his mother could do was to threaten to give him away. I discussed his behavior with him, showing him that he was endangering others and getting himself into trouble. His answer was: "I'm not afraid of anybody. I'm even stronger than a cop, and no one can do anything to me." I told him he was getting me into trouble too because I, after all, was responsible, having asked his mother to take him home and keep him. Since his mother was incapable of doing it, I had to teach him the fundamental restrictions and rewards of social behavior. Robert understood that I was serious, that he could not affort to lose me, and that he would have to control his aggressive impulses. After the interview, the social worker found him sitting on the curb, refusing to go home with his mother. The mother, in the presence of the social workers, spoke to him in endearing tones and promised to buy him a toy, but he refused to go with her, saying that he would wait and go home with me to live, showing clearly his need for security and a firm, consistent attitude. With much work, the mother was made aware of her ambivalence. She came to understand that she wanted to prove that Robert was impossible and could not be kept at home and that instead of encouraging temper tantrums, countered by threats, she would have to be firm and consistent in her attitudes in order to help him gain control of himself. This change in the mother's attitude had an amazing effect on the boy, whose reaction altered very considerably in every respect. From enjoying his parents' quarreling about him and the urge to separate them, he now began to show concern about them, at times even assuming the role of mediator. His father had difficulty with his work, became upset about it, and quarreled with his wife. Robert insisted that his father come to talk to me about it. Previously he had squandered money he got on candy and toys; he began to save and took pride in doing so. He showed a new interest in books and stories and drawing with color crayons. He became interested in other children, made friends, and played outdoors with them.

His physical symptoms had disappeared, and plans were made for him to go to the country with his mother while I went on vacation. When I returned from my vacation, I learned that he had had a relapse while away with his mother. He had been acutely ill for two weeks with vomiting, bloody diarrhea, and high temperature. His vomiting was so severe that he could hardly retain any food. The pediatrician who examined him advised immediate hospitalization and blood transfusions. Robert was desperate and implored me to keep him out of the hospital. Although I had prepared him before I left for my vacation, his attack represented his reaction to my leaving him. He complained that he had felt very unhappy in the country and that he could not get along with his mother. He seemed to understand my interpretation that "Little Robert" (as we spoke of his unconscious impulses) had been so furious at me for deserting him that he wanted to destroy me and in this way destroy himself. He said, "I know what you're telling me; I promise I'll stop it. I'll make him stop it if you keep me out of the hospital." With this agreement, Robert went home. After a few days his mother telephoned me to say he had stopped vomiting, his temperature had dropped, and the bloody diarrhea had disappeared. He was eating well and improving rapidly.

Treatment was resumed at the clinic once a week. Robert started school and did well, which was the more remarkable since he had shown very little interest in intellectual activities during his illness or before it. Our contacts became more infrequent, but I continued to see him once every month or two because I felt that he needed support since the family situation had remained almost unchanged. His father had increasing difficulties with his employment (a displacement of the marital difficulty) and conceived the idea of leaving home and taking work out of town. For a time Robert took this situation very well. When I discussed the problem with him, wondering how he would manage without his father, he said, "I told him to go and I'll show you that I won't get sick. And besides he got me a puppy."

The father came to visit the family every other week end. After a few weeks, the child showed a peculiar reaction to his father's leaving when the week end was over. He became restless, looked at the clock, and developed a temperature of 102 to 103 which would last for a day or two without any other symptoms. When his father came home for the New Year's week end, Robert was more than usually excited. On New Year's Day, when his father was to leave, he became very restless, kept looking at the clock, and began to run to the bathroom. But there was no bloody diarrhea. He developed a temperature of about 104 with no other symptom. His father decided to remain at home (he told me he preferred not to go back).

In an interview with Robert it transpired he had had an agreement with his father that he might keep his job away from home until the end of the year; and Robert felt that he had kept his part of the bargain. Although the family remained a very unsatisfactory one, he did not have a recurrence of ulcerative colitis, but reacted to the difficult environment with the peculiar symptom of elevated temperature for which no organic explanation was found.

At present he is doing very well, attending school, and has become an enthusiastic collector of stamps. His weight is seventy-six pounds which is about double his weight when treatment began. He has made an excellent social and intellectual adjustment during the past two years.

Barbara (7½)

Barbara was seven and a half years old when she developed ulcerative colitis. She first began to complain about cramps and diarrhea shortly after her father was inducted into the army. She was put immediately on a diet. Her stools became bloody; and developing an elevation of temperature, she was admitted to the hospital. Medical and proctoscopic examinations, x-ray and laboratory tests established the diagnosis of nonspecific ulcerative colitis.

Barbara had one brother, four years her junior. He was described as a friendly and outgoing boy. Barbara never smiled. She had had a much closer relationship with her father than with her mother, and his leaving her was obviously a psychic trauma. Shortly after her father's induction, her mother went to work and Barbara was left to herself. She was described by her mother as being a very moody, "bossy," and sensitive child. The mother had been very strict in her upbringing of Barbara, adhering strictly to rules and letting her cry for hours. She had trained her very early and put much stress upon cleanliness. She was openly dissatisfied with her daughter, complaining that she displayed all the unpleasant characteristics of her husband's family which she hated intensely. She was determined not to let Barbara grow up to be like this family. Barbara had always been afraid of her mother and used to shrink whenever she came near her.

In my first interview in the hospital ward, Barbara told me a dream she had had the night before she was to go to the hospital in which her entire family was killed by a witch. She felt completely helpless and unhappy in the hospital. She wanted to go home but feared her mother would refuse while she was ill. As I was to leave for my vacation, arrangement was made to have the child remain in the hospital until my return. Instead the child was discharged, and after two days at home was taken, acutely ill, to another hospital where she remained for three months. Her condition became much worse, she had no control over her bowels and soiled herself in bed. During the first ten days, she did not take any food. She ran a high temperature to 106 and had bloody diarrhea. She refused to see her mother. Her father was given an emergency furlough to visit her.

When her condition improved somewhat, but still with fever and bloody diarrhea, she was discharged and referred to our psychiatric clinic for treatment. Barbara was very suspicious of me and feared that I might talk to her mother about her. It soon became apparent that she was very much afraid of and angry with her mother whom she blamed for having sent her father away. She reproached her mother for not having cried when her father left, and after his furlough, she was quoted by her mother as saying, "No one even cries for Daddy. I am the only one." Barbara had always felt protected by her father, and when he left she was left entirely and helplessly in her mother's power. In addition to the projection of her own unconscious hostility toward her mother, there was justification in reality for Barbara's feelings. Her mother was very ambivalent towards her and, at the time, besides working and being "wrapped up in herself," she was interested in another man. Meanwhile Barbara was transferring some of the feelings she had for her mother to me. This may be illustrated by a dream she had when her father had just left.

"There are soldiers and sailors in line. She asks me, 'What's that all about?' I say I do not know. She asks her mother and her mother does not know either. Then she asks her mother's friend (the only person for whom Barbara had friendly feelings at the time), and the friend tells her that these soldiers are on a furlough and will not have to go back. Then she vomits and I say to her that she will have to come to the hospital for a couple of days. She stays five days, goes home, and vomits again; then I tell her she will have to come to the clinic."

It was possible to convince Barbara of her resentment, anger, and frustration; and simultaneously the symptoms of colitis began to diminish. The development of intermediary symptoms consisting of facial tics and blinking of the eyelids were reported by her mother as having existed previous to the onset of the colitis.

Barbara was now doing well. She gained about sixteen pounds in weight, had no diarrhea, nor elevation of temperature, was going to school, and was fairly happy, perhaps happier than she had ever been before. In the meantime her father had been discharged from the army, and treatment was discontinued after about five months.

Two months later, her mother called to say that Barbara was very ill, had a high temperature, was complaining of pain in her knee, and had bloody diarrhea. This was almost exactly one year after the onset of her illness, just before her brother's birthday, and also, as we learned later, shortly after her best and only friend had moved away from the neighborhood. She appeared to be very ill, and she was much afraid that her mother would send her to the hospital. She told me (confirmed by her mother) she had squeezed a turtle, belonging to her brother, so that a greenish liquid oozed, to which she referred as "the guts coming out"; then, apparently in a quite sadistic manner, she had dismembered the turtle, put stones on it, and buried it. Barbara was so sick that she could neither be kept at home nor brought to the office, and she was admitted to the hospital with the understanding that I would see her there. At the hospital she proved herself to be a very disagreeable patient about whom both the nurses and the doctors complained.

In the ward she began immediately to tell me how unhappy she was and begged to be allowed to go home. When I said that "little Barbara" (as we spoke of her unconscious impulses) was responsible for her plight because she was so angry that in her attempt to "get even" with everybody she did not care what happened to "big Barbara," the child screamed, "Stop it! Stop it!" She writhed and called for the bedpan. While she sat on the bedpan, straining to defecate, I continued to talk of her rage and destructiveness, adding that she now included me in her anger because I was telling her these things.

I now reassured her that I could and would help her if she wanted me to and if she herself would fight "little Barbara." She became calm and we parted with my promise to get her some concessions in the matter of food and other liberties in the ward. When next I saw her, she was much quieter and an arrangement was made, with her approval, that she be taken in a wheelchair to the clinic to see me regularly twice a week. She was running a high temperature, despite sulfonamide medication, was very weak, and was receiving blood transfusions regularly. She had bloody diarrhea, severe anorexia, and had lost much weight. There was a question of a complicating rheumatic fever because of pain in her knees and wrists and swelling of her wrists and fingers. All laboratory examinations including electrocardiograph and repeated sedimentation rates were negative. Proctoscopic examinations revealed an extensive ulcerative process in the colon.

I promised Barbara, regardless of her fever, to let her go home as soon as she could walk. One day when she was wheeled into my office, she got up from the wheelchair and staggered to a chair, looking at me triumphantly. I felt obliged to say that although she had "walked," she was still not well enough to go home. She flew into a rage, screamed and shouted, "You're a witch. I wish you were dead!" and then began to cry. That I remained calm and described to her her feelings impressed her strongly. I said we both wanted to get her out of the hospital permanently but that this was not yet possible. I explained further that I would have to prepare her mother to make certain that she not only would take her home but would be willing to keep her there and bring her to me for treatment. Barbara's gloomy face lit up, and I had the feeling that for the first time she accepted me as an ally. The subsequent change in her condition, and especially in her prevailing mood, was striking. She began to eat, the diarrhea stopped, and her temperature began to drop. An x-ray of the bowels repeated before her discharge showed no changes.

Barbara came to see me several times at my office. The colitis symptoms disappeared entirely. She still had some pain and swelling in her wrists and fingers for which she received salicylates. She was playing with children and enjoying excursions to a beach. On my return from a holiday of one month, I learned that she had been well, was starting school, and planned to attend a dancing school.

One month later her mother called to tell me that Barbara was very sick. She was complaining of abdominal cramps, had bloody diarrhea, and elevation of temperature. It later transpired that the mother had disposed of Barbara's dog which had been bought for her after her discharge from the hospital. Although the mother thoroughly disliked dogs, she had promised Barbara, when she was acutely ill in the hospital, to get her one when she came home (unconsciously she did not expect Barbara ever to come home).

Barbara was carried wrapped in blankets to my office by her father. She began immediately to tell me how much she hated her brother. She had asked her mother to remove him from the house. She could not sleep in the same room with him. When it became clear that "little Barbara" wanted to destroy Jim, Barbara began to complain about her aching knee and lay down on the couch. She was afraid to fall asleep with Jim in the room because she feared what she might do to him in her sleep. The pains of which she was complaining had to do with "little Barbara's" wish to break Jim's bones, much as she had dismembered the turtle. I reassured her by telling her that she could not cause anything to happen to Jim just by wishing it and that she therefore did not have to punish herself by becoming sick. Jim after all, I said, was running around playing happily while she was sick. She retorted, "But he does have sore throats." For her, the destruction of Jim was an accomplished fact, justifying her sickness. Her fantasy of omnipotence caused Barbara to wonder why her mother never got sick: periodically, however, she would keep her mother up nights and upset her during the day, finally getting the satisfaction of hearing her mother complain that she would collapse soon and that she was so dizzy she could hardly stand on her feet. After the session, as Barbara walked without aid out of my office, she asked me not to laugh at the way she walked. It was a peculiar kind of zigzag gait. Next morning her mother called and told me in amazement that Barbara had got up in the morning, dressed herself, and was walking around without complaint.

This phase of the analysis is reported in more detail because (1) it lends itself to a clear understanding of the mechanisms involved in the production and dissolution of somatic symptoms and (2) the initial reaction to interpretation, as in this particular interview, brought on an immediate disappearance of all the symptoms (fever, bloody diarrhea, pain, swelling, sleeplessness, and anorexia)—an effect comparable to the effect of surgery in an acute surgical condition. Unfortunately such results do not last until this understanding has become an integrated part of the child's personality.

Barbara's reaction to frustration with rage quickly followed by somatic conversions can be best illustrated by an episode. She came for the first appointment after her discharge from the hospital to the clinic where, having to wait for me, she saw two patients admitted to my office before her. She was moody and uncommunicative. Although realizing that she was angry with me for keeping her waiting, I was unable to devote sufficient time then to analyze her feelings. That afternoon her mother called me to tell me that while Barbara had been quite well that morning, she had returned from the clinic very much upset, complaining of stomach ache, having bloody diarrhea, vomiting, and repeating, "I don't care what happens to me."

When I next saw Barbara, she looked very ill, had to be carried by her father, and was trembling. I interpreted to her her reaction of disappointment in me, indicating that she must have been very angry with me. This she confirmed, telling me that the fact that I saw other patients before her proved to her that I did not care for her. This discussion had a very beneficial influence on her. She left feeling and looking much better. She got up next day and again the physical symptoms disappeared.

At the next session Barbara complained of difficulty in chewing her lamb chop. She then related that she often had to get up at night and have her mother sleep with her. To my question, "So that mother cannot sleep with father?" she replied, "'Little Barbara' gets angry when they sleep together. She doesn't want them to be so close." Once, when she got up at night, she "saw what they did together." "Mother was on top of him," she said. Barbara then spoke of an occasion when in play the boys took pictures of the girls' genitals with toy camers. She said her brother calls his penis "cookie," doesn't like it, and wants to cut it off. "He even tried to do so today. Father tells him it will fall off if he touches it. It can't fall off, can it?" she asked. "He says he doesn't want it. He wants mine," she continued, "He wants to urinate on me when he plays with it." Barbara was covering up her penis envy by denying it. "Some girls would like to have it," I ventured. She replied, "I know a girl; she's in the hospital because she wants to be a boy and urinate like a boy. My cousin wants to be a girl. He puts my dresses on."

I suggested, "Sometimes a dream can wake you up." She said, "I had a dream last night and I woke up. I saw 'little Barbara' and she looked just like me. She worked on Jim but then she also worked on me. She said something—I don't remember what." "What does this mean, 'she worked' on you?" I asked. "She broke his bones—no, she cracked his bones. But then she cracked mine too. I woke up and I had to go to the bathroom."

Barbara had the habit of cracking her finger joints. She said she liked the noise of it. "A little girl showed me how to do it when I was four years old [her age when her brother was born]. She had to have both her hands bandaged up." While speaking, she alternately cracked her fingers and pulled at the bandage that covered a little sore on her knee.

During this period Barbara revealed her fantasies about pregnancy, childbirth, and intercourse. Her predominant fantasy of impregnation was an oral one. Mother gets the baby by eating a certain food that father gives her. Birth was conceived as an act of defecation. Barbara had a ritual for undressing—a defense against exhibitionism: the doors had to be locked, the shades down, and no one was permitted to enter the room, especially her brother. Suddenly, on occasion, she would appear almost nude, especially when a certain male friend of the family was visiting. Later she became very casual about these things, abandoned the dressing ceremorial and behaved quite naturally, although for a long time she preferred to wear slacks instead of dresses.

Barbara called me, crying into the telephone, "I can't stand Jim. Take him away." When I saw her she said, "Jim did disappear, but only for one night." When I reminded her that she wanted to have Jim out of her way completely, she laughed hysterically, cracking her fingers. She asked, "Can you keep a secret? You know, I'm really scared of her ['little Barbara']. I'm afraid to fall asleep. I feel choked when my mother wants to put on my hat and tie the ribbon. I'm even scared to do it myself." After a pause she said, "That's what she wants to do," and she made a movement with her hands like squeezing or choking. "She wants to make mush out of him. I just don't sleep. I keep on going to the bathroom but I don't always have a bowel movement although I try."

Although her condition had improved considerably, when she next came she was carried by her father like a baby and was scolding and criticizing him for not handling her carefully enough. The moment he had left the room she said proudly, "How often do you think I got up last night? Ten times! And I made sure everybody was disturbed." Asked why she continued to employ this method of keeping her parents separated she said, "Mother doesn't want to sleep with him anyhow. He's kicking her; so she sleeps with me." At the end of the session, she first agreed to walk out by herself but then complained of a stomach ache. After some discussion, she said, "I'll make her walk," and she did.

At the next visit Barbara walked into my office with a staggering gait. She volunteered, "You know 'little Barbara' doesn't want me to walk; but I am fighting her. When I want to walk stairs she wants me to fall. That's why I have to hold on to the banister. I'd rather not walk stairs at all." Her mother said that Barbara was afraid of climbing stairs.

As Barbara improved, her mother became more and more impatient to get her out of the house and off to school. To this Barbara reacted with a compulsive need to cling to her mother whom she simply would not let out of her sight. Sensing the hostile, aggressive impulse in this behavior, and resenting it, the mother in turn reacted sadistically, thus creating a vicious cycle. In addition, the analytic therapy was releasing Barbara's aggressive impulses which was essential for her physical improvement, and these encountered great opposition from her mother who began to feel that she could not endure the situation any longer.

Soon a telephone call came from the mother stating Barbara was sick with an abscess of her foot and high temperature and was being treated with penicillin. At this point it was deemed necessary that the mother be given some understanding of her own destructive impulses towards Barbara and of the effects of the reciprocally hostile, unconscious rapport between her and the child. It was essential to try to enlist the mother's aid in helping her daughter develop a sense of confidence and trust which she had so far not been given the opportunity to develop. Only if she could feel more secure with her mother could she develop emotionally and learn to tolerate psychic tensions instead of discharging them in a neurotic way.

In this interview, Barbara's mother was sufficiently ambivalent and guilty that she could hardly face me. She said, "I have done everything but it doesn't help. Everybody says there is no hope for the child. Aren't you giving up? Barbara said to me today, 'You are not a mother. You are a nurse.' I said, 'Don't I do everything for you?' and Barbara answered, 'A mother doesn't do these things. Nurses do.' [Barbara hated nurses intensely.] The other night, when I was looking at Barbara, my husband said, 'Why are you looking at her like that? You think it would be better if she were dead.'"

I continued to see the mother while the child was confined in bed. Barbara's behavior, as described by her mother, was very characteristic. She made a great fuss when the wound was dressed, and the doctor could examine her only by force. She always wanted to look at her foot, asking frequently whether it would leave a permanent deformity and whether she would ever be able to walk again. This illness was her solution of the conflict whether to remain a baby and cling to her mother or to grow up and go to school.

Besides cracking her fingers, Barbara also had the habits of biting and picking her nails and pulling at her skin and scabs. Such habits are well-known expressions of strong unconscious sadism. The infection of her foot she had acquired by picking and scratching. She wanted to think this infection was "accidental" but her doubtful questioning about whether "little Barbara" could bring on such a thing gave proof that she had some vague awareness of the deep and hidden ways in which her unconscious was working.

Over two weeks later, Barbara was carried into my office, her leg still swollen and bandaged. She looked very pale and ill. "I'm afraid," she said. "I want to get well but, I'm afraid 'little Barbara' won't let me." Then she asked, pointing to a plant in the room, "When is that plant going to die? Before, I wanted to be sick; then I could be like a baby, but now Mommy says she can't lock herself up with me and she can't sleep with me." "The more reason," I said, "for 'little Barbara' to be angry with mother." "Yes," she said, "I had a big fight with her. I called her names and tore her dress. She had to change it before we came here."

A week later her mother called to tell me that the child was behaving surprisingly well and had improved physically. She quoted her as saying repeatedly, "I want to get well and go to school like other children," and she was also eating much better.

Barbara looked much better and offered to let me take the bandage off her leg and look at it when I next saw her. She told with satisfaction that her brother had an infection of his finger and he could neither use her typewriter nor play with her things. "Perhaps he will have to be cut," she said, "I would like to cut him to pieces. But mother wouldn't let me." With satisfaction she reported the many times she had awakened her mother at night. She was quite conscious of her sadistic behavior: "I scratched my father on his face. He has to pull away from me." She continued to be very jealous of her father and resentful of his attentions to her mother. After talking pleasantly in my office, just after she had been carried out by her father there was a loud outcry. It was Barbara shouting at her father for not being careful with her.

Barbara was improved and only occasionally ran a temperature. Her parents were now convinced that her illnesses, including the colitis, were emotional in origin. The mother approached me with the request that I see her daughter three times a week until she was ready for school.

During the succeeding weeks Barbara learned further to understand her needs, her conflicts, and also her defenses. She was growing up almost visibly. One day she came in saying jokingly, "I am a big girl now. I am eating by myself and I am also sleeping at night now." She had, until recently, been disturbed at night, sometimes talking to herself in her sleep, once being overheard by her mother saying repeatedly, "It's got to be done. It's got to be done." She was much

more pleasant and friendly than ever before, and her mother was
pleased with her conduct. The mother did not understand what had
wrought the change and felt it had to do with something I discussed
with Barbara. The degree of the mother's acquired insight into her
daughter's continuous emotional struggles was remarkable. For
instance, when Barbara whose foot was still bandaged but much better
said, "I want to walk," her mother replied, "All right." When Barbara
objected, "But I can't," her mother said, "Then don't walk."
Whereupon Barbara began to cry, "But I want to walk." Formerly the
mother would have become very angry and have screamed at her,
"Leave me alone." Barbara, of course, was looking for the opportunity
to externalize her conflicts, so that instead of having to fight "little
Barbara" she might have a fight with her mother. The mother, better
than ever before, was still sufficiently ambivalent to ask such
questions as "Will Barbara ever really change? I don't mean the colitis.
You know what I mean. She is just like his whole family [the father's
family which she considers 'crazy']." She worried no less about
Barbara when she was doing well, fearing a relapse as if she could not
believe the child could so remain or, unconsciously, not wanting her to
be well.

Barbara had never been as pleasant as she now was. She helped with
housework and one day surprised her mother by making breakfast for
her. Her mother commented, "I didn't know she had it in her." She
became protective of her brother and started to play with him. When
he became sick Barbara said to her mother, "You know, mother, 'little
Barbara' thinks that she made Jim sick. Isn't that silly?" Visiting a
family toward whose little daughter Barbara had previously been
very hostile and assaultive, the little girl hit her in the face. The
mother of the little girl wanted to punish her daughter. Barbara said,
"Don't hit her. She's only a little girl. And you don't make her better by
hitting her."

In discussing her return to school, she was frankly frightened.
Having missed almost two full terms of school, there was some
justification for her apprehension that she could not compete with
other children. Immediately after she came home from her first day at
school, she called me to break the news. She was in a complicated
emotional state, torn between her resentment toward her mother,
who was urging her to return to school, and her wish to break this
dependence. The mother, as usual whenever the child improved,

became irritable and knew "something was going to happen." The tension grew and one day when the mother insisted that she stay home from school because of a cold, Barbara flew into a rage accusing her mother of wanting her to be sick and threatening to "get even with her." She took food, demanding that her mother look on while she took one bite and crumbled the rest. If her mother started to leave the room, she would either hold her or run after her. She threatened her with a recurrence of an attack of ulcerative colitis, saying she would make her mother empty the bedpan for her. Although she was up all night with the bedpan at her side, she could not produce bloody diarrhea nor any of the other symptoms of ulcerative colitis, but had only one formed stool in twenty-four hours. For the first time she displayed severe anxiety, screaming that she was going blind. She developed a swelling of the previously infected foot, and when I saw her again, she was bandaged and had to be carried in. She looked very fearful and began to cry and call for her mother. I called her mother in and Barbara held on to her hand in a phobic manner. I said, "You are afraid to lose your mother." Barbara nodded her head. It became clear to her that she had to hold on to her mother physically in order to protect her from her own death wishes. Barbara then permitted her mother to leave the room. She described her fear of the destructive impulses she felt towards mother and brother, understanding that because it was impossible to achieve them or get rid of them, she was releasing the destructive anger against herself. She had been up for several nights listening for noises from the parental bedroom. She was reliving the trauma of Jim's birth. "And worst of all," she added, "he was a boy." When she left she was composed, almost cheerful.

To reassure her I had stated to her that she had no need to fear "little Barbara" since she could not give her bloody stools any more. She had a single bloody stool that day after she returned home from the visit. The interpretation to her of this symptom as a transference reaction she understood very well. She said, "You see you said I don't have to be afraid of 'little Barbara' any more."

She avoided looking at her foot and refused to let me see it. In our last session, while discussing her destructive impulses, I suggested that her sore leg seemed to represent Jim whom she wished to destroy like that. She became anxious and pleaded, "Don't let me do that!"

The physician who treated her foot advised hospitalization because he suspected an osteomyelitis. With this Barbara complied in a reasonable and sensible way. The x-ray examination did not show any bone pathology, and the ulcer cleared quickly with penicillin. When I visited her in the hospital she said, "'Little Barbara' doesn't have much to do with this now. She only started it."

In these and other similar cases from which conclusions are drawn, we found an extremely ambivalent mother who subjected her child to very early and deep frustration. All these mothers showed strong unconscious destructive impulses towards the child with a wish to rid themselves of it, rationalized in every case by the opinion that the child would do better away from home. To such ambivalent and therefore inconsistent mothers the children reacted with hostile attachment and an intense need to hold on to the position of a baby with extremely strong oral and anal sadistic tendencies. All these children showed a fixation on an oral sadistic level due to early frustration. The personality of these children is characterized by an extreme inability to tolerate any psychic tension. Failure in resolving the Oedipus Complex and in achieving a genital level of development leads to pregenital regression.

The symptoms, eating difficulties, vomiting, stomach ache, and diarrhea are very common in children as a neurotic reaction to disappointments and frustrations and are somatic expressions both of the child's inability to control the situation and a defense against and release of painful psychic tensions. The difference between such cases and those who develop ulcerative colitis shows itself in the initial phases and especially in the attitude of the child towards the illness. In ulcerative colitis the complete absorption of the child in the illness and the symptoms are striking and indicative of a narcissistic orientation. The bleeding occurs quite early in the illness and that differentiates, not only somatically but also psychologically, such cases from all other forms of diarrhea. One gains the impression that the amount of bleeding can be determined by the individual child. There is no ulceration in the initial phases, proctoscopic examinations revealing a diffuse inflammation and edema of the mucous membrane with transudation of blood. Later, after a number of recurrences, a secondary ulceration takes place. I observed in many instances, by comparing the proctoscopic

findings upon discharge and readmission, that the inflammation had subsided while the child was at home, increased during
hospital residence, and cleared after a second discharge from the
hospital. This confirms my impression that hospitalization
represented a traumatic experience to which these children
reacted in a specific way. It disrupted their narcissistic
equilibrium. They could accept such an environment only after
they had decided that they could live again, so to speak. The
corresponding reaction of the mothers was guilt and anxiety as
their unconscious wish to get rid of the child was fulfilled. To
the child it meant loss of the mother and being helplessly left to
destruction, a fate which could be avoided only by setting into
motion the archaic mechanism of oral sadistic incorporation of
the needed object with all the destructive somatic consequences
of the defense mechanisms.

These children are in a state of permanent frustration that
results in a state of unconscious rage with an irresistible urge
for immediate discharge. The slightest additional frustration
such as medical procedures and dietary restrictions provokes
exaggerated reactions. The destruction and elimination of the
object through the mucosa of the colon (bleeding) would seem
to be the specific mechanism in ulcerative colitis. As the object is
incorporated sadistically, it is a hostile inner danger and has to
be eliminated immediately. The feces and blood (in severe
attacks, only blood and mucus) represent the devaluated and
dangerous objects. In all cases with much bleeding, observed
and analyzed, it appeared as if the quantity of blood was directly
proportional to the intensity of unconscious rage (oral and anal
sadism) present at the time. Although essentially it is the degree
of regression that differentiates ulcerative colitis from conversion hysteria and mucous colitis, I believe that it is the quantity
of sadism that perhaps determines the depths of the regression
itself.

The severe form of ulcerative colitis shows great resemblance
in behavior and personality structure and dynamics to
melancholia, and seems to represent the somatic dramatization
of the same conflict, with relatively little mental pain, that in
depression is expressed psychologically. Wittkower states,
"Sometimes the patients notice a decline of the mental

symptoms during the period of the increased bodily symptoms."
Similarly in Daniel's case, with a decline of the physical
symptoms the patient developed depression with strong
suicidal tendencies. Cullinan writes, "There are few diseases in
which a patient may become so ill and emaciated and yet
recover."

It is a known fact that sometimes a severe depression clears
up when the patient becomes physically sick or suffers a great
physical loss. Like depression, ulcerative colitis is a process
aimed at reparation. But because the introjected object becomes
part of the patient, the outcome will depend upon the quantity
and quality of the sadism that now is turned within towards the
introjected object. Only after the sadism has been satisfied and
has been exhausted or changed by treatment can the individual
recover. This perhaps explains spontaneous recoveries in
depression and ulcerative colitis, and also why some cases of
depression inevitably end with suicide and some cases of
ulcerative colitis are fatal.

While in depression the ego is attacked by the superego, in
ulcerative colitis the organism is attacked by the aggressively
incorporated object and tries to free itself by immediate
discharge anally. The gnawing of the conscience in depression is
represented in ulcerative colitis by abdominal pain and bleeding.
These observations of sadistic devouring tendencies employed
in the service of the ego as an act of self-preservation (but at the
same time detrimental to the physical economy) are in
accordance with Simmel's concept of a primary gastrointestinal
libido organization, the prototype of all pregenital libido
strivings. Psychodynamically, ulcerative colitis is an organ
neurosis with pregenital conversion symptoms. The choice of
the organ is determined by oral and anal fixations—the colon
being the eliminatory organ. The anorexia, vomiting, abdominal pain, diarrhea, and bleeding represent expressions of and
defenses against aggressive incorporation of the frustrating
object.

Since psychoanalysis is difficult in these cases and has to
include the mother, prophylaxis would be the best treatment.
Prophylaxis in such cases should start with the treatment of the
mother, or even better, with the prospective mother.

PART 3

MUCOUS COLITIS

Observations from the Treatment of Children Suffering from Nonbloody Diarrhea or Mucous Colitis

These are observations from a study which deals with the psychoanalytic investigation and treatment of fourteen children between the ages of two and a half and thirteen years, suffering from the syndrome medically known as "mucous colitis." The presenting symptoms were persistent or recurring attacks of nonbloody diarrhea and abdominal cramps associated or alternating with difficult or neurotic behavior. The onset of the diarrhea occurred typically between the age of one and a half to two and a half. In those cases where the symptoms existed from early infancy, an acute intensification of them occurred at this age. The significance of this phase for character formation and personality development is well known from psychoanalysis. During this phase when the child is attempting to overcome his dependence, it would seem that he is particularly sensitive to any interference with his strivings for independence. Even with a very accepting and encouraging attitude of the mother, some conflict about whether to let go of her as the sole object of dependence or whether to hold on to her is unavoidable.

The turning of the aggressive impulses toward the outside world is a characteristic manifestation of the anal phase and an essential step toward overcoming dependency. It will depend largely upon the attitude of the mother whether she becomes so much an obstacle in this process that control over her comes to stand for independence. In his struggle for control, the child uses all available means, and consequently since this struggle sets in or is at its height during the anal phase, the components and derivatives of the anal instinct will be fully employed in it. These lend themselves particularly well both for the overt and for the symbolic somatic expression of this conflict, which the child, because of his actual helplessness, is not capable of resolving in reality. Temper tantrums and destructive behavior are the most common overt manifestations of this struggle. The unconscious identification of the frustrating object (mother) with feces leads to the giving up of the object in the symptom of diarrhea. In the cramps and diarrhea, control over the frustrating object (mother) is achieved omnipotently through the unconscious equation of object equals feces.

It has long been known that diarrhea is somehow associated with tension, fear, rage, and instability, and these findings have been confirmed by such investigators as White, Cobb, and Jones (1939). More specific are the concepts of diarrhea of Franz Alexander (1950) and his co-workers, who emphasize the factor of restitution in the symptom of diarrhea.

It is my experience that diarrhea is an attempt on the part of the patient to separate himself from the mother to whom he clings but whom he gives up in the diarrhea. The patient solves the conflict somatically, that is, he separates himself from the object on which he is dependent, but the conflict continues in reality in attitudes of helplessness.

The impotent rage at his helplessness leads the patient to a need to assert himself emotionally. This he reenacts in the stormy diarrhea, destroying the object which he can neither control nor escape from by reducing it to feces and expelling it repeatedly and forcefully.

All the children of this study had a complete medical workup before referral; some of them had had unsuccessful medical treatment for several years. Two cases from the group of children of preschool age consisting of four children aged from two and a half to five years have been selected for this presentation. This group seems to me of particular interest because some of the mechanisms which were already firmly established in the older children can be studied in the state of formation. Also, the phases preceding the onset of the manifest psychosomatic symptoms and the behavior associated or alternating with the diarrhea can be observed more directly while it has to be reconstructed in the treatment of the older children (see chapters 9 and 10).

Michael (5)

Michael was nearly five years old when referred for treatment. He had been suffering from abdominal cramps and severe diarrhea for the past three and a half years. He had been under medical treatment during this time, and the diagnosis of mucous colitis had been established after careful medical observation and repeated x-ray and rectal examinations. He had been on a very limited diet since the age of eighteen months, and there were continuous fights between Michael and his mother about food.

He was also a behavior problem, prone to severe temper tantrums. The onset of this behavior dated back to the phase of toilet training. The onset of the diarrhea could also be traced back to the same period of his life. According to the mother, there was a continuous battle going between Michael and her, except for the times when he was sick with diarrhea and cramps. At such times he was good and obedient and she found it easier to care for him. Both parents were high-strung, the mother particularly would lose her temper quickly and punish Michael severely at the slightest provocation. She could not understand why he would not obey her. She said, "I give him such terrific beatings, that if somebody did that to me I would be terriby scared." The father, on the other hand, tended to overindulge him because Michael was the younger child (he had a sister five years his senior) and a boy.

Michael was a skinny, hyperactive boy, obviously insecure in his relationship with both parents. His provocative behavior was found to be an overcompensation of his fear of his parents, but particularly of his mother. His exaggerated need for control over his mother was a reaction to early and repeated injuries to his narcissism by his mother. In this struggle for control Michael had adopted a masochistic mechanism in his dealings with his mother. The dynamics of his behavior could be understood, as follows: "I upset her whenever I want to, and I make her punish me. She can't punish me if I don't want her to." This mechanism proved to be an effective regulator of his mother's behavior. She always responded to his provocations in the expected way, namely, by punishing him. His need for love and care from his mother remained unsatisfied at the times when he misbehaved. When he had diarrhea and cramps and was sick and not bad, his mother cared for him and paid attention to him. Thus, at the price of illness, Michael could gratify the need for love from the mother inherent in every child.

There were, however, deeper motives than this secondary gain from illness involved in the dynamics of his diarrhea. It was found that the mother had been unable to accept any adequate overt expression of aggression and strivings for independence on the part of Michael. This had been evidenced particularly in the forceful way in which she had handled Michael during the period of toilet training. The sadistic elements stemming from the anal phase, which had been a particularly traumatic one for Michael, could be seen still in operation in both the child and the mother. The mother had used the rigid execution of the diets prescribed by the physician as a means of punishment and deprivation for Michael. When, for instance, during Michael's treatment, she was advised by me to relax this rigid regime, she would often complain, "Now that I let him eat whatever he wants and don't beat him up, he has no diarrhea, but his behavior is still bad, perhaps worse, than before."   In his temper tantrums and in the destructive behavior, Michael openly rebelled against his mother. This rebellion and his struggle for control over mother was expressed in a disguised way in his diarrhea and cramps. Thus the destructive behavior, on the one hand, and the diarrhea and cramps, on the other hand, represented two different ways in which Michael attempted to free himself from his mother's domination. At such times, when he felt most helpless and dependent upon his mother in reality, he would have cramps and diarrhea, because only when he was sick could his dependent needs be gratified by his mother. At the same time the diarrhea served to release his repressed destructive impulses instantly through the body without being punished for it by loss of love from his mother. In the diarrhea, Michael succeeded in giving up his mother symptomatically, while, in reality, he could not free himself from her. Thus, in the sadistic struggle for control, he proved himself victorious at the price of illness (M. Sperling, 1948).

It was necessary to work with the mother and to help her to meet Michael's provocations differently and to enable her to tolerate some overt expressions of his aggression without restricting him too severely, so that he would not be forced to repress these destructive impulses abruptly and then release them in the cramps and bouts of diarrhea. It was also necessary to help Michael to learn to tolerate his destructiveness without releasing it immediately in temper tantrums or converting it into illness.

Jerry (3½)

Jerry was three-and-a-half years old wen he was brought for treatment because of difficult behavior. I learned from the mother that Jerry had been suffering from diarrhea since infancy. He had been a colicky baby who never slept through a night without disturbance. According to his mother, Jerry was a high-strung, nervous child from birth. The mother had had a bad pregnancy with him and had vomited up to the last day. Jerry was a bright boy who had walked and talked when he was nine months old, and his mother, therefore, had expected him to perform similarly in his toilet training. Whenever he wet or soiled himself, she would hit him. He was fully bladder trained at fourteen months. His bowel training was more difficult because of the diarrhea. Also because of the diarrhea, he had been on a very limited diet since infancy.

His behavior had become increasingly difficult, especially since the birth of his brother three months ago. Jerry would shout and scream, throw things, spit, and hit, especially smaller children. The mother had resorted to hitting him, which, she claimed, had helped in the past, at least, for a short time. Now, after the birth of his brother even severe beatings did not help. Jerry was beginning to speak baby talk and occasionally would wet his bed deliberately, shouting, "I'm the baby." The mother could not help but see how jealous Jerry was of his younger brother. He constantly sought reassurance from her, asking her whether she loved him, and promising not to be a bad boy. She would often, because she was "fed up with him" and "couldn't stand it any longer," threaten to leave him.

It was found, in his treatment, that he was very attached to his mother and caught in an insoluble conflict with her. On the one hand, he wanted very much to be a big boy and to excel and to please his mother, who put so much emphasis on the acceleration of his development. On the other hand, he had a fear of losing his mother if he were to become self-sufficient and independent of her. This fear had been reinforced by the birth of the baby brother. His behavior characteristically alternated between periods when he acted very grown-up and would play outside with the children without his mother and even be annoyed when he caught her watching him through the window and periods when he could not leave her and would follow her around in an almost phobic manner.

In his play sessions, he would frequently enact a scene in which a child, who was having a good time playing outside with the children, suddenly had to stop playing and run into the house because the mother was angry and didn't want the child to play outside. Another scene of this repetitive game showed a mother busy with her baby. The mother did not want to be bothered by the older child, at whom she shouted, "Go away and don't come back." He often finished the game by having the older child run away so that the mother could not find him. In this game he was doing in play what he would have wanted to do but could not in reality. In reality he was worried that he would find his mother and that she would leave him, as she already, according to his feelings, had abandoned him for the sake of the baby.

Following this phase of play therapy, there was a very marked improvement not only in Jerry's behavior but also in his diarrhea. At this point (after three months of treatment) the medical treatment and dietary regime were discontinued with the consent of his pediatrician. It did not have to be reinstituted because Jerry's diarrhea stopped completely and has not recurred since. I heard last from Jerry when he was seven years old.

In work with the mother it was found that she felt guilty about her handling of Jerry. She felt that she had pushed him too much and that she had not allowed him to be a baby. She had always felt very tense with Jerry and exhausted from taking care of him. She was much more relaxed with her second child. It was found that the mother had very strong unconscious dependent needs which had been reinforced by Jerry's birth. She had fought these needs by denying their existence in herself and by trying to suppress them in her child. She would therefore not allow him to be a baby. At the same time because of her unconscious identification with Jerry, she projected her own unresolved dependency conflict onto him. It would seem that the effects of this conflict of the mother upon Jerry had already manifested themselves in his early feeding difficulties and colics (see chapter 4).

Jerry had always required much care and time from his mother because of the complicated formulas and diets prescribed for him. Furthermore, the diarrhea in necessitating much bodily handling allowed for close physical contact between Jerry and his mother, which she did not permit herself to enjoy openly. Actually, she had never complained about the diets nor the diarrhea. She was bothered by his overt behavior, but only about those aspects of it which in her mind were associated with infantile demanding behavior, for instance, his waking her at night, his clinging to her, his demands for attention from her, and the display of temper when she refused him.

On superficial observation, the behavior of Jerry and Michael appears to be similar, yet there was a distinct difference in the quality of it as well as in the quality of the mother-child relationship in each case. There was also a distinct difference in the personality types of the parents. Michael's parents, particularly his mother, showed definite psychopathic traits. There were no standards of behavior set for him by his parents. Michael's mother rejected him and treated him at times with outright cruelty and neglect. She openly frustrated his attempts for self-assertive and aggressive behavior and demanded submission and slavish obedience at all times. Michael, in turn, showed little concern for other people's feelings. This was apparent also in his relationship with me and evidenced itself in the way in which he played and in which he handled play material. In his games, people would always fight (the actual behavior of his parents) and kill each other in openly sadistic ways. Michael hated and feared his mother; he was contemptuous of his father, who, he felt, submitted to the mother. This was very different from Jerry, who was a warm and affectionate child, with a capacity for love. In his struggle, particularly with anal-sadistic and phallic impulses, he was in the process of developing a phobic attachment to his mother, as the psychologic equivalent of the diarrhea (see chapter 9).

Michael can be regarded as a case arrested in a transitional phase in which his behavior still alternated between somatic symptoms and overt destructive behavior, that is, the state before repression, reaction formation, and other defenses have led to the establishment of reaction formation, and other defenses have led to the establishment of such definite clinical pictures as phobias, early compulsion, neurosis, or severe character disorders. Such a situation is often encountered in the treatment of older children and adults who suffer from mucous colitis during the period when their aggressive impulses are liberated from the symptom and before they have gained enough ego and superego strength to enable them to control and use their aggression more adequately.

These observations would seem of particular interest for the understanding of the personality structure of patients with mucous colitis and of the nature of the etiological traumata in their early childhood.

Psychogenic Diarrhea and Phobia in a Six-and-a-half-year-old Girl

Ellen (6½)

Ellen was six and a half when her mother consulted me because the behavior of the child worried her greatly. Ellen clung to her mother, was afraid to go out and play with other children, and was disturbed about school. I learned that Ellen had also suffered from diarrhea since infancy. She had been on a very limited diet for that reason, and as she could not eat what she would have liked, she was a very bad eater and much underweight. The mother had observed that Ellen's diarrhea would flare up at times and at other times be less marked, but neither she nor anyone else had ever linked Ellen's phobic behavior with the diarrhea. The mother had always attributed the acute aggravation of the diarrhea to dietary mistakes and therefore added more and more restrictions, frequently changing these diets and the doctors who prescribed them.

There was another child in the family, a little girl one and a half years old, of whom the mother was very fond. She felt guilty in relation to Ellen, because she did not have the same feelings toward her. She had never noticed any envy or jealousy on the part of Ellen, who seemed to like her sister, nor any change in Ellen's behavior after the arrival of the other child. She stated that Ellen had always been a very moody and rather withdrawn child, but that this had become more apparent as she grew and particularly since she had started school about half a year before. The mother, who appeared to be a tense and compulsive person, was in conflict about her feelings for Ellen and her handling of the child. She was aware that she had always been very strict and impatient with Ellen and in retrospect felt guilty that she had toilet-trained her early and firmly. According to the mother, Ellen had been fully toilet-trained at one year of age but because of the diarrhea had not been able to achieve regularity of bowel functions. Ellen's diarrhea was particularly bad between the ages of two and two and a half, during which time she had frequent soiling accidents because of the diarrhea. She had been fully bladder-trained at one and a half years and had never had any relapse. Like all compuslive mothers, Ellen's mother too had carried out rigidly all prescriptions and suggestions and had always asked for blueprints.

Ellen was a very inhibited little girl who obviously could not afford any open expression of aggressions and hostility. Although of superior intelligence, she did not do well in school, where she behaved very timidly and was day-dreaming most of the time. She told me that she often had very bad abdominal cramps and diarrhea, particularly in the morning, so that she was unable to go to school. In the therapeutic relationship with me, she was enabled to express herself freely and gradually began to bring out very hostile and sadistic impulses directed particularly toward her little sister and her mother. I learned from Ellen that her sleep was very much disturbed, that she had fears at night before falling asleep, and that she was awakened by nightmares practically every night and then would lie awake for hours. Her parents did not know about this because Ellen would not dare to disturb her mother. She felt very distant from her father, who seemed to keep himself aloof from the family. Ellen's dreams and nightmares were very helpful for the understanding of her feelings, and in associations to these dreams her repressed feelings and her fantasies were brought out. She was preoccupied with death and revealed fantasies of being buried alive and crushed to death; she liked to play "choking" with her friend and thought she could easily choke "somebody" if she wanted to. ("Somebody" was her little sister, as emerged later.)

I should like to report one nightmare which seemed particularly illuminating: "Kidnappers came. She was just a skeleton, bones and skin, but they insisted on putting her in a pot and boiling her." In this connection it came out that Ellen had the idea that her mother wanted to starve her to death deliberately and that this was her interpretation of her mother's dietary impositions. But it also revealed Ellen's own sadistic impulses toward her sister, whom she would have liked to see kidnapped and dead and starved by the mother. This was brought out especially clearly in another recurrent nightmare. In this nightmare her little sister is stepping on a yellow cloth attached to a stick underneath which a bee was hidden. When her sister steps on it the bee comes out and stings Ellen's friend. She tells her sister not to step on it, again, but her sister steps on it and the bee stings another one of Ellen's friends. This is repeated until all the girls in her class have been stung and then the bee comes toward her and she awakes in fear.

The analysis of this dream led to an understanding of Ellen's quite intense "insectophobia." She was afraid of all insects which sting and bite but also very much afraid of ants. The symbolic significance of insects as representing rival siblings is well known from psychoanalysis. The analysis of this nightmare revealed that the bee represented Ellen's own deeply repressed oral-aggressive impulses which were reactivated and intensified by the experience of observing her sister nursing. By the mechanism of projection in the nightmare, as in the phobia, the repressed aggression is displaced and projected outside. In this way the danger from within is transformed into an outside danger which can be avoided. In Ellen's nightmare, the little sister by stepping on the yellow cloth (sucking on the nipple) mobilizes the dangerous bee which in the end, after all the substitutes have been stung, comes toward Ellen who saves herself in the last moment by waking.

Ellen now began to complain openly about her mother, that she gave her many lickings, that her mother had no time for her, never took her to the movies, etc. The awareness of her resentment toward her mother and her hostility toward her sister brought on a very marked change in Ellen's behavior. She gave up her phobic clinging to her mother and was able to go out by herself in the street, to make some contacts with other children, and to accept school much better. With the working through of her unconscious sadistic impulses, her cramps and diarrhea disappeared and she developed a remarkable appetite and gained weight. Ellen, who by this time had become quite aggressive and outgoing, was able to accept separation from her mother to the extent that she readily accepted the suggestion that she go to camp that summer. This was the first time in her life that she had stayed away from her mother for any length of time. She had been under treatment then for about a year.

I had little contact with the mother, who was seen by our psychiatric social worker. It seems that the mother had difficulty in accepting Ellen's growing independence all along, yet at this point she appeared to be particularly disturbed. I learned that, according to the mother, this was due to the attitude of her husband, who had decided to leave the family and to go to live with his mother in another state. It seems that there was a very tense atmosphere in the home and that the mother directed her irritability and impatience toward Ellen. I had not seen Ellen for several months because of the summer vacation and her being away at camp. I learned that she had a recurrence of the abdominal pain and diarrhea, that she had lost weight, and that her mother had gone back to the dietary restrictions. When I saw Ellen again, she looked very unhappy and told me that her mother intended to take her to a specialist in celiac disease and that she was here today upon her own insistence. She complained that her mother was very irritable and that she had severely restricted Ellen's diet although she really did not have much diarrhea but had merely complained about abdominal cramps. At this point I felt it necessary to see the mother myself.

I learned from the mother that she herself had felt deprived as a child and that she had carried much responsibility from early youth. The maternal grandmother, who suffered from tuberculosis, died when the mother was twelve, and the burden of the house and the care of two younger children fell to her. Her father never remarried. She always had to manage on very little and prided herself on the fact that she was very thrifty also with her husband's small income. Her husband spent a sizable part of his earnings on his hobby of working on mechanical inventions. In addition to the money, he also invested most of his free time in this hobby, which took him away from his family. She had never asked him to mind the children so that she had never gone anywhere at any time without the children, which meant that she spent all her time at home. She therefore had the need for Ellen to grow up very quickly, and recognized now that she had been much too strict and impatient with her. She knew that she was much easier on the younger child, who nevertheless was also becoming a problem to her. This child was then about three years old, a severe thumb-sucker, enuretic, and also suffered from diarrhea. Her condition had been diagnosed as celiac disease, and she was kept on goat's milk and a banana diet.

In the therapeutic interviews with the mother, I found that she had always felt very insecure in the relationship with her husband and that she had overcompensated for this by trying to make herself indispensable to him. She therefore had never made any demands upon him and in fact had always been overindulgent with him so that he occupied the place of the spoiled child in the family. She had been completely unaware that she was identifying Ellen with her husband, particularly in the objectionable aspects, and the younger child with herself. She also had been unaware that she was compensating for her frustrated need to control and to keep her husband dependent by exercising this control over Ellen nor that she was releasing on Ellen the resentment which belonged to her husband. Nothing Ellen ever did pleased her mother. Ellen was awkward and very clumsy with her hands according to the mother, and she had therefore never encouraged Ellen to use crayons, paints, and the like. In her therapeutic sessions with me, the mother came to understand that she had also acted out through Ellen her feelings about her husband's hobby. She had never allowed herself to recognize that she considered his hobby child's play and that she felt furious at him because he preferred "playing" to giving his attention to her. She was amazed and pleased to find that her tendency toward severe headaches and her allergy which consisted of severe sneezing attacks (both conditions had developed since her marriage) cleared up as a side effect of her therapy with me.

The fact that Ellen in the course of her treatment not only overcame her clumsiness but developed a very remarkable ability for drawing and painting and later on for playing the piano, which she had started upon her own wish, seems of particular interest. It was my impression that without the change in the attitude of the mother brought on by her awareness of her feelings toward her husband, Ellen could not have achieved this sublimation of her pregenital (mainly anal) impulses. In my opinion, the unconscious attitude of the mother plays a decisive part in both the retardation and the development of certain ego functions of the child.

In Ellen's case only the prompt psychoanalytic interpretation of the mother's behavior stopped her acting out and prevented the abrupt termination of Ellen's treatment. Had I not seen Ellen's mother in time, withdrawal of Ellen from therapy would have been the result. The withdrawal from treatment is then rationalized by the mother with the aggravation of the child's physical condition, which, to the mother and the environment, proves the ineffectiveness of psychotherapy. Actually, in such a case the child's aggravated condition is due to the increased unconscious resistance of the mother toward the child's treatment. I find it necessary particularly in the treatment of the more severe psychosomatic disorders in children to work closely with the mother so as to give her sufficient understanding of the motivations of her behavior and her role in the illness of the child and thus to modify her attitude toward the child. Without this, I do not think that lasting therapeutic results can be obtained for the child. Close contact with the mother is necessary in order to prevent sudden acting out on her part which causes exacerbations in the child's symptoms and may result in sudden withdrawal of the child from treatment.

The change in the attitude of the mother was reflected in Ellen's rapid improvement. Although the change in the mother's attitude was consistent, her ambivalence toward Ellen had not been resolved and came out in many instances. I should like to report one rather amusing episode to illustrate this. Ellen felt that she was gaining too much weight and began to cut down on certain foods. Her mother urged her to eat more by telling her, "You know Dr. S. would like you to eat more." Ellen made an appointment with me. She wanted to find out whether this was so, because she did not think I wanted her to get fat, particularly since she was in competition with another little girl for the attentions of a boy in her class.

I should also like to give some information regarding Ellen's sexual fantasies and fears, because they were related to her phobic behavior and the diarrhea. We know from psychoanalysis that the fixation of the libido to a pregenital level inevitably colors the course and outcome of the oedipal conflict and with that the ultimate sexual development of the child. In the case of a pregenital fixation, overt sexual activity may be completely missing and sexual impulses will be then expressed in a disguised form as oral or anal activity. Diarrhea for instance, in such a case, serves not only as an outlet for repressed aggressive and hostile impulses and as a means of dealing unconsciously with feelings of dependence and helplessness but also as an outlet for the repressed sexual impulses, which in accordance with the pregenital level of fixation are of a sadistic nature (see chapter 11).

After the freeing of the repressed hostile and aggressive impulses and the consequent improvement of her condition, Ellen began to reveal fantasies of a sexual nature. This resulted from the fact that through the analysis the diarrhea had become unusable as an outlet for these impulses and their gratification in reality was not permissible because of their frank sadistic nature. I should like to illustrate this. Ellen's fantasies centered around sadistic tortures; she claimed she had heard about and also seen pictures of tortures. For example: "The breast of a nude girl is cut around, honey is smeared on it and boulder ants are crawling on it."; or "A nude woman or a nude man were thrown into a cave where there were man-eating rats." She talked about her sexual fears and wishes. A girl had told her that in the park in the neighborhood where Ellen lived there were boys with knives who were holding up girls and dragging them into the bushes. In one of her sessions, she drew a boy with a knife and then drew a knife with blood on it as he pulled it out of the girl's body (her concept of intercourse). She then confided that she had a problem, namely, that she was very much ashamed of her breasts. They were developing too early. She drew the body of a naked woman with breasts and in place of the genital a big leaf which looked like a penis. She also revealed her fantasies about wanting to have a baby and asked me, "Do you think I could have a baby with my father?" After I explained to her the facts of sexual development and the need to wait for masturbation for the satisfaction of such desires she said, "But what if I don't get a husband when I'm grown up? I read in the paper that an eight-year-old- girl had a baby. Do you think she did it with her father?" Ellen was then eight and one half years old.

In the fantasy of the man-eating rats which she elaborated upon with an obvious thrill, as well as in the fantasy of the skeleton being boiled and eaten, the oral sadistic elements are quite apparent. Because of her own very strong oral and anal sadistic tendencies, the sexual act was imagined as a cruel and sadistic attack, as brought out in the fantasies about the boys cutting the girls up with knives. In the fantasies of the man-eating rats, the boulder ants, and in the nightmare of the skeleton, her own oral envy and desires to eat everything up so nothing would be left for her sister are brought out. Her original eating difficulty had been due partly to an inhibition of these very intense oral sadistic impulses. The idea that her mother wanted to starve her to death, grotesque and paranoid as it appeared at first glance, was not entirely a projection of Ellen's own oral sadistic impulses upon her mother, but had a kernel of truth in reality. Her mother actually because of her ambivalence had difficulty in feeding her properly. Ellen's mother, coming from a home where, as she claimed, there was often not enough food for the children, had an ambivalent attitude toward food. She had been very (ambivalently) attached to the maternal grandmother, who had died of tuberculosis "because of too much work and too little to eat."

After the working through of these sadistic fantasies, the change in Ellen's personality was very striking. Although she had overcome her phobic clinging to the mother, she had still been suffering from a number of fears which she tried to conceal and about which she only spoke in her treatment. She was particularly afraid to go to the bathroom, fearing that a burglar or kidnapper would come in through the window. She lost her fears; she was able to move around freely and even go through the park herself, where she had acquired a garden plot which she took care of herself. As mentioned before, she also showed a good ability for sublimation which evidenced itself in her scholastic achievements and interests. All in all she now led a full life for a girl her age (nine—ten). When I discontinued therapy, we had the understanding that Ellen would call me for an appointment should she experience any difficulty. Ellen did not call me, and I learned from the mother that her development proceeded very satisfactorily although the family situation was not a good one.

In conclusion I should like to question the role of the constitutional and hereditary factors in this case. The thought of a hereditary factor suggests itself readily because both children suffered from similar symptoms. The treatment of both children (I supervised the treatment of the younger child) and the work with the mother, however, showed that the transmission of the attitude of the parents and particularly the unconscious feelings of the mother were a basic factor in their condition. It may be of interest and certainly amusing to learn that after the mother became more relaxed in her relationship to the children, and also more aware of her insecurity with her husband and therefore better able to assert herself with him, the father developed an episode of diarrhea. When the mother reported this, she laughed and said, "Does he also have diarrhea because of me?" In the treatment of Ellen and also from the mother, I had learned that the father used to spend hours in the bathroom, where he would read his paper and magazines and practically set up a workshop for himself. The mother also was an anally fixed person, very compulsive and with a great emphasis on anal functions. It would seem obvious that such an attitude on the part of the parents would intensify the anal tendencies in the children.

The age level at which Ellen's diarrhea manifested itself and became increasingly worse I have found to be typical for the onset of this symptom (Prugh, 1961). This age of one and one half to two and one half, as we know from psychoanalysis, represents the height and passing of the anal sadistic phase in the psychosexual development of the child. As in other cases, in Ellen's case the mother had toilet-trained Ellen early and strictly. This and the other circumstances, as we have seen, contributed to an intensification of Ellen's anal impulses and to the abrupt repression of them. It would seem to me, however, the one very important psychological factor characteristic for this phase lies in the fact that it represents a phase during which the object relationships of the child undergo definite changes. The physiological growth of this age and the developing motility, coordination, sensory perceptions, speech, etc. produce a marked change in the child's behavior, leading from the passivity characteristic for the infant of the oral phase to the activity and assertiveness of the child of the anal phase. In other words, there is correlated with the physiological development and the accompanying changes from passivity to activity also a psychological development with accompanying strivings toward independence and a change in quality of object relationship.

The child of this phase who is attempting to overcome his dependence and to separate himself as an individual from his environment and particularly from his mother is very sensitive to any interference with these strivings. He cannot be deceived by his mother's overt attitude but invariably senses and reacts also to her unconscious feelings and wishes. He needs, as it were, his mother's permissions both conscious and unconscious to develop as an independent being. Even with a mother who accepts and encourages her child's strivings for independence, some conflict on the part of the child as to whether to let go of his mother as the sole object of dependence or to hold on to her

is unavoidable. This phenomenon of ambivalence is a characteristic of all instinctual life, and the fact that it becomes so
apparent during the anal phase is not entirely due to the special
quality of the anal instinct but, as I believe, is related also to the
dependency conflict which ensues at this age. Actually it is only
during this phase that we can observe the phenomenon of a
dependency conflict, while during the oral phase the manifestations of the infant's dependent needs and of his reactions to
gratification or frustration of these needs predominate.

The turning of the aggressive impulses toward the objects in
the outside world, which is most apparent during the anal
phase, we can regard as an essential step toward turning away
from and becoming independent of the mother. How much of
an obstacle to the child she will become in his struggle for
independence will to a considerable degree depend upon the
attitude of the mother. From this in turn it will depend in part
also on how intense the hate impulses directed against the
mother will be and what means the child will adopt in coping
with these impulses (see chapter 8). In Ellen's case it became
quite obvious that, because of the personality of her mother and
the child's relationship to her, the mechanims of repression
would have to be chosen as a main defense mechanism by Ellen.
The components and derivatives of the anal instinct lend
themselves particularly well both for the direct expression and
for the symbolic somatic dramatization of his dependency
conflict, which the child because of his actual helplessness is not
capable of resolving in reality. Temper tantrums and destructive behavior are the most common direct expression of it, while
the unconscious identification of the frustrating object
(mother) with feces with the elimination of it (mother) in the
symptom of diarrhea is the symbolic dramatization of this
conflict. This devaluation and symptomatic giving up of the
mother is counteracted by the child in the phobic clinging as if
by the actual holding on to mother, the child were protecting
her from his unconscious destructive impulses.

These points it would seem to me were well illustrated by
Ellen's case. Through her manifest attitude Ellen's mother
clearly indicated her wish for Ellen to grow up quickly and to be
a more independent child. She was annoyed and disturbed by

Ellen's phobic behavior and in fact it was for this behavior that she brought Ellen for treatment. Yet in the treatment of the child and in work with the mother it became evident that Ellen had perceived and carried out her mother's unconscious need and wish for Ellen to remain dependent upon her. This was brought out particularly by the mother's attempt to remove Ellen from treatment when she felt threatened by Ellen's growing independence. Also the interrelation of the phobic mechanism with the diarrhea could be observed very well during treatment. Periods of clinging to her mother and diarrhea alternated with periods during which Ellen was able to assert herself; she became more aggressive and less dependent with a clearing up of the diarrhea. While in reality she was holding on to her mother in the phobic clinging, she was giving her up (unconsciously) in the diarrhea. When Ellen was helped through analysis and through the changed attitude of the mother to resolve her dependency conflict and to free herself in reality, she no longer needed the phobic clinging nor the diarrhea as the symptomatic expressions of an unresolved (dependency) conflict.

10

Mucous Colitis
Associated with Phobias

Boy (12)

A twelve-year-old boy had been suffering two years from severe diarrhea of unknown origin. A series of tests and examinations established the diagnosis of mucous colitis. All treatment was ineffective, and his condition became progressively worse. He also had many phobias which, with the diarrhea, prevented him from attending school.

A very fearful and inhibited child, he came for analytic treatment accompanied by his mother. He was afraid of his father who, he felt, looked down on him. He stated he could not go anywhere without his mother. Whenever he attempted to leave the house without her, he got cramps and had to run to the bathroom. Before he had to stop attending, he had been doing poorly in school because of the diarrhea and because he worried so much: a little cut or scratch would throw him into a panic for fear that he would die of septicemia; the slightest cold threatened him with pneumonia. He could not concentrate on his studies, worried about his poor grades, and feared that he would be left behind. His belief that his classmates and the teacher were laughing at him caused him to withdraw from children altogether. He sat alone at home, listening to the radio or modeling airplanes which was his only hobby.

Whenever we discussed his relationship with his mother, he reacted with an immediate urge to move his bowels: "It seems that I can't talk about my mother without having diarrhea," he remarked one day. This was then interpreted to him as indicating that he was very angry with her. "Well," he said, "she does prefer my brother." He then complained that his mother held his brother, who was five years his senior, up to him continually as a model boy and superior student; also that his mother gave a great deal of attention to his younger sister. He recalled that he had had a severe attack of diarrhea right after his sister was born (he was then about seven years old), and that he had been very unhappy because shortly before his sister was born, his grandmother, who lived with the family and who took care of him, had died; he had been very much attached to her. His sister had actually replaced him in the affection of the mother who had always wanted a girl and had made no secret about it; hence, the birth of his sister was a particularly severe trauma because he had then lost both his mothers: his grandmother through death, his real mother to his sister. The diarrhea and increased phobic dependence on his mother at that time were his reactions to this trauma. He also had lost his pet dog at that time. He had had attacks of diarrhea before that too, when he started school. He did not want to go to school and leave his mother. His father had brought him there by force and remained outside to make sure that the boy did not leave the classroom to run home. He remembered that when he was between three and four years old his brother showed him a picture of the world (a globe). He suddenly had a terrible fear of being separated from his mother and ran panic-stricken to look for her. He pleaded with her to promise him that if he should have to die, she would hold his hand and die with him, and if she should die he wanted to hold her hand and die with her. When he was still younger, he had temper tantrums for which his mother hit him; so he gave them up.

He reported a nightmare which he had dreamed many times prior to the analysis: "My mother was tied to a big bell and the bell drove her crazy and she became a monster that looked terrible. She came into my house and started to beat me up." His mother constantly criticized and nagged him for being clumsy and slow; he had long since reacted by exaggerating this very behavior, and by calling himself "a moron and crazy." At the beginning and just prior to his analysis there was a period when he was in a constant state of panic, unable to do anything for fear that he was going out of his mind. In this self-depreciation, he was actually depreciating his mother. In his dream the boy permits himself to say, "Mother is crazy and a monster." His mother often said to him, "You're driving me crazy with your dawdling," but he never had admitted to himself that his mother was driving him crazy with her constant pushing and nagging. The sexual meaning of this dream was later analyzed when other dreams related to the oedipal situtation made clear his sadomasochistic conception of intercourse. "Crazy" meant his (sadistic) sexual impulses directed toward his mother and also his masochistic sexual identification with her. "Crazy" also signified losing control and giving vent to his destructive impulses.

Although exaggerated and neurotically distorted, the boy's feelings toward his mother were a reflection of his mother's attitude toward him. The mother admitted that she had not wanted a child at the time her younger son was born. She had wanted still less another boy, and she had had some sort of "nervous breakdown" as a reaction to his birth. She disliked the child intensely, was very impatient and punitive with him, thought him homely, and was hurt narcissistically by his protruding ears. She had put great emphasis upon toilet training. During his first year, he was mostly in the care of his grandmother. When the mother took over his care, he would soil himself occasionally. She beat him for this and he became "clean" very soon. Between one and a half and two years of age, he had attacks of diarrhea alternating with severe temper tantrums and was generally a difficult child. He had many colds and, when he was about two and a half, he contracted pneumonia after which he changed and became a "quiet" and "good" boy. His mother was then annoyed with him because he would not go to sleep unless she lay with him on his bed and because he clung to her all the time. In retrospect, she could see how her attitude had affected the boy, and she felt guilty and greatly worried about him. Looking through his books, as was her habit, she found a paper on which he had scribbled, "I'm afraid I'm going crazy."

In proportion to the growth of his awareness of his repressed hostility and of his death wishes, directed primarily toward his mother, he was better able to tolerate frustration, and his general behavior and particularly the diarrhea improved. Psychoanalysis made him aware of the satisfaction he derived from the behavior which was so disturbing to his parents. He liked to scare his mother by telling her about an irresistible urge to kill his brother. He once sprained his brother's wrist in a fight, and in fights with boys he became very violent. Once he almost killed a boy who teased him. This murderous hostility gave vent to both his hatred of his mother and his implacable jealous rivalry with his brother.

Phobic clinging to his mother had the aim of protecting her from his unconscious impulse to destroy her. The common association of a phobia with somatic symptoms indicates failure of the phobic defense. The destructive impulses warded off by the phobia broke through and found somatic expression in diarrhea, in which, by devaluating his mother to and identifying her unconsciously with feces, he separated himself from her somatically. Since he felt very helpless and dependent on his mother in reality, he could give her up only symptomatically.

When he was ten years old, the paternal grandfather came to live with the family. Up to that time, the boy had shared a room with his older brother with whom he very much enjoyed roughhousing every night and morning. The patient first recalled that he was chosen to share a room with the grandfather, whereas his brother now slept in the parents' bedroom. The grandfather was a cardiac invalid. The boy was required to be quiet; he often remained awake to determine whether the old man was still breathing or already dead. Later this was found to be a retrospective falsification (confirmed by the mother) and that it was he, not his brother, who had first moved into the parental bedroom. He had had severe nightmares which kept him up most of the night and was for this reason moved after several weeks into the room with his grandfather. These events were followed by acute emotional disturbances and recurrence of diarrhea.

During this phase of analysis he had frequent nightmares: "I had a stomach-ache and thought I had to have my appendix taken out, but I found I didn't really. I tried to get out of the hospital, but I didn't" and, "I was bitten by a mad dog on my arm and when I went to the hospital, it was so crowded that I couldn't see a doctor. There were little squares where the dog had bitten me and more and more came." The father had often warned the boy that if he "touched himself," he would become sick. He believed that, if after touching his genitals he should accidentally touch his eyes, his sight would be impaired. This worried him because it would thwart his wish to become an airplane pilot. He had started modeling airplanes when he was about eight, imitating his brother who then gave it up. He would walk daily several miles to an airport, and once he parachuted with an open umbrella from a tree, narrowly escaping serious injury.

A recurrent nightmare appeared in various versions. Of the two versions which follow, the first he had dreamed the previous night.

"I saw a mummy in a box in my closet and became very scared. I got up and awoke my mother. I went into my parents' bedroom. I went into my mother's bed and she went into mine. I saw my little sister. She was carrying a mummy like a toy and she was playing with it. She did not show any fear. I was very much afraid, especially when I saw that the box had a crack and I thought that I might see a mummy through this crack. My mother opened the box and I was looking on. Inside was a brown wallet. When I opened the wallet, it enlarged to about the size of two feet. While opening the box, I scratched my finger and I was afraid of it.

"My brother brought some mummy cases home and my mother put them into the cellar; then I found myself in the cellar and was very frightened. I didn't know how to go out, being all surrounded by mummy cases." He exhibited a scratch on his finger which he had noticed upon awakening, and which must have occurred in his sleep. He was very much disturbed about it, and it revived his hypochondriacal fears about injuries and septicemia. He had once read about a curse on those who disturb mummies and about a man who had died as a consequence. It appeared that he had been seduced by his little sister into sexual play. He had observed his sister masturbating without signs of fear, while he felt very guilty for having touched her genital.

In an almost hallucinatory way he visualized a scene in the house in which he lived when he was four years old. It was a warm summer day. He was in his room with a little girl, his cousin. They were masturbating each other when his mother suddenly entered the room. In reproducing this memory he reexperienced the severe shock he had felt at being caught. He remembered his mother's threat that he would become very sick. He knows that he stopped masturbating abruptly after this. It would seem that this threat, coming from his mother when he was at the height of the oedipal conflict, had profoundly influenced his psychosexual development to the exclusion of all genital activity. Part of the dream reproduces events of his third year when he could not fall asleep without his mother and when almost every night he went frightened to his parents' bedroom to look for his mother and remain there the rest of the night. The father's later threats of punishment for masturbation only added weight to the mother's much more effective threat. (It is my observation that the boy reacts to the mother's threat of castration more severely than to the father's, perhaps because the mother is herself a castrated object who demonstrated the reality of such a threat.) His terror of seeing a mummy through the "crack" expressed his wish to see a penis where there was none (mother's, sister's genitals). Inability to resolve his fear of the castrating woman and failure to resolve the oedpius led to a partial unconscious acceptance of castration and the wish to take his mother's place.

Although an unwanted child, the first year of his life was comparatively unaffected because he was cared for by his grandmother. When he began to react to his mother's hostility by soiling and having temper tantrums, a struggle for control ensued.

Rejected and at the same time overstimulated by the mother (sleeping with her), her threat (castration) when she caught him playing with his little cousin put an abrupt end to this and seems to have precluded any sexual activity including masturbation. Very much afraid of his father who, he thought, always looked down upon him, he could neither compete nor identify himself with him. He also hated his brother as the rival for the mother's love; besides which, according to his mother's wishes, he should have been a girl. Utterly frustrated, he regressed to the anal level of libido development; hence the recurrence of diarrhea when he was about four years old (oedipal phase), at the start of school (separation from mother), at the birth of his sister (resentment toward mother), and at the age of ten when, overstimulated by sharing the parental bedroom, he found himself caught in a violent masturbatory conflict. All his thwarted aggressive and sexual impulses he released anally in the diarrhea.

During the first four months of treatment he was seen three times a week. He was able to resume his studies in school, and soon worked himself to the top of his class. He came and went without his mother, made friends, and participated in school activities and outdoor play. The diarrhea had disappeared completely. For the first time in his life, his mother went on a vacation with his little sister without him. He commented: "I hope she will not interfere and make me depend on her again when she comes back."

He was seen less frequently at greater intervals to help him achieve the emotional independence and detachment from his mother necessary for mature (sexual) functioning and to resolve the transference. During the earlier part of this phase of the treatment, he became moderately depressed. He once had a prolonged cold which kept him away from the analysis for several weeks. One day he called for a special appointment because he was very much disturbed about a dream he had had the previous night: "I was with my best friend and suddenly someone plunged from a fifth floor window. My friend called out, 'It is your mother.' I ran over crying, 'Mother! Mother!' She got up and said, 'Nothing happened.'"

That week he had felt very sad and, whenever anyone talked to him, felt like crying. He recalled again with much emotion the episode with the globe which occurred when he was three or four years old. He understood that at present these feelings related to me. To him to get well meant to lose the analyst, just as to grow up meant to lose mother through her death.

He began to show interest in girls. He was masturbating without any fear, bur rather infrequently. The shift in his sexual interest was illustrated by a dream.

"It was dusk and I was up on the roof of my house. The Japs were coming. They wanted to do something sexually to my mother. I came down with a machine gun and they were all standing in a circle around her. One in the center, an officer, said, 'She's too old for me, anyhow.' I was turning my machine gun and shot them one after the other, so they fell down dead. Then I thought that if the Japs were at my house, they probably were also at Stella's house [his girl]; so I went to Stella's house to help her. When I arrived there, there were no Japs and she was all right."

He was defending his mother, as well as his girl, against his own sadistic impulses.

The analysis ended when he was fourteen years old. He had just finished the first term of a high school for aeronautical training, where he had been awarded a scholarship, and worked during his summer vacations in an airport.

The psychoanalysis of a boy of twelve is reported to demonstrate the interrelation between a somatic symptom (diarrhea) and an anxiety hysteria (phobia). The phobia was a fear of being separated from his mother, protecting her against his unconscious death wishes. In the diarrhea he was giving her up by identifying her unconsciously with feces. At the same time, however, the conflict whether to keep mother or to give her up continued in reality, expressing itself in these very symptoms— the phobic clinging and the diarrhea. The overdetermined psychodynamics of the diarrhea would seem to be as follows: (1) a retreat from the genital to the anal-sadistic level of libido organization which provided the possibility of discharging aggressive and sexual impulses (masturbatory substitute) (2) the direct release of sadistic impulses in an effort to protect himself from the overwhelming anxiety stemming from his own destructiveness (conversion on a pregential level), (3) devaluation of the frustrating object (mother equals feces) and getting rid of her—therefore, sadistic control over mother realized in the secondary gain derived from the illness (he could stay home with mother, take her away from the others, and have her accompany him wherever he went), (4) punishment through physical suffering and the restrictions imposed upon him by the diarrhea and his fears.

PART 4

ANOREXIA NERVOSA

11

Introduction

Although I do not consider anorexia nervosa a psychosomatic syndrome, I have decided to include it in this volume so that some of these issues can be discussed and clarified on the basis of clinical material. I regard anorexia nervosa as an impulse disorder occurring in certain types of pregenitally fixated patients. At present, the knowledge, and consequently, the treatment based on it is so inadequate that an attempt to improve it should be made. Forced feeding, drug therapy, and brain surgery are still the prevalent treatment in anorexia nervosa.

A survey of the literature reveals that with few exceptions most contributions to this subject during the last ten to fifteen years are by investigators who have studied their material from a phenomenological rather than from a dynamic point of view. With regard to therapy, some investigators (Bruch, 1962, 1971; Crisp, 1969; Dally, 1969) hold the view that a psychoanalytic approach should be avoided. Bruch, for example, advises that "motivational analysis and insight should be avoided" and states that anorexia nervosa patients do not associate freely, do not bring material, and do not report dreams.

My experience with anorexia nervosa patients as well as that of other psychoanalytic investigators, Lorand (1943), Thomä (1967), Jessner and Abse (1960), Blitzer (1961), Waller (1942), Margolis and Jenberg (1960), to name only a few, most certainly disprove the validity of such a position. It would seem to me that a preconceived attitude on the part of the investigator is neither therapeutic nor rewarding in terms of gaining insight into the dynamics of the illness and the personality of the patient. In this connection, a brief paper by O. Fenichel (1945) is of interest. It shows the wealth of information and insight one can gain in two psychoanalytic interviews with such patients. In the woman patient, he recognized the role of the mother-daughter relationship and the role of food in this family. He also recognized the basic differences in the dynamics between male and female in anorexia nervosa. The female starts off by not wanting to eat on a conscious level.

Dally (1969), in his treatment recommendations, puts the emphasis on weight gain (two pounds per week) to be achieved by all means, that is, with the patient confined to bed under strict hospital regime. Chlorpromazine treatment is given as a routine procedure to anorexia nervosa patients. He reports that many of these patients shed the enforced weight gain as soon as they leave the hospital and that this procedure in some cases is repeated several times. His report is instructive from various points of view. A number of these patients turned into compulsive eaters, one committed suicide, and there were several suicide attempts. An important aspect that can be fully understood and appreciated only in careful psychoanalytic study is the fact that these patients suffer from intense but very vulnerable narcissism. All their lives they have felt manipulated by their mothers, and they are extremely sensitive to any manipulation, especially by the therapist. Hospitalization is recommended also as a means of separating the patient from the family. The emphasis, as can be seen, is on physical separation and not on emotional separation. Those who practice physical separation, that is, removing the patient from the family without providing psychoanalytic therapy for the patient, do not realize or do not accept the fact that the anorexia patient is dealing also with internalized objects and conflicts and that the struggle with the internalized mother will go on no matter where the patient is. Unless this can be made conscious to the patient, there is no possibility for a more realistic solution of this conflict. Even though the patient may give up the anorexia nervosa, other neurotic, psychosomatic, or psychotic symptoms will replace the anorexia nervosa.

Dally's report and those of others about the outcome of untreated or inadequately treated patients with anorexia nervosa confirm this statement. D. W. Kay and K. Shapiro (1965) found a 17 percent mortality in their earlier material. The duration of anorexia nervosa is no less than two to three years and in 25 percent it is longer. These patients remain more or less permanently undernourished and their sexual adjustment is impaired. Crisp (1969) gives a poor prognosis when there is rejection, overprotection, or ambivalence in the parents. The best prognosis he states is when the attitudes of the parents are normal. He seems to overlook the fact that, with "normal" attitudes of the parents, children do not develop anorexia nervosa and even what might appear as an appropriate attitude to the untrained observer on the surface often conceals the unconscious pathological rapport between the patient and her parents. Emotional separation, that is a basic change in the relationship with the mother, can be achieved only in psychoanalytic psychotherapy. Hospitalization is recommended in spite of the experience that as soon as the patient leaves the hospital she returns to starvation and that improvement, if it occurs, comes about by unknown reasons, perhaps by external factors, time, etc., but not as a result of the hospital treatment. In these cases, then no real changes in the personality of patients have occurred except that this particular behavior, anorexia nervosa, was given up, or more correctly was exchanged for other pathological behavior. Into this category belong also the so-called spontaneous recoveries. Another sizable percentage (40 percent) of these patients reported by Dally (1969) turned into compulsive over-eaters as a result of the hospital treatment. Electric shock treatment and brain surgery, especially prefrontal leucotomy, was performed in more resistant patients and in some patients more than once. As far as psychotherapy is concerned, Dally recommends the anaclitic type of treatment in which the therapist makes himself available to the patient as a substitute parent. This attitude is reminiscent of that taken by Margolis and Jenberg (1960) some years ago in the treatment of patients with psychosomatic diseases except that anaclitic treatment then was introduced as a parameter to precede psychoanalytic therapy. The effect was that it produced such severe states of regression that these patients not only became unsuitable subjects for psychoanalysis but suffered severe aggravations of their symptoms, psychotic breaks, and other unmanageable behavior, Sperling (1957a, 1960b and 1967c).

A brief review of some of the presentations at the Symposium on Anorexia Nervosa in Göttingen by J. E. Meyer and H. Feldman (1965) might be helpful in assessing the more current views on this subject. K. Tolstrup recommends isolation from home and considers hospital treatment as essential in any case of anorexia nervosa. The treatment he practices is a kind of superficial supportive therapy. The emphasis is on eating with discussion of daily problems. With children, Groen et. al. (1966) advise education of the family for the purpose of allowing more expression of aggression and freedom. The role of sexual identifications, repression of sexuality, with displacement to the oral zone and eating are ignored.

Another point to be considered is that many of those who report on cures and good results have no long term follow-ups and do not consider the personality changes which occur subsequently to hospital treatment, such as the breakdown of obsessional compulsive defenses and the transformation of compulsive noneaters into acting-out patients and overeaters as the psychiatric result of that very treatment. The nonanalytic interference with the mechanisms of defense by untrained or inadequately trained personnel can have the most deleterious consequences for the maintenance of an emotional balance in such a patient.

Of particular interest in this connection are the discussion remarks of Cremarius in response to H. Frahm who uses forced feeding and medication like Dally and Sargent. The discussant felt that the use of large amounts of phenothiazines in tube feeding could be regarded as a kind of chemical leucotomy.

Phenothiazine is not a specific chemical for the treatment of anorexia nervosa. Tolstrup, who relies on encouraging the patient to eat, overlooks that the noneating has an important unconscious dynamic function for the anorexic patient. It is the main pathological defense against loss of control. To give up their right to control their own food intake, without understanding the unconscious meaning of surrendering impulse control causes severe anxiety. This in turn leads to acting-out behavior affecting various symptoms in the patient.

Bruch, in her discussion at this symposium, stressed that the disturbance of body image is of delusional proportions in these patients. My point of argument follows: There is a difference of whether we deal with a deficiency of perception or with the results of repression. Repression can be lifted with psychoanalytic treatment. This pertains also to sexuality. Bruch maintains that there is a lack of sexuality. There is a difference whether there is a lack or whether there is a repression of sexuality with displacement from the genital to the oral level and with the equation of food with sexuality. Deficiency is not corrigible analytically. Her explanation for the anorexic behavior is faulty learning, but she leaves out the concept of the unconscious and of the drives and, with that, the role of unconscious fantasies and conflicts as well as the vicissitudes of pathological development of aggression and sexuality in the genesis of anorexia nervosa. She falls back on neurophysiology and behavioral concepts.

H. Thomä, whose monograph "Anorexia Nervosa" (1967) I consider the most valuable and informative contribution on this subject during the last decade, reported on his analytic approach in the treatment of anorexic patients. Of the fifty patients, most were treated in the hospital, at least in the initial stages. In thirty-seven patients a psychoanalytically oriented psychotherapy and in thirteen patients psychoanalysis with interpretation of resistances, defenses, etc. were used. He was aware that these patients lie or refuse to talk about anything that could disturb the precarious equilibrium and that the analyst has to take a more active stance. The hospitalized patients were treated in conjunction with other medical personnel, a treatment which in my opinion makes the application of the true psychoanalytic method rather difficult. There are split transferences with other doctors and hospital personnel and contamination of the transference because the analyst is at times compelled to actively intervene in hospital and other real life situations of this patient. This lends reality to the patient's transference feelings and requires then more time for working through and eventual resolution of the transference. Another discussant, who recommended that the therapist make himself the parent substitute, then went on to say that the more successful the therapist becomes in intervening for the patient, the more demanding the patient becomes. Selvini in her paper, "Interpretation of Mental Anorexia," stressed the patient's struggle against hunger and experience of the nourished body as a threatening, indestructible force. This is her explanation why the patient's food intake is reduced to absurdity. She does not consider anorexia nervosa as a defense against oral-sadistic impulses but points out that at puberty anorexia nervosa is a defense against depression and schizophrenia.

She takes the position that the body represents the mother and must therefore be kept in check. She minimizes and perhaps even overlooks the role of instincts. The body in my opinion represents the instincts, especially sexuality. There is a lot of concern with the body and with bodily functions on the part of the patient, for instance, with constipation or with the flat belly where "nothing must stick out." This behavior indicates the patient's preoccupation with unconscious pregnancy fantasies (wishes and fears). According to Selvini, impregnation fantasies cover more primitive fantasies of being invaded by the mother. There is hardly any mention of sexual conflicts, masturbation, and sexual identifications.

The body must be kept in check because from it emanate all the dangerous impulses, especially sexuality. If there is no body, there are no sexual feelings. These patients make a negative exhibitionistic display of themselves with shock effect: One of them took pride in looking like bones and skin and felt that no boy would want to take her out and that he would hurt himself by touching her. Another felt that the nourished body, especially the fat body, represents the pregnant mother. Food equals different objects on different levels: on the oral level various part objects or mother, on the anal level, feces or devalued part objects. These can be poisonous and dangerous, sperm and urine, fecal penis and a fecal baby; on the oral level it is the breast, penis, and mother that the child wants to devour. On the phallic level, it represents pregnancy in identification with mother as a female, which the anorexic patient cannot accept because of her hostility against mother. The anorexic patient, because she actually has received gratification from the mother and others, has more object libido available for cathexis than the depressive or schizophrenic, which represent a regression beyond anorexia nervosa.

In this connection, certain behavior in adolescent girls who do not suffer from anorexia nervosa is of interest. These girls alternate between asceticism and sexual indulgence (excessive masturbation) or, in displacement of the sexual conflicts to the oral level, between a dieting and overeating. They react to overeating as to a sexual transgression, with orgastic feelings and severe guilt. Like Bruch, Selvini (1965) too considers anorexia nervosa a special psychosis, midway between schizoid paranoid psychosis and depression, and in treatment, she too is against interpretation and insight treatment.

12

Case Histories
of Anorexia Nervosa

Feeding Disturbances in Small Children

Feeding and eating disturbances are the earliest and most frequent disorders in children. These disturbances can be considered as the first indications of something amiss in the mother-child relationship, but they seldom come to the attention of either the analyst or even the child psychiatrist. The work of Spitz, especially on hospitalism (1945) and research in child development by psychoanalytic investigators such as Benedek (1938), Brody (1956), Escalona (1954), Rank (1948), and Ribble (1944) are of importance in this connection.

Even if very young children, especially infants, were brought to a psychoanalyst for the treatment of an eating disturbance, it was not thought possible to study such a young patient directly by the psychoanalytic method. Therefore the work of the investigators referred to above consists of observations and conclusions derived from them.

I devised a method which enabled me to study and to treat young children psychoanalytically. The main feature of this method was the inclusion of the mother into the treatment. In the case of children of pre-verbal age, the child was treated indirectly by treating the mother (Sperling, 1949, 1950d, see also chapter 3). In the case of children of verbal age, simultaneous treatment of mother and child (in separate sessions but by the same analyst) or successive treatment (mother treated first and later if necessary the child) was the treatment of choice (Sperling, 1959a). Even in cases where direct psychoanalytic treatment was possible, a positive relationship and occasional contact with the mother were necessary to support her and to insure her willingness to allow her child to resolve the pathological relationship existing between them. In my paper, "Equivalents of Depression in Children," (1959), I could demonstrate clinically that some eating disturbances leading to starvation and illness are the consequences of a disturbed mother-child relationship and represented the equivalents of a depression in these children.

I would like to summarize briefly some of the findings from my research which are most relevant to the subject under discussion and in particular to the genetic aspects of anorexia nervosa. The analytic exploration of the mother in cases of severe eating disturbances in infants invariably revealed highly ambivalent feelings and in some cases unconscious rejection of the child by the mother (Sperling, 1970). Making the mother aware of her feelings and at least of some of the unconscious sources of these feelings in a brief kind of "analytic first aid" approach was strikingly sucessful in many cases. I found that these feelings frequently stemmed from unresolved ambivalence conflicts from the mother's own childhood which she had transfered to her child or from unconscious identification of the child with repressed and rejected aspects of the mother's own personality (Sperling, chapter 3, 1949, 1951, 1959d). Follow-up studies revealed that the changes in the feelings of the mother affected by this brief technique were sustained in many cases during the important developmental stages of the child (Sperling, 1970).

In children of pre-latency age, where the personality of the child had already been molded according to the unconscious expectations of the mother and the eating disturbance had become a focal point of the conflict between them, simultaneous treatment was the method of choice for quickest and best therapeutic results. At the same time, this method was proven to be the most rewarding approach for a fuller understanding of the dynamics of the mother-child relationship and their role in the child's psychopathology. Clinical vignettes from the psychoanalytic treatment of young children and of adolescent girls suffering from anorexia nervosa will be presented to illustrate this point and the dynamics which I consider essential in anorexia nervosa.

Simultaneous Treatment of Anorexia Nervosa and Paroxysmal Tachycardia: Linda (2)

Already in young children the basic dynamics characteristic of the pernicious type of anorexia as seen in some cases of adolescent girls are clearly discernible. Fortunately, however, at this early stage, this pathology can be reversed by simultaneous treatment of mother and child. One brief clinical vignette taken from a case report published in 1952a may serve as an illustration. Linda developed a severe eating disturbance at age two. At twenty-two months she had been referred to me because of nocturnal attacks of paroxysmal tachycardia by the hospital where she had been hospitalized twice for this condition. Among other symptoms indicative of a disturbed mother-child relationship were states of withdrawal, excessive sucking of her tongue and lips, and disturbed sleep. Linda had also suffered from eating difficulties since infancy with an intensification following a tonsillectomy at nineteen months and an acute exacerbation after the birth of a brother when she was two years old.

Linda had reacted to these traumatic events with feelings of abandonment and loss—feelings aggravated because the birth of the brother occurred during my summer vacation which had interrupted her play therapy of two months' duration. The repression of oral and anal sadistic impulses initiated earlier by the premature weaning and toilet training became more intensified now. The use of primitive defense mechanisms against a breakthrough of the repressed impulses, in particular, the mechanisms of externalization, projection, and displacement, led to the formation of phobic symptoms with a disturbance in the sense of reality and with a slight but definite paranoid taint.

The depressive and paranoid features and the disturbance in the sense of reality, which make the treatment of anorexia nervosa in adolescents more difficult and which cloud the prognosis, were clearly observable in Linda's case. If not for the referral for paroxysmal tachycardia, Linda's anorexia nervosa would certainly not have come to the attention of a child analyst. Her play therapy enabled her to bring to the fore and to resolve her repressions, as well as her oral greed and envy and the depressive and paranoid feelings associated with them. The concomitant treatment of the mother revealed that Linda's feelings, though distorted and exaggerated, were founded on reality, that is, on her mother's psychic reality. We found that the mother rejected Linda because of her sex and because of her personality. She considered her weak and a "cry baby." This rejection was based upon the mother's feelings about herself and about her own mother. She had repressed these feelings about herself and displaced them onto Linda. The essential, beneficial factor in the treatment of the mother, the change in the quality of her relationship with Linda was brought about by the mother's ability to come to terms with her own mother and to accept herself and her daughter as female.

The Psychoanalytic Treatment of Anorexia Nervosa. Karla (7)

Seven-year-old Karla, referred to me because of a severe eating disturbance which had not responded to medical treatment, displayed all the classical symptoms of anorexia nervosa, except amenorrhea. Since the onset of the anorexia nervosa a year ago, she had lost ten pounds, and in addition to a general refusal to eat, she had marked aversions to certain foods. She would frequently force herself to vomit after eating, and her attitude towards food and her mother had a paranoid quality. We found that the acute onset of the anorexia nervosa followed the birth of a brother when Karla was six years old. At that time she also developed a fear of cats and a suspicious attitude toward her mother. In her treatment, she expressed ideas that her mother was not giving her the right food, that she did not care for her, that she disliked girls, and that she was too preoccupied with the baby brother. As with Linda, the birth of the brother had been particularly traumatic for Karla because of the highly ambivalent relationship between Karla and her mother. The birth of the brother was experienced by Karla as a rejection by mother on various levels. Karla, who had been in competition with her mother for her father's attention, became more possessive and demanding of her father after the baby's birth.

Oral impregnation and anal birth fantasies dominated her fantasy life. Because Karla had also become very constipated, the mother was giving her frequent enemas. This was an added stimulation to her already strongly developed anality and became a factor in the distortion of her psychosexual development which remained bisexual with definite leanings toward a homosexual orientation. This manifested itself in her somewhat paranoid attitude toward her mother and in a cat phobia, as well as in hypercathexis of the anal zone. Karla's analysis provided an opportunity to study the oral, anal, and phallic roots of food symbolism and its role in her anorexia nervosa. She had strong cannibalistic impulses which had to be repressed, leading to an inhibition of biting and chewing. She had wishes to eat something "alive." These wishes expressed her fantasy of the baby getting into the mother's belly by being swallowed alive. These repressed impulses were, in part, externalized and projected onto cats as manifested in the cat phobia. Her coprophagic impulses played a part in her paranoid attitude towards food which at times she treated as if it were dangerous, like poison, which in her mind equaled feces, breast, penis, and baby. Karla worked well in her treatment which could be brought to a successful conclusion after one and a half years with a follow-up into late adolescence. The mother was able to avail herself of the guidance offered to her and credit for the success fo the treatment and the sustained therapeutic results should be given also to her understanding and cooperation.

Such an attitude towards food as displayed by Karla is so frequent in patients with anorexia nervosa that it deserves closer investigation. A few comments about some of the similarities and differences between food aversion and food phobias in anorexia nervosa and food idiosyncracies and other types of neurotic eating difficulties in children without anorexia nervosa seem to be indicated.

Neurotic Food Idiosyncracies other than in Anorexia Nervosa: Ted (7), Paul (8)

Such food idiosyncracies in children usually develop also in response to maternal attitudes; however, in these cases, we found that the attitudes of the mother relate more to her own feelings concerning certain foods which she passes on to the child. The usual complaint met with in these cases is that the child is very selective and limited in his choice of food. This refusal of food is not because of a need to starve oneself, although in some cases this selectivity may lead to undernourishment secondarily. Such food idiosyncracies occur with equal frequency in both sexes, while true anorexia nervosa is predominantly an affliction of females.

The case of seven-year-old Ted is a good illustration to show how such idiosyncracies can be determined by the mother's own food predilections. Ted did not eat red meat, liver, eggs, butter, most vegetables, especially those which had strong colors, or chocolate or anything that contained chocolate or fish or seafood or anything that smelled. While giving me the history, his mother said, "If you can get him to eat these things, you are a wizard, I can't eat them so I can't make him eat them." In this case, the mother was fully aware of her own idiosyncracies but not of their origin which related to her own unresolved anality nor of the part this had played in her handling of her son's anal phase development.

In some cases, the mother has an unconscious ambivalence about food and about feeding stemming from unresolved conflicts in her own childhood. This is frequently covered up by an overly indulging attitude and by offering a great variety of choices to the child. Such an attitude is confusing and the child senses the mother's ambivalence and responds with finicky eating. This situation can be corrected by making the mother aware of her ambivalence and its role in feeding her child. It has been my experience that once this was overcome, the child would eat any food which the mother prepared without objection.

In some cases, the mother may use food as a sadistic weapon against a particular child. Although this may not be apparent to others, the child invariably senses it and responds to it in his own way, not with anroexia nervosa nor even with food idiosyncracies, but usually with behavior and characterological difficulties. Such behavior and characterological problems were the cause for the referral of eight-year-old Paul. His mother told me that she was actually aware that she did not want her son to eat in the morning and that by rattling off a list of foods, she was confusing him, as if, "I was hitting him with my tongue." He finally would leave for school without breakfast. For dinner she would often prepare food she knew he did not like and would not eat. The ensuing arguments ended with Paul being sent to his room without dinner. Paul would take money from his mother's purse, stay away from school and make up stories. He also was a bedwetter and liked to make fires. In this case, it was necessary to work with the mother first to induce her not to discharge her resentment of her husband on her son and to help her to resolve her hate of men stemming from her relationship with her brother and father.

Neurotic eating disturbances in children other than anorexia nervosa often associated with other neurotic behavior are as frequent in boys as in girls, while true anorexia nervosa is restricted to girls. This point will be taken up more fully later in the discussion.

Food Phobias and Aversions in Anorexia Nervosa

Food phobias, frequently encountered in anorexia nervosa, usually make their appearance during the anal and phallic phases of development when the repression of oral and anal impulses takes place and symbol formation becomes operative and available to the child for the symbolic expression of pregenital and phallic impulses via food and anal excretion. The specific unconscious meanings of such food aversions can be established only by psychoanalytic investigation where the separation of the unconscious meaning of the food from the food itself can be accomplished. Pronounced food phobias and food aversions in anorexia nervosa are usually an indication of a coexisting strong anal fixation.

It is a well-known fact that patients with ulcerative colitis frequently also suffer from severe anorexia. This anorexia is usually considered to be a consequence of and a symptom secondary to the ulcerative colitis. While there can be no doubt that anorexia is a frequent secondary symptom in severe somatic illness, the similarities with true anorexia nervosa in the behavior towards food and in other aspects, such as amenorrhea and bouts of hyper-activity were so striking in the adolescent girls with ulcerative colitis, whom I treated, that it deserves closer investigation. Like anorexia nervosa, ulcerative colitis is a syndrome frequently afflicting adolescent girls, and the combination of the ulcerative colitis with anorexia nervosa in some of these cases presents special problems in clinical management and also raises the question of whether these are two different coexisting syndromes serving different pathological needs or whether they are interdependent and both fulfill similar needs through a disturbance of different organ systems and functions.

Usually by the time a patient with ulcerative colitis is referred for psychoanalytic treatment, the ulcerative colitis has been in existence already for a considerable period of time and anorexia and weight loss are readily accepted as symptoms belonging to the clinical picture of ulcerative colitis. Experience from the treatment of adolescent girls suffering from ulcerative colitis and severe anorexia have made me question the validity of this assumption and prompted me to investigate such cases with this view in mind.

A correct assessment of the dynamics and of the economic function of each of these two syndromes in the psychopathology of the patient is important both for adequate treatment and for prognosis. The presence of anorexia nervosa points to a predominance of oral fixation and to a disturbance in the mother-child relationship on this early oral level. Such a fixation may predispose the child to severe psychotic depressive reactions with disturbances in the sense of reality in situations of separation and object loss, real or imagined. This fixation also aggravates the prognosis while a predominantly anal fixation, especially to the second anal phase, makes for a better prognosis. I shall try to illustrate some of these points clinically with a case of ulcerative colitis and anorexia nervosa in an adolescent girl referred to me shortly after the onset of her ulcerative colitis. In this case these two syndromes and their different functions as well as their different genetic roots could be clearly distinguished. This patient had many food phobias and food aversions, and their symbolic meaning and dynamic functions in her anorexia nervosa could be studied and resolved in her analysis.

The Role of the Father-Daughter Relationship in Anorexia Nervosa: Paula (12)

The emphasis in this presentation so far has been on the role of the mother-child relationship in anorexia nervosa. A few remarks about the father-daughter relationship and the dynamic role it plays in this condition seem indicated. I had an opportunity to study these relationships directly in my therapeutic work with the parents of patients with anorexia nervosa in some of my own cases and in collaborative and supervisory work. I made the observation that frequently the onset of the anorexia nervosa symptoms was preceded or coincided with a change in the overt behavior of the patient towards her parents. In the analytic treatment, it was found that the change in the overt behavior reflected a change from a positive oedipal to a negative oedipal constellation in these patients. Instead of competing with mother for the attention of the father as before, these patients now exhibited a competitive rivalry with the father for the affection of the mother with a possessive-controlling, homosexual attitude toward her. This regression from the oedipal to the pre-oedipal (oral-anal) relationship with the mother was often associated with a negation of the genitals and of heterosexuality. The anorexia nervosa in these cases also serves to defeminize the girl and to make her unattractive to her father and to men.

This change in feelings and behavior, as well as the onset of the anorexia nervosa, often follows a disappointment and rejection by the father or an experience which the patient interprets as a rejection by the father. The case of Paula may serve as a brief illustration. At age twelve, Paula started a rigid diet which later developed into anorexia nervosa, following a remark of her father's which concerned her weight and her preference for fattening foods. She had interpreted this remark as a rejection of her developing femininity. Of course, this is only one factor in a chain of pathological developments and traumatic experiences which help to precipitate the manifest symptoms of anorexia nervosa in these girls. In the case of the patient just mentioned, it was found that she had correctly interpreted her father's remark. He had a decided preference for slim, boyish-looking women but even more importantly, as long as she was bodily still infantile, he could be close to her without guilt. I want to emphasize, though, that this was only one contributing factor among many which precipitated her anorexia nervosa. At that time, the patient was approaching adolescence and had acute conflicts about her femininity and growing up. These feelings were particularly intense because of her relationship with her mother and had been reinforced by a traumatic experience with an older boy. Paula had interpreted this experience as a warning against growing up and being female. She went into analysis at fifteen years of age and her analyst later referred her mother to me. He felt that Paula was not making sufficient progress because of her relationship with her mother. This assumption was fully confirmed in the analysis of the mother, which clearly revealed that the patient was taking her cues for the anorexia from her mother. To any improvement of Paula, the mother reacted with irritation, depression, and renewed attempts to retain control over her daughter. When Paula gained weight, the mother would starve herself, rationalizing that her husband wanted her to be thin. The analysis of the mother not only facilitated Paula's successful treatment, but prevented the complete breakdown of the whole family which had been held together by the anorexia nervosa of the patient.

Even where the father appears to be missing in the family constellation or his influence is devalued or denied by the patient, psychoanalytic investigation reveals such attitudes as defensive maneuvers against powerful positive oedipal strivings. I should like to focus on these and on some other aspects more closely and I have selected for this purpose some fragments from the analysis of an adolescent girl with anorexia nervosa and that of her mother.

Mother and daughter were treated for a brief period simultaneously and then intermittently for longer periods of time. This case is of interest for several reasons. Judging from the literature, few investigators have had the experience of concomitant or intermittent psychoanalytic treatment of such patients and their mothers. This method of treatment made it possible to study the dynamics in the behavior of the mother and the daughter and their mutual interaction and to follow the vicissitudes of the mother-daughter relationship in a case of anorexia nervosa during adolescence. Of interest also is the observation that indirect treatment, that is, modification of the attitudes of the mother, had a marked therapeutic effect upon the illness of the child even in adolescence. This case serves also as a good illustration of the point made before, namely, that even if the father seems to be insignificant or nearly missing in the family constellation, he, nevertheless, constitutes an important factor in the anorexia nervosa of his daughter.

The Psychoanalytic Treatment of an Adolescent Girl with Anorexia Nervosa and of Her Mother: Helen (15)

Helen was referred to me when she was fifteen years old, following a nine-month period of illness during which she had been hospitalized three times in different hospitals because of severe anorexia, vomiting and a low-grade fever for which no organic basis was found. In the hospital, her condition would improve but the cycle repeated itself as soon as she returned home. I saw her three times and I realized that she would not

accept treatment then because of her relationship with her
mother. The latter's overeagerness for Helen to start therapy
concealed opposing unconscious wishes, and it was to these that
Helen was reacting. I did not exert pressure upon Helen when
she indicated her unwillingness for therapy. We agreed that she
should return to school in spite of her mother's apprehension
and that she would contact me should she experience any
difficulty.

Without Helen's knowledge, I arranged with the mother for
psychoanalytic therapy for herself because this seemed the best
way in which to help Helen at that time and also, perhaps, to
render her more amenable to psychoanalytic treatment in the
future. The mother revealed very strong guilt feelings
regarding her daughter's illness. She had felt intuitively that
her child's condition was in some way related to her, although
she did not know how. She had expressed this feeling to the
attending physicians, and it was actually through the mother's
prompting that Helen was finally referred to me. She had been
very much aware of the fact that Helen had been able to eat and
that her condition improved whenever she was away from
home and that she vomited and stopped eating when she
returned. Helen was her only child and she had always given her
much attention and care. Until Helen was about thirteen, they
had been very close to one another. At that time, Helen had
begun to detach herself from her mother and become very close
to a girl friend. Upon her mother's instigations, she broke off
this friendship shortly before her fourteenth birthday. The
mother now blamed herself for having destroyed this relationship and connected this event with the onset of Helen's illness.
She tried to rationalize that the friend was not a good influence
on Helen but came to realize that she had actually resented the
friend for taking her daughter away from her.

Later, in Helen's analysis, it was found that in her attempts to
separate herself from her mother in early adolescence, she had
transferred her pathological relationship from mother to
friend, upon whom she became as dependent as she had been on
her mother. For some time preceding the onset of the acute
anorexia and vomiting, Helen's mother, who previously had
been overindulgent with Helen (reward for dependence), had

become very critical and disapproving of her (rejection for strivings for independence). During her analysis, the mother was able to understand that she had been unable to differentiate herself from Helen and to accept her as a separate being and an individual on her own. The relationship with Helen made up for an unsatisfactory marriage, and she could not bear to lose her to a girl friend or, even worse, to a boy friend. When Helen began to show interest in boys, her mother blamed the influence of Helen's girl friend for what she considered a premature interest. She managed to bring about the social isolation of her daughter who, instead of having a birthday party to which she had no one to invite, got sick on her fourteenth birthday.

Helen improved remarkably during the first few months of her mother's treatment. She lost her symptoms and gained twenty pounds, and her menses returned. I had arranged with the mother that Helen was not to be coaxed by her but should be permitted to take her food herself and to eat her lunches in school. Helen also had made up with her girlfriend and made a number of other friends at school. She spent very little time at home.

Helen came for psychoanalytic treatment at the age of sixteen and a half, after her mother, who had gained sufficient understanding of her relationship with her daughter had discontinued analysis. The precipitating event was a disappointment by a boy friend, to which Helen had reacted with somatic symptoms, developing a sore throat and persistent fever which resisted medication. Mononucleosis or any other infection or diagnosable cause for her condition had been ruled out. She accepted readily the suggestion of her doctor, who knew of her past history, to see me. She told me that she had been seeing a young man and that shortly before she became ill they had a quarrel. She had expected him to call her and for two days before she became sick, she had stayed home to guard the telephone, constantly expecting his call. Because they had had an argument, she was not certain that he wanted to see her again. It was on the second day of her anxious waiting that she fell ill.

Helen was able to understand and to overcome in her treatment her psychosomatic mode of reacting to disappointment, separation, and loss. She learned to tolerate consciously painful feelings without getting sick physically. In the course of her analysis, it was possible to explore in retrospect the deeper dynamics of her anorexia which now was a matter of the past. She told me that even as a child, she had been aware that her parents were not happily married and also that her mother was monopolizing her by excluding her father. Her mother had always belittled her father and portrayed him as inconsiderate and as interested only in sexual exploitation. She felt that her mother had a low opinion of men in general. The mother seemed to have conveyed to Helen a masochistic concept of the female role. Her father's attempts to get closer to her were experienced by Helen as seductive attempts which she both enjoyed and feared. Up to about fourteen years of age, she had been overweight and had masturbated excessively with only barely concealed incestuous rape fantasies. At that time, boys were beginning to make passes at her, and her father would frequently remark that she was now developing into a real woman. She was preoccupied with sexual fantasies and temptations and the close friendship with her girl friend served also to protect her from these heterosexual dangers. At the same time, it made it possible for her to continue in a more acceptable form with her friend the type of relationship she had had with her mother. She had been her mother's confidante and favored by her at the expense of her father.

Her menses had been irregular since her menarche at thirteen and a half. Shortly after her fourteenth birthday, she decided to stop masturbating and at the same time, put herself on a reducing diet and lost weight rapidly. She vomited when she transgressed her self-imposed dietary restrictions. She also developed amenorrhea. Her amenorrhea preceded the weight loss and lasted for exactly nine months. Analysis revealed that she had displaced her masturbatory conflicts and her pregnancy wishes and fears from the genital (overtly sexual) to the oral sphere. Instead of being preoccupied with sexual thoughts and temptations, she became preoccupied with controlling or rather "overcontrolling" her food intake. This is a mechanism so frequently found in patients with anorexia nervosa that it has to be considered as typical for such patients.

Another feature typical of patients with anorexia nervosa is the feeling of "either-or" which is particularly threatening to the patient in regard to sexuality. This tendency, too, Helen had displaced to the oral sphere. She had the feeling or rather the fear that unless she stopped certain dangerous urges or activities completely, she would be unable to control them at all and would be totally at their mercy. This latter tendency to lose control and to act out her impulses became more apparent after she had given up the anorexia. She made innumerable friends, superficially, spent little time at home, and let herself be picked up by strange boys, thus playing with the very danger she feared most. Also she had periods of overeating.

Helen could be diagnosed as a cyclothymic personality, with a tendency to alternating depressive and mild hypomanic states. In her psychosomatic pattern of response, the depressive aspects manifested themselves in the somatic symptoms— physical pain and forced inactivity—and the hypomanic aspects in her acting out behavior. In her anorexia nervosa, the depressive tendencies were expressed in the refusal to eat and to enjoy pleasure by cutting off of all sexual fantasies and activity and the hypomanic tendencies in the vomiting and general hyperactivity.

When Helen was nineteen and became engaged to be married, her mother had a recurrence of insomnia with depressive feelings. She returned for more treatment, this time with the knowledge of her daughter whose analysis had been successfully terminated (Sperling, 1970).

Further Remarks on the Father-Daughter Relationship in Girls with Anorexia Nervosa

Such an attitude on the part of the mother to portray the husband to her growing daughter as a sexual exploiter and the need to devalue him and men in general, I have found to be a prevalent feature among mothers of adolescent girls with anorexia nervosa. Particularly instructive is the following example: The mother of an anorexic adolescent girl complained incessantly about her husband's sexual demands upon her. Later, in her treatment, when she overcame her frigidity and her envy and resentment of men, she realized the distortion and exaggeration of her complaints. In fact, it was now she who seemed to have more sexual libido than her husband. She could now even acknowledge some of his positive qualities since he had become less of a threat to her. The daughter, who up to the time she developed anorexia nervosa had had a good relationship with her father, had stopped talking to him and even refused to be in the same room with him. At the time when both the mother and daughter had progressed in their respective analyses and the daughter no longer would run out of the room when her father entered, the mother had a significant dream. In this dream, her daughter came nude into the room where her father was waiting for her. The mother recognized herself the meaning of this dream as portraying the danger of letting her daughter and husband get together and as a warning not to relax her vigil and to keep them apart.

Some Comments on Anorexia Nervosa in Males

Like that of other investigators, my experience with male anorexic patients is limited. Of the three male patients I have analyzed, one had, in addition to the anorexia, ulcerative colitis and the other two had spastic colitis and hemorrhoids. All three were adolescent boys, none came for analysis because of the anorexia as the presenting symptom, although it was severe in each case. An unconscious identification with the mother was a prominent feature. This observation has been made also by other investigators (Falstein, 1956). In addition, in two of my patients an identification with an envied and hated sister was an important dynamic factor. It was my impression, however, that the feminine identification was primarily in defense against intense castration anxiety, stemming from an unresolved positive oedipal conflict manifesting hate and fear of the father. All three patients had marked bisexuality with feminine wishes and pregnancy fantasies which were symbolically expressed in the pregenital conversion and somatic symptoms from which these patients suffered (Sperling, 1957). The male patient, too, may use anorexia as a means of controlling sexual impulses and activities with displacement via food. There are certain qualities, however, characteristic for true anorexia nervosa in girls missing here. The refusal of food in the girl is also a declaration of independence from mother and often expresses a reversal of roles, especially in the power of controlling lives by feeding or eating. In the male, the anorexia made the patient actually more dependent on the mother or her substitutes and was used to get special food which equaled special attention and love from the mother. Also, the other cardinal symptom of true anorexia nervosa in girls, amenorrhea, is missing. The feminine wishes and identifications of the male patient are usually expressed, as mentioned before, in pregenital conversion symptoms of the lower gastro-intestinal tract in such various forms as colitis and hemorrhoids. This was the case with the three patients I have treated. Constipation may or may not be present. In my cases, there was both constipation and diarrhea as well as abdominal cramps, hemorrhoids, and rectal bleeding. All these were used for the symbolic expression of infantile feminine concepts and wishes, such as pregnancy, menstruation, and birth. Also, the girl with anorexia nervosa wants to be thin consciously. She does not want any roundness and is exhibiting her thinness. The males with anorexia which I have treated, were concerned about the thinness and were making conscious efforts to gain weight. In this connection the observations of Blitzer et al. (1961), and more recently, those by Taipale et al. (1972), are of particular interest. These authors consider anorexia nervosa in boys to be a more or less feminine way of reacting which occurs in boys with a particular predisposition.

13

Discussion

I have reported my case material in some detail primarily as the basis for convincingly developing my concepts and views on anorexia nervosa and for a critical evaluation of views held by other investigators in this field. There are few cases of anorexia nervosa patients reported in the literature who have been treated solely with psychoanalytic methods without the aid of hospitalization, medication, and the help of other medical specialists. Several of my patients had been hospitalized prior to analysis without deriving any benefits from the hospitalization or medical treatment. Surprisingly, in my critical review of the literature on anorexia nervosa, I found, particularly in the more recent literature, warnings against the application of psychoanalytic methods in the treatment of such patients. At the same time, the treatment and prognosis of anorexia nervosa is regarded with pessimism, and the therapeutic approaches in some centers and hospitals are short of barbaric.

Some of my patients have been studied by the method of simultaneous psychoanalytic treatment of mother and patient, and in some cases the mother was in psychoanalytic treatment with me while the patient was treated by a colleague in collaboration. These methods of treatment provided insight into the complex dynamics of the unconscious interaction between the mother and the patient and made it possible to understand some of the otherwise unexplainable, bizarre behavior of the patient. Having both partners of the pathological relationship in treatment was also an important factor in the therapeutic success.

The understanding of anorexia nervosa is still limited and there is controversy regarding classification. Some investigators consider it a psychosomatic disease, some a special type of psychosis, and others a neurosis in which obsessional compulsive features predominate.

Let us start the discussion with the issue of classification and see what psychoanalytic understanding can contribute to the solution of this problem as well as to the other problematic issues raised in the introduction. In psychosomatic disease, it is assumed that psychological factors, such as unconscious affects, conflicts, and fantasies, are using for their expression various organ systems whose functions and tissues are demonstrably affected and altered. In conversion hysteria, according to the classical concept, the function of the affected organ is altered (usually but not always it is inhibited), but there are no demonstrable tissue changes or damage. In anorexia nervosa, the organ and function affected in adolescent girls are the uterus and menstruation. There is an inhibition of menstruation but without demonstrable tissue changes in the uterus. The amenorrhea is a neurotic inhibition of a physiological function acting through the hypothalamic structure. Amenorrhea is a symptom observable also in other neurotic conditions of adolescent girls and females, especially those of the hysterical type. The weight loss and the bodily changes are sequelae of the starvation but not the amenorrhea. Amenorrhea also is an essential criterion in the diagnosis of anorexia nervosa and sometimes may even precede the onset of the anorexia nervosa itself. Another organ and function affected is the gastrointestinal tract and here too the function is usually inhibited and leads to constipation and preoccupation with the processes of evacuation. These patients frequently used vomiting and the refusal of food as a means of torturing the parents. In many instances, the vomiting although it appeared spontaneous was willfully induced psychologically or even manually. Some cases had another symptom, a feeling of coldness which disappeared during the analysis. Morton in 1689 noticed subnormal temperatures in these patients and Gull in 1888 suggested that the diagnosis of anorexia nervosa be based on a slow pulse and respiratory rate, slightly subnormal temperatures, and the absence of any internal thoracic or abdominal disease. He considered the emaciation the result of the chronic starvation. The fact that there are also psychological factors involved in the temperature regulation and in the subjective feeling of temperature has not been considered by any investigator thus far. That such factors do play a part in producing this feeling is well illustrated by Anita. After the birth of her brother when she was five years old, long before the onset of the anorexia nervosa at age fourteen, she began to feel "cold" and the house became a cold place to her. The cardinal symptom from which the term *Anorexia* is derived, however, is the refusal of food intake. There is actually no organ or function affected in this. The anorexic patient is fully capable of eating and does so under her own very special conditions. The refusal of food is not related to a disturbance of appetite. It is a conscious hunger-strike, the patient can turn on and off her hunger at will; it is a conscious rationing of food intake. Nausea and vomiting are used as means of regulating food intake. There are no observable changes in the physiological equipment of the patient serving the food intake nor any physical obstructions which would interfere with the swallowing and eating of food. In the anorexic patient, food intake is inhibited consciously by rationalization since the true reasons are unconscious and not known to the patient. This is typical neurotic behavior, similar for instance to that in phobia. The phobia patient for example is consciously avoiding phobic situations and objects by using a variety of rationalizations but is not conscious of the true reasons for this behavior. Unlike the patient with globus hystericus and fears of choking (Sperling, 1953), the patient with anorexia nervosa does not refuse food because of fear of choking on it. Some patients with anorexia nervosa may also have aversions to certain food items. This aversion relates to the symbolic meaning attributed to this food by the patient. Most patients with anorexia nervosa however avoid carbohydrates and "rich" foods even at times when they are not starving themselves. The emphasis is on thinness and appearance. Most anorexia nervosa patients have the ability to "cut off" that is to deny their hunger because to feel hungry entails not only the danger of eating but of over-eating. The latter actually occurs in those cases of anorexia nervosa in whom episodes of anorexia nervosa alternate with bulimia (Wulff, 1932; Berlin, 1951).

My investigations also revealed that a very important dynamic factor operative in the anorexic patient's behavior is a disturbance in object relationship. This disturbance in object relationship is significantly different in quality from that which I have observed and described in psychosomatic patients (Sperling, 1955b). In the psychosomatic patient the actual dependence on mother or her substitute is increased in reality by the patient's illness. In psychosomatic patients, to be sick and dependent on mother equals to be a good and obedient child who is rewarded by the special care and attention given to him during the illness by the mother (or her substitute). In the psychosomatic type of relationshp, the mother does not tolerate overt expressions of aggression or strivings of independence. Therefore the rebellion and aggression is not expressed overtly by these patients but is converted into somatic symptoms and discharged bodily without conscious awareness. In anorexia nervosa, the rebellion against mother and the attempts to establish independence from her are expressed more openly in the rejection of food, especially when prepared by mother, and in accusations such as that mother does not give the proper food or even that the food is bad or poisoned. Anorexia nervosa patients want to handle, prepare, and ration their food themselves. They prefer to eat alone instead of with the family, by this attitude expressing a rejection of mother. Anorexic patients are usually hyperactive even if they are emaciated and prefer to feed others rather than to be fed.

While anorexia nervosa is not a psychosomatic syndrome, it can occur in patients who also have psychosomatic symptoms. I found that in such a case the anorexia nervosa and other more manifestly neurotic behavior usually preceded the onset of the psychosomatic symptoms. It is my impression that the anorexia nervosa in these cases has the economic function of protecting the patient from developing psychosomatic symptoms and that the onset of the psychosomatic symptoms (in such a case) signifies a failure of this defensive function of the anorexia nervosa and indicates that a further regression in object relationship, namely to the psychosomatic type of reaction, has occurred.

I am in agreement with those (Palmer, 1939; Sours, 1969; Thomä, 1967) who consider anorexia nervosa a neurotic symptom complex. It can occur in a variety of pregenitally fixated character disorders such as borderline, depressive, obsessional, or hysterical types. I would like to draw attention to other dynamic factors, which although they may not be immediately identifiable are always present in the psychopathology of anorexia nervosa patients. One dynamic and genetic factor is the anorexic patient's relationship with her mother. Most generally this could be described as an unresolved, ambivalent relationship. I should like to elaborate on this because an unresolved ambivalent relationship with mother is a frequent finding in various character disorders and neurotic patients without anorexia nervosa. It is my impression that in anorexia nervosa the child has been conditioned very early to regard food as a means of controlling life. Peculiar attitudes toward food in the parents of anorexia nervosa patients have been generally noted. On closer observation, I found that the parent's feelings about food in many cases were very similar to those of the patient but manifested themselves in more subtle ways. There is usually great emphasis on food in general and more specifically upon the safety of food prepared by mother. Other food is regarded with suspicion. The dangers of overeating and eating wrong food are stressed, and the skipping of meals, especially after having eaten "too much" is recommended. Some of the mothers behave in a way that could be described best as "latent anorexic" and remain latent as long as the anorexia nervosa is carried out by another member of the family. A good example is one mother who at the time when her anorexic daughter began to eat, went on a diet and began to look like an anorexic herself. I should like to make clear that when I am talking here of "the mother," I am including the father and other members of the family too. In these cases the mother assumes the leadership and gives the cues as far as the food and eating is concerned. In the case just mentioned, when the anorexic daughter was beginning to eat again, the mother on several occasions did not prepare dinner for her as she had for the rest of the family, rationalizing that her daughter would not eat this particular food. The daughter rightly accused her mother of not wanting her to eat. Food for the anorexia nervosa patient becomes unconsciously equated with the life-controlling, omnipotent mother. Some investigators who consider anorexia nervosa in adolescent girls as the central syndrome of the anorexia nervosa group underestimate the seriousness of the psychopathology in those adolescents who develop anorexia nervosa. They maintain the attitude that these patients "outgrow" their disease. Unfortunately this is not the case in neurosis. What happens are changes in the manifest symptomatology, where the anorexia nervosa may be replaced by severe character and personality disorders. Dally (1969) believes that anorexia nervosa is but an "exaggerated" adolescence, not recognizing that it is the culmination of a specific pathological psychosexual development in certain girls starting with a specific pathological relationship with the mother in early childhood and that it can be promptly influenced or resolved only by psychological intervention.

There are some dynamic similarities between anorexia nervosa and addiction which are of interest here. In addiction the life-controlling mother is symbolically represented by the drug, food, alcohol, smoking, etc. However, in anorexia nervosa, the mechanisms of defense against dangerous impulses are different from those employed in addiction. In anorexia nervosa, the main mechanisms of defense are denial, repression, reversal of affect, reaction formation, overcompensation, displacement, and projection. These are mechanisms belonging mainly to compulsion neurosis which indicates a fairly advanced stage of ego and superego development. In addiction, the patient cannot resist incorporating the dangerous substances which symbolically represent the destructive mother and thereby harming or even destroying himself in the process. In addiction, the inhibition against incorporation, which operates in the anorexic's refusal of food intake, is lost. If therefore in a patient with anorexia nervosa, the anorexia, that is the tool by which the anorexic achieves control of food intake, is removed before a sufficient modification in the object relationship and in the personality structure of the patient has occurred, the defensive structure breaks down, and the patient may resort to dangerous acting out not only in the area of control over food intake, but in the area of impulse control in general.

This is a point to be kept in mind in the therapeutic management of such patients, especially when considering forced or other coercive procedures. A case in point is that of an adolescent girl whom I saw in consultation. Her anorexia had improved considerably after a few months of analysis but she had not yet achieved any significant changes in personality structure. At the time of an anticipated separation from her therapist for which she was not ready, she began to ingest large quantities of aspirin, resorted to wrist cutting, and had a psychotic episode. She thus dramatically demonstrated that to her giving up control over food intake had equaled loss of control in reality as expressed in her self-destructive irrational behavior.

This change from excessive control (exercised in the noneating) to loss of control (binges of overeating) can be seen in those cases in which episodes of anorexia nervosa and of bulimia alternate in the same patient (Sylvester, 1945; Wulff, 1932; Berlin, 1951; Dally, 1969). My material indicates that the strongest fear of a patient with anorexia nervosa is the fear of losing control altogether, that is, of gratifying impulses without restraint. This does not pertain only to eating but particularly to sexuality since these patients deal with their sexual impulses by displacement from the genital to the oral level.

Another important dynamic aspect of the anorexic patient's dealing with food is that it represents a reversal of the early childhood situation when mother was in control of food and thus of the patient's life. By assuming control over food intake herself, the patient puts herself in the place of the mother and assumes control over not only her own life but also that of her mother. Some of these patients like to feed, or rather overfeed, others especially their mothers, while not eating themselves. This makes the patient a better mother than her own mother. As with every neurotic behavior, the behavior of the anorexic patient is overdetermined and serves the gratification of various needs from various levels of development. This was particularly clear in the case of Anita whose starving herself also represented her way of killing her grandmother-mother (the hated female aspects in herself). To be able to go without food is also to prove that life is possible without mother. It proves the opposite if carried to the extreme. The patient's compromise is to reduce food intake to a minimum and in addition to renounce essential instinctual gratifications—the pleasures of eating, excreting, and sleeping properly (many of these patients suffer from disturbed sleep) and of a sex life. By doing this, the patient both rebels against and declares her independence from mother at the same time expiating her guilt for the hate and murderous impulses against her mother.

The patients with anorexia nervosa carry within themselves a deep rooted feeling of being rejected by mother which in part is due to a projection of their own hatred but in part, as the joint treatment studies of mother and patient have revealed, is founded on reality, at least on the psychic reality or unconscious feelings of the mother. These mothers are ambivalent towards this particular child whom they tend to identify with some rejected parts of their own personality. These mothers also suffer from unresolved infantile conflicts particularly in regard to their own sexual identities and their impulse control. Such feelings of the mother partly reinforce similar feelings and conflicts in the daughter who later may develop anorexia nervosa under certain precipitating conditions. One adolescent girl said that she "closed up her throat so she would not swallow her food." She would do this when food which she liked such as ice cream and cake were served. She knew that otherwise she could eat the whole cake and all the other food. Then with a burst of anger she cried, "My mother never wanted me to eat food I liked. She never wanted me to do things I wanted to do. She controlled my life." The pervasive feeling was "my mother never wanted me." Later in her analysis, we found that she had felt so rejected because of her female sex. In this case, the mother and grandmother lived together and dominated the father and the entire household.

Together with the struggle against eating in the anorexic, there is also a struggle against accepting the female role and a feminine identification. Because of the hate and murderous impulses against the mother, the female role and genital sexuality are dangerous and are shunned by the patient. I found that penis envy and the competition with men in these patients (Sperling, 1950f) is not so much prompted by the wish to please mother as a male as some investigators assumed (Masserman, 1941; Leonard, 1944) but that it resulted from the wish to be able to possess and to control mother sexually, as the father does. Father's sexual power and control over mother are attributed by the patient to his having a penis. In all other areas, the father and males are usually devalued by the family of such a patient. In the patient's mind, possession of a penis thus becomes the symbol for ultimate control over mother (Sperling, 1950f).

The dynamic factor which I consider *essential* in the genesis of anorexia nervosa in adolescent girls is the revival or persistence of an intense, positive oedipal conflict during puberty and adolescence. Puberty and adolescence, critical developmental stages, are also the preferred time of onset of anorexia nervosa. Unresolved oedipal conflicts are a frequent finding in a variety of neurotic patients and in character disorders with a variety of psychopathology. What makes the difference however is the specific way in which an individual patient deals with these conflicts. This in turn depends on the patient's early, acquired, premorbid dispositions involving specific fixations and object relationships. It is the ego and the superego which determine the choice of the mechanisms of defense, and both structures contain the incorporated parental attitudes towards instinctual demands.

From the psychoanalytic point of view, anorexia nervosa can be considered as a *specific pathological* outcome of unresolved oedipal conflicts in a female who by her preoedipal relationship with her mother is predisposed to this particular reaction under certain precipitating circumstances. Masserman (1941) and

Leonard (1944) stressed the role of the inverted oedipal conflict and of the anorexia nervosa as a defense against growing up and assuming the adult female role.

The unresolved preoedipal fixation to the mother contributes to the difficulties in psychosexual development and to the intensity of the oedipal conflict in these girls. These difficulties become particularly apparent during puberty and adolescence when the reliability of a proper sexual identification, of the ability to separate from love (need) objects, and of making peer and especially heterosexual relationships is tested. Anorexia nervosa is initiated by a regression from the genital to the oral level and is associated with a deemphasis of manifest sexuality and instinctual pleasures in general. In these girls sexual and masturbation conflicts are displaced from the genital to the mouth, and food and eating become equated with forbidden sexual objects and sexual activities. Depending on the degree of libidinization, the picture of the anorexia nervosa is either more hysterical, more obsessive, depressive, or psychotic.

The amenorrhea in anorexia nervosa is not a secondary symptom but is as primary as the restriction of food intake even though it may occur in some cases during the course of the illness. Thomä (1967), and others also believe that the amenorrhea in anorexia nervosa is not a primary endocrinological but a primary psychological disorder. Of interest in this connection are the following observations. During the last war, 60-70 percent of women capable of menstruation developed amenorrhea immediately after they were captured and interned in Hong Kong (Sydenham, 1946). This psychological amenorrhea was then reinforced secondarily by weight loss. In most cases amenorrhea precedes or occurs simultaneously with the anorexia. This symptom too is highly overdetermined. Amenorrhea on the one hand supports the patient's unconscious pregnancy fantasies and on the other hand serves to support the wish to regress to an infantile level before a definite sexual role is established (Berlin, 1951; Waller, 1942; Lorand, 1943; Sylvester, 1945.)

These dynamics could be observed particularly clearly in one of my cases who wanted to be a baby, a boy and to be pregnant as his sister and her mother had been, all at the same time. When she decided to be a girl (of her age) she started to eat and to menstruate.

Vaginal bleeding is unconsciously associated by these girls with internal injury, castration, and birth, all of which are dangerous and have to be avoided. Menses are also something that only girls have and anything that is manifestly an indication of femininity has to be avoided. One of the patient's aims in the pursuit of thinness is the avoidance of roundings such as breasts, buttocks or a protruding belly, all indicative of femininity. The constipation is as important a symptom to these patients as the amenorrhea. The constipation in anorexia nervosa patients is psychologically motivated and maintained. Some patients are more preoccupied and concerned with the constipation than with amenorrhea because on the infantile level impregnation, pregnancy, and birth are associated with the digestive systems and with excretory functions. That anorexia nervosa and the accompanying constipation are particularly well suited for the expression of infantile oral impregnation and birth fantasies has been noted long ago by various psychoanalytic investigators (Lorand, 1943; Masserman, 1941; Leonard, 1944; Sylvester, 1945).

In some patients with anorexia nervosa, the admixture of anality may show in overt obsessional compulsive, phobic, and paranoid features. In the latter case, paranoid feelings manifest themselves in the patients' attitude toward certain food which may become equated with poison and in their relationships with people. These features and their management have been dealt with in some of the relevant case presentations.

Summary and Conclusion

I should now like to examine what this study has contributed toward the answers to the question raised in the introduction.

1. It seems to me that we were able to clear up some of the problems surrounding classification. It is my suggestion that anorexia nervosa should be classified as a neurotic symptom complex which can occur in a variety of character disorders, ranging from borderline to hysterical. It is not a psychosomatic syndrome.

2. Should the term *anorexia nervosa* be restricted only to adolescent girls and only to females? Intensive psychoanalytic study of adolescent girls with anorexia nervosa and in some cases also of the mothers revealed that the conflicts in these patients are of a sexual nature centuring around sexual identifications and resistance to accepting the female sexual role. My investigations led me to consider anorexia nervosa in adolescent girls as a special outcome of intense unresolved oedipal conflicts. These conflicts were particularly intense and difficult to resolve because of the preoedipal fixations and the relationship with the mother. I would be inclined to reserve the term *anorexia nervosa* to this eating disorder in adolescent girls or at least its onset during adolescence. I would also be inclined to think that it is a syndrome typical to an anatomic female who refuses unconsciously to accept the female role. While as we have seen in these patients control over food intake came to represent impulse control, that is, self-control in general, this is not the primary dynamic. This need for control could be worked out in a variety of psychopathologies other than anorexia nervosa. Anorexia nervosa is a specific outcome of an unsuccessful attempt at solution of an unconscious sexual conflict concerning sexual identity.

3. In the male patient with anorexia, feminine tendencies and feminine identifications are a major dynamic in the anorexia. However, the situation in males is different; the nature of the oedipal conflict is different, and anatomically they do not possess female genitals and the capacity for procreation. Such unconscious wishes and fantasies do not necessarily need to be worked out through anorexia. In my opinion the anorexia in these cases is an indication of the pathological relationship with the mother and belongs more in the area of neurotic or even psychotic eating disturbances than in the category of true anorexia nervosa.

4. Does true anorexia nervosa occur in children? It seems to me that there are infantile forms of anorexia nervosa which should be differentiated from other eating disturbances which may appear to be similar. True anorexia nervosa even in children indicates the primary difficulty of the child to accept her femaleness. While the child unlike the adolescent or young adult does not have to make a decision about functioning

sexually as a female, the child indicates already at an early age during the oedipal phase, or even perhaps before, that she is unwilling to accept the female role with this particular behavior. This behavior is also an indication of the pathological relationship with mother and her conditioning in this direction. I should like to state here that it is not always necessary to find a manifest eating disturbance in childhood preceding the onset of anorexia nervosa in adolescence. As in any neurosis, the infantile neurosis may remain latent until a trauma in later life mobilizes it and revives it in a manifest form. This manifest form has been predetermined by the earlier relationship with mother and early experiences. This traumatic origin of anorexia nervosa is particularly relevant in adolescence which even without the addition of precipitating situations represents a traumatic situation for such a girl. Nor does any anorexia nervosa in a child have to continue or be revived in adolescence unless there are specific traumatic life situations at work. H. E. Richter (1965) considers prepuberty and childhood anorexia as forms of anorexia at this particular developmental level. The dialogue between child and mother as he postulates it for anorexia nervosa is already recognizable then.

5. There is considerable controversy concerning etiology with those who believe that anorexia nervosa is a psychosis or a deficiency and therefore hold to a constitutional etiology. This outlook of course affects also their attitude towards treatment. The early mother-child relationship in my opinion acts like an early acquired constitution in these cases. The emphasis on food and deemphasis of sexuality also play a part in determining the choice of symptoms.

6. The dynamics, as in every neurosis, are very complex. Nonanalytic investigators who do not work with the concept of overdetermination in illness and symptom formation and need to simplify everything, reduce everything preferably to one formula such as oral fantasies or aggression or pregnancy fantasies. Nonanalytic or antianalytic investigators also assess only the manifest behavior without considering the underlying unconscious motivations for this behavior, and they take verbalizations and rationalizations of the patient at face value. The fact for instance that the affect of depression is missing consciously is taken as an indication that there is no depression

operative in the patient (Crisp, 1969). These observers do not
realize that these patients do not feel capable of tolerating
consciously painful affects such as depression or feelings of
sexuality or even hunger because of fear that they would
succumb to these feelings and act them out in reality, by
becoming depressed, going insane, committing suicide, acting
out sexually, or becoming prostitutes (Goitein, 1942), or by
overeating and becoming fat and pregnant. In such a case, the
symptoms of anorexia have to be considered as depressive
equivalents (Sperling, 1959b) to protect the patient from
experiencing her true feelings.

7. Is there a specific type of anorexia nervosa personality and
if so what are the characteristics of such a personality? The
concept of specificity of personality and symptom choice did not
hold up. I found that patients with the alleged specific type of
personality for developing one specific symptom can develop
other symptoms in addition or substitution when the symptom
had been given up without resolving the underlying conflicts
and other important dynamic factors which are at work in the
production and maintenance of the symptoms. Certain
unconscious conflicts are universal but can in some individuals
assume pathological proportions. The specific mechanisms of
defense especially which an individual chooses or has at his
disposal to deal with these conflicts determine the symptomatology and choice of illness. An important factor has been
already stressed on many occasions, namely the role of the
mother-child relationship. As in the other syndromes with
anorexia nervosa, it occurs in families where there is great
emphasis on food. There may be more than one member of the
family afflicted by it, as in the case of twins. A sibling may
develop anorexia nervosa after one sibling has given it up, or in
some cases the mother may develop anorexia nervosa when the
daughter has given it up. This resembles other neurotic or
psychosomatic syndromes such as asthma, diarrhea, or ulcers
which run in families and are considered by some as familial
diseases. What happens in these cases is an overemphasis on
certain organs and organ functions by the parents which is
passed on to other members of the family and offspring. Such
overemphasis is transmitted through attitudes rather than

genes. As we have seen, anorexia nervosa can occur in a variety of character disorders some of which are close to psychosis, depression, or obsessional neurosis and hysteria. This leads us to another point.

8. Which are the factors which determine the severity and outcome of anorexia nervosa? One important factor is the level of fixation. The more orally fixated, the poorer the prognosis. The closer the phallic, that is hysterical, the better the prognosis. We are dealing here with patients with pregenitally fixated character disorders who have retained a high degree of narcissism and omnipotence which interferes with reality testing and the ability to cathect objects reliably.

9. Is anorexia nervosa a neurosis caused and maintained by psychological factors or is it an organic disease in which psychological factors are used secondarily or is it a combination? What is the most effective treatment? It was my intention to show that I consider anorexia nervosa a specific neurotic syndrome which occurs in females, especially during adolescence, who by their relationship with their mother and earlier experiences have been predisposed to such a reaction. It is an indication that these patients have not reached true genitality but have remained fixated at earlier levels of development and are therefore unable to establish proper sexual identification and heterosexual relationships. There is no specific anorexia nervosa personality, although these patients do show some common features. Depending on fixation and the degree of regression, the pregenital characteristics of narcissism, omnipotence, ambivalence, some degree of bisexuality, and a low frustration tolerance will be more or less evident. They are present to a pathological degree in all patients with anorexia nervosa. This also points the way to what would be the most effective treatment for such a patient.

10. A survey of the literature discloses that the treatment methods presently used and recommended are inadequate to say the least. The method which the psychoanalytic pioneers used some thirty and twenty years ago now seems to be in disrepute. Today as then such patients were not considered by some analysts to be suitable objects for psychoanalytic treatment. Since then our knowledge and our techniques have greatly improved, and as my work and that of other shows, the

psychoanalytic method has been successful. One has to realize though that the reconstruction of a character disorder is no easy task. It requires a particular skill and determination on the part of the analyst to establish and to maintain a workable, that is, uncontaminated transference. This can be achieved only by persistantly analyzing and frustrating the patient's need to turn the analyst into the mother, because in this way the analyst will be treated with the same ambivalence and distrust as the mother. It is only in the transference, that the patient can gain some insight and learn to separate the analyst and others from the mother. I do not have in mind here positive transference reactions or transference cure because these don't last. They are not based on analytic insight nor on changes in the ego structure of the patient and change rapidly with the patient's feelings. What I have seen in the literature described as achievements in treatment were in many instances only a shift of the patient's dependence to the therapist or to medication. Unless a modification of the relationship with the mother and some insight for the deeper motivation of the patient's behavior can be brought about, treatment even if it results in the patient's putting on weight and functioning better in some areas cannot be considered successful because the patient cannot make a realistic adjustment in her sexual and social relationships. The only change is in the manifest psychopathology and sometimes it is questionable whether the new is preferable. In the analytic treatment I have been conducting and recommending to others, we begin by analyzing superficial defenses and resistances, avoiding content interpretations, in particular of a sexual nature, until a reliable transference is fully established.

The physical separation of the patient from her parents, as I have tried to show, also misses the point, because the patient will always find someone with whom she can act out the mother transference.

Only psychoanalysis or psychoanalytically oriented therapy can bring about the personality changes and growth which enable the patient to cope with instinctual drives and conflicts in a more appropriate way than anorexia nervosa. Psychoanalytical treatment aims at enabling the patient to separate from the mother or mother substitute while those who recommend superficial psychotherapy or anaclitic treatment are in fact encouraging the patient to maintain the pathological tie to the mother by transfering it to the therapist.

PART 5

PSYCHOLOGIC DESENSITIZATION IN BRONCHIAL ASTHMA

14

Asthma in Children: An Evaluation of Concepts and Therapies

There has been increasing psychiatric interest in bronchial asthma of children during the last two decades. In this chapter, I am attempting to survey and bring together our present knowledge on this subject and to add some of my own views based upon twenty-five years of clinical experience with asthmatic children and their parents. The major advance in the medical treatment of bronchial asthma in children in the last decade has been the introduction of corticosteroids. Although these provide immediate symptomatic relief from asthma in many cases, the gains from long-term use of steroids in asthma are questionable. The phenomenon of steroid dependency in asthmatic children and the difficulties in withdrawal of the steroids as well as the undesirable side effects of prolonged steroid treatment, especially the retardation of growth and development in children, are well known. Less well known is that the increase in death rate is attributed to the use of steroids. Mueller (1961) states that since 1949 when steroid therapy was introduced, the death rate which had previously been rather constant has multiplied two to three times. Mueller cites three asthmatic children receiving steroids who died subsequent to an infection. He stated, "All were similar in that what seemed like a simple respiratory infection progressed to an overwhelming illness and, in spite of heroic medication with antibiotics, chemotherapy, and all manner of supportive treatment, they went rapidly into shock and died."

Clinicians with long experience in this field (Abramson, 1961a, 1961b, 1963; Peshkin, 1963) maintain that in every case of asthma, regardless of the established etiology (whether allergic or not) the psychological factors are of great importance in the course and proper treatment of this syndrome. Gerard (1946) demonstrated that asthmatic children with an established immunologic etiology, that is with a constitutional allergic sensitivity, have become and remained free of asthma after psychotherapy even when exposed to these allergens, although their constitutional sensitivity remained unchanged. In my own work extending over more than two decades I have been able to confirm Gerard's findings and the fact that asthmatic children develop a resistance to allergens in psychotherapy, although they remain sensitive to them on skin tests. This would indicate that the constitutional factor, even when present, is not the decisive factor, but that various factors (extrinsic and intrinsic) are operative in producing the complex syndrome of asthma.

Well known is the classical experiment by MacKenzie (1886) of the production of "rose asthma" by an artificial rose. In this connection the experiences reported by Long et al. (1958) are of interest. In one experiment, for example, a group of asthmatic children when in the hospital, removed from home, failed to respond to heavy exposure of house dust which had been incriminated in their asthma. This is also of interest concerning the nature of the therapeutic factors in removal of asthmatic children from home to hospital or residential treatment centers, particularly in view of the fact that separation from the home and especially from the mother is considered a major problem in children with asthma. The therapeutic separation of the child from his parents has been referred to as "parentectomy" by Peshkin (1963). He and Jessner et al. (1955) have dealt with this problem, to which I shall return later.

One of the phenomenon which comes up in connection with allergic sensitivity is the phenomenon of children "outgrowing" asthma. Lamont (1963), in dealing with the problem of predicting which children will or will not outgrow asthma, mentioned a case which is of particular interest here. On questioning a former patient, who had been seen ten years previously, about how and under what circumstances he had lost his asthma, Lamont obtained the following story, which was confirmed by the patient's mother. This boy had wanted a cat, to which he was demonstrably allergic, for a long time and the mother had refused. She finally gave in and let him have the cat. At first he would wheeze each time he patted the cat, but then he gradually stopped wheezing and never has had an asthmatic attack since. This raises the question of whether there could be such a phenomenon as self-desensitization.

In 1949, I reported fragments from the indirect treatment of an asthmatic child (see chapter 3). These observations seem to me to be most pertinent for the understanding of the phenomenon of self-desensitization. As soon as the mother of this asthmatic boy gained insight and could understand how through her behavior she had transmitted to her son the expectation of allergic reactions culminating in severe asthmatic attacks, previously forbidden foods and inhalants as well as physical exercises were gradually introduced with excellent results. Allergic reactions or asthmatic attacks which previously had required emergency treatment with prolonged bed rest and absence from school no longer occurred. All these changes took place within less then half a year and concomitant with the cessation of all medical treatment. This boy who had been demonstrably sensitive to animal hair could later own first a hamster and then a dog and was able to go horseback riding. Prior to his mother's and his own treatment, he would have severe wheezing culminating in asthmatic attacks when he came even close to a horsetrack or stable (see chapters 4 and 15).

The essential point I want to make here is the significance of the mother's permission or prohibition relating to the child's insinctual activities (oral, anal, phallic, and indeed the entire aggressive and sexual spheres) in sensitizing or desensitizing the child's reactions. In the child's mind these prohibitions become associated with his own fear and guilt for instincutal activities and may assume the role of taboos, the transgression of which is punished with the expected symptoms. I have dealt with this subject, especially as it relates to food taboos and food transgressions (1950, 1953, see also chapters 2, 3, and 4).

I should like to proceed now with the discussion of the two

factors that I consider most significant in the genesis of bronchial asthma in children: (1) the role of a specific mother-child relationship and (2) the role of the anal phase and of anal fixations.

The role of the mother-child relationship as a factor in the etiology of psychosomatic diseases in children has received considerable attention in the last twenty years. Most investigators have emphasized the factor of maternal rejection (Gerard, 1946; Miller and Baruch, 1948; Ribble, 1943; Spitz, 1951). My own investigations, particularly those conducted by the method of concomitant analysis of mother and child (1955c), revealed that the specific quality of this relationship, which I have termed the "psychosomatic type" of relationship, is that the child is rejected by his mother only when he is healthy and evidences strivings of independence but is in fact rewarded for being sick and helpless by the special care and attention given to him at such time.

The validity of the concept of the psychosomatic relationship is borne out in the therapeutic process, especially in the transitory phases when the child's rebellion and aggression come out in his manifest behavior. The mother's response, if not anticipated, can make treatment impossible. The work of Coolidge (1956), Jessner et al. (1955), Mohr et al. (1961), and Fries (1944) is of particular interest here. Coolidge (1956) refers to the asthma as a special form of communication between mother and child. Jessner et al. (1955) stress the conflict between wishes to fuse with and to separate from mother; and Mohr et al. (1963) are impressed with the use of the child's asthma in the service of intrafamilial tensions, stating that "the families of asthmatic children appear openly hostile until the asthmatic attack appears." Abramson (1961a) refers to the mothers of asthmatic children as "engulfing." I found that the child's illness is in compliance with the mother's unconscious wishes and her need for control over her child, who by his illness becomes manifestly dependent upon his mother. The child's aggression and rebellion against the controlling mother is not expressed overtly but is discharged together with other forbidden and dangerous impulses through the somatic symptoms (Sperling, 1950, 1955; see also chapters 3 and 15).

Acceptance and understanding of this concept will be most helpful in clinical work with asthmatic children. It will prepare the therapist for the changes in the manifest behavior of the child and for the fact that cessation of asthmatic attacks will be followed by such overt aggressive and often objectionable behavior as soiling episodes (even in older children), the use of dirty (toilet) language, and openly rebellious behavior. It is necessary during this phase of treatment to provide more appropriate physical outlets for the child's freed aggression and in particular to prepare the parents, and more specifically the mother, to accept these necessary transitory changes in the child's behavior.

The mother of an asthmatic boy of eleven, who during this phase of his treatment became openly rebellious against her, is a good illustration. This mother, who previously had been overindulgent and seductive with her son, now openly rejected him. She expressed conscious death wishes toward him to me, telling me that she wished he had asthma rather than behave toward her in this way. She now found him obnoxious and impossible to live with. She went through a phase of severe depression with strong suicidal impulses. The murderous impulses against her son were now turned against herself until, supported by the therapeutic relationship with me, she was able to relinquish this highly pathological relationship with her son. He had no recurrence of asthma during the four years I followed the case.

In the case of a twelve-year-old severely asthmatic, steroid-dependent boy, I had to treat his mother first for one and a half years before I felt that she could accept treatment for her child. I want to make it clear that when I speak of acceptance of treatment I am not refering to acceptance on a conscious level in reality. In fact this mother appeared very eager for treatment for her son. Before coming to me her son had been in therapy for a year, but his condition had worsened so that she had to attend to him day and night. They had become inseparable. She had explored the possibilities of residential treatment, but the mere mention of it provoked severe asthmatic attacks in her son, and her husband also was opposed to it. But it was really the mother, and this was brought out later in her treatment, who could not accept separation from her son. It was necessary to work first with the mother, especially on her own phobia which was so well covered up by her child's illness and dependence upon her. (I deal more fully with the interrelated dynamics of asthma and phobia in the next chapter.)

It is essential to work with such a mother during these phases of treatment of the child; otherwise the gains from treatment not only will be lost, but the child may become even more severely ill than before treatment due to the mother's resistance to treatment. In psychosomatic diseases of children the resistance of the mother comes out in an aggravation or exacerbation of the child's illness, which may necessitate hospitalization and withdrawal from treatment at a time when it is most needed (Sperling, 1959d). In a child with asthma, such a severe aggravation may even result in a fatality. In this connection, "The Death of an Asthmatic Child," reported by Schneer (1963), is of particular interest. I had an opportunity to discuss this case at the Asthma Symposium held at the State University of New York, Downstate Medical Center in 1961. This was a severely asthmatic, steroid-dependent child, who appeared to be very dependent upon her mother. During the treatment she had become quite aggressive with a release of oral- and anal-sadistic impulses. It was my impression that this mother was not prepared for the changes which were taking place in the child's behavior. The child died in an asthmatic attack the day before she and her mother were to resume treatment after vacation. In the case of severe asthma in a steroid-dependent child, my approach is to start with the treatment of the mother first, and only after an appreciable modification in the mother-child relationship has been achieved through this preparatory treatment of the mother should direct therapy of the child be attempted.

With older children it is preferable that mother and child be treated by different therapists who have a similar approach and who collaborate closely. In one such case when I had treated the mother first for one and a half years, the early phases of the boy's treatment, conducted by a colleague with whom I worked in close collaboration, were difficult for the son and the mother. This mother too found it more difficult to tolerate the self-assertive behavior of her son during the period when his aggression was being freed than she had during his asthmatic attacks. At one point, when the mother's marital problems, her ambivalent relationship with her husband, and her use of her son's illness as a means to keep the marriage together were dealt with, she became very resistant. Her resistance was reflected in an immediate aggravation of her son's asthma. In this case it was possible to analyze successfully the mother's resistances and to enable her to resolve her own neurotic problems which had profoundly affected her marital life and her son's health.

I would now turn to the role of the anal phase in the etiology of bronchial asthma in children. During the anal phase of development, which extends roughly from the end of the first to the third year of life, very important transformations take place. From a passive-dependent infant of the oral phase the child develops into the toddler of the anal phase with a turning outward of aggression and with strivings for self-assertion. It is during this phase that the conflict of clinging to and separation from mother is present in every child to some degree. During this time the child also has to acquire sphincter control and to learn to repress crude anal-erotic and anal-sadistic impulses. Conflicts arising between mother and child during this phase and the following phallic phase, in which sexual impulses are added to the struggle, can lead to various disturbances in early childhood. With a mother who because of her own personality is in need of the psychosomatic type of relationship with her child, the outward manifestations of aggression and self-assertion will have to be repressed severely by the child and the conflicts of clinging to and separating from the mother cannot be resolved. Jessner et al. (1955) have particularly emphasized these conflicts in asthmatic children. In fact, the onset of childhood asthma occurs most frequently between the ages of two to four. Abramson (1961a, 1963) believes that the closer the onset of the asthma is linked to the anal phase, the more intractable the asthma will prove to be later. Mohr et al. (1961) found that the change from infantile eczema to asthma in the children they studied also occurred at age two to three at the time when the assertive drives became manifest with a concomitant diminution of the need to be infantilized.

But why asthma in these children and not some other psychosomatic disorder? This brings up the problem of specificity and the role of inherited constitution. Are there psychological factors which determine the specificity of somatic symptoms or does this depend entirely on the somatic constitution? Allergic sensitivity is a definite constitutional factor in bronchial asthma. However, we find that, on the one hand, individuals without this constitutional allergic sensitivity can have asthma and that, on the other hand, individuals with constitutional allergic sensitivity who had asthma and have been successfully treated with psychotherapy will not develop asthma when exposed to these allergens, even though they retain their constitutional sensitivity (Gerard, 1946; M. Sperling, 1953; see also chapters 4 and 15). In this connection, studies of asthma in identical twins are of interest. Lieberman and Lipton (1963), reporting such a study, found that one twin, although he too had had an asthmatic attack in early childhood between age three and four, developed a manifest phobia later, while the other twin became a severe asthmatic. The authors related this development to the difference in the maternal attitude. Benjamin et al. report on identical twins in whom there was striking variation of both maternal attitudes and the severity of asthmatic symptoms (see Knapp, 1963). In my own twin study (see chapter 15), I found that, although both twins had asthma, it was of a different nature in each of them and the attitude of the mother toward them was also different. She wanted to have only one of them treated, the one whom she considered neurotic and by whom she felt dominated.

The fact that asthma or allergies are often present in other members of the family of the asthmatic child would seem to support the belief of a constitutional etiology. In some cases the mother of the asthmatic child either had been or, less frequently, may still be suffering from asthma. But here again, a psychological rather than a heredity mechanism must be considered, namely, the identification of the child with the asthmatic mother. In this connection the work of Coolidge (1956), Knapp (1963), and others (Dunbar, 1938) is of particular interest. Although in the cases reported by Coolidge (1956) mother, maternal grandmother and child suffered from asthma, his observations bear out the impact of the emotional attitudes of the mother upon her child and the transmission of these attitudes from mother to child through the generations.

This intricate dynamic interaction between mother and child can be observed best in the simultaneous analysis of mother and child. My studies revealed that the pathological effects of this interaction manifested themselves in a variety of disturbances in the children. The factor which I consider of utmost importance concerning specificity of symptom and choice of organ is the mother's unconscious morbid preoccupation with certain functions and organs of the child, often projected from herself onto the child. I have demonstrated this factor in operation in a variety of eating, sleeping, bowel and bladder disturbances of children (Sperling, 1950, 1955a, 1959, 1965, see also chapters 2-4 and 9). The mothers of asthmatic children have a morbid preoccupation with breathing and the respiratory system. Early and frequent respiratory infections are found to precede, to predispose, and to precipitate asthma. Here again the constitutional and the psychological factors seem to be intertwined, with an overvaluation of the physiological conditioning and an underestimation of the psychological factors. The frequent colds and respiratory infections of the child not only tend to increase the mother's preoccupation and anxiety but actually help to rationalize such a preoccupation.

The case of a five-year-old girl with intrinsic asthma, attributed to bacterial allergy and precipitated by respiratory infection, is of interest here. This child had been on steroids since the age of two and a half. The mother of this child reported that her observations made her feel that cause and effect in the asthmatic attacks of her child could be the reverse of what the attending allergist thought. When her child's asthma was controlled with steroids, she did not get respiratory infections. The mother knew that cortisone was not a deterrent to infection. When the child was not using steroids, she would wheeze and when it was bad enough to call the doctor he would diagnose the condition as infection. This observation, plus her child's increasingly difficult behavior, prompted her to seek psychiatric consultation.

Asthmatic children are usually overprotected and kept from physical activity and climatic exposure. One can observe that when the preoccupation and anxieties of the mother and of the child are dealt with and lessened, exposure to previously forbidden activities not only is well tolerated but has a very beneficial effect on the course of the asthma. Lamont (1963) in his paper "Which Children Outgrow Asthma and Which Do Not?" mentions a case followed up who reported that he lost his asthma when he started vigorous physical exercises in early adolescence.

The views of French and Alexander (1941) concerning the dynamics of asthma, namely, the "suppressed cry of fear and rage" as a specific dynamic factor in asthma, are well known. This concept is certainly valid, but it is only one factor in the complex dynamics of the syndrome of asthma. It would seem to me that the concern of a mother with the respiratory system and her anxiety over breathing, which the child senses, could make this system vulnerable from the start. A mother who herself has or had asthma will watch for it in her child. In this connection, the observations of Coolidge (1956) regarding the feelings of the mother preceding and shortly after the birth of the child who develops asthma are of interest concerning the role of early acquired psychological predisposition versus that of inherited organic constitution.

It is not possible to discuss within the framework of this chapter the psychoanalytic theories of symptom formation, but it should be stated that, as in conversion symptoms, the factor of somatic compliance is essential in the structure and dynamics of psychosomatic symptoms. The role of unconscious fantasies expressed in the specific symptoms of asthma can be explored only in careful psychoanalytic study. I am referring in this connection to the studies of Fenichel (1931, 1943, 1945) who dealt with fantasies of respiratory incorporation and the displacement from below upward (that is, from the anal to the respiratory system) to those of F. Deutsch (1939), Dunbar (1938), Knapp (1960), and to my own studies of bronchial asthma in children (see chapter 15). I regard bronchial asthma as a pregenital conversion neurosis. This is in full accordance with my findings in other psychosomatic disorders which I have studied psychoanalytically. On the basis of these investigations I was able to formulate the concept of pregenital conversion neurosis in psychosomatic diseases. It should be stated here that there is neither a specific asthma personality nor one type of asthma. Just as the clinical manifestations of asthma can range from mild and episodic to severe, chronic, intractable, and steroid-dependent asthma, so can the spectrum of the underlying psychiatric disorders extend from the neurotic to the borderline or even to the psychotic.

I want to draw attention to a phenomenon which I think is not sufficiently known or considered by many who work with bronchial asthma in children. The phenomenon to which I am referring here is that of reverse reciprocity between somatic and psychological symptoms in psychosomatic diseases. That is to say, the sicker the patient is somatically, the less apparent will be the underlying personality disturbance and vice versa (Fenichel, 1945a, 1945b; M. Sperling, 1955b; Wittkower, 1938; see also chapter 2). Kerman (1946) reported on two patients who had asthma before the onset of psychosis and again after shock treatment, when the manic-depressive psychosis disappeared.

With special reference to bronchial asthma in children, the disregard of this phenomenon and the consideration of the manifest attitudes of the parents and the child only lead to a misinterpretation of observable, clinical, and psychological test data. Purcell et al. (1961) divided asthmatic children admitted for residential treatment into two main groups: the rapidly remitting and the persistently steroid-dependent. The group labeled rapidly remitting consists of those children whose asthmatic symptomatology disappeared shortly after admission and who remained symptom-free without regular medication of any kind. The steroid-dependent group consists of children whose asthmatic symptomatology persisted after admission to a degree that required continued maintenance on corticosteroids for symptom control. These authors believe that among the rapidly remitting children asthma more often serves as a means of coping with conflict and anxiety. Asthma among steroid-dependent children, on the other hand, is viewed primarily as a response to genetic, infectious, and allergic rather than to psychogenic factors. Their hypothesis, however, does not preclude the possibility of a significant degree of psychopathology in the steroid-dependent children.

Baraff and Cunningham (1965) are impressed with the role of the father in the life of the asthmatic child and feel that the relationship with the mother had been overemphasized. Using psychological tests and the division into rapidly remitting and steroid-dependent children, they found that the fathers of the steroid-dependent children scored significantly higher on the healthy father scale than did the fathers of rapidly remitting children. From this they deduce that for the steroid-dependent children, asthma appears to be more dependent on physiological stimuli and that these children either have less psychopathology or that their psychological difficulties are unrelated to the particular symptoms of asthma. To come to such conclusions on the basis of psychological test data is not only fallacious but dangerous. In conformity with the phenomenon of reverse reciprocity between somatic and psychological manifestations, we would expect to find more overt neurotic symptoms in the rapidly remitting child and his family than in the severe asthmatic steroid-dependent child and his family. This would indicate, however, that the severe psycho-pathology in the case of the steroid-dependent, that is, more severely asthmatic child, is masked, while the somatic pathology is more in evidence.

This thesis also explains why symptomatic treatment of asthma can bring only temporary relief and does not alter the course of the illness. In order to treat asthma in a child effectively one has to take into consideration that the asthma is one aspect not only of a personality disorder of the child but also of a pathological family situation which needs to be changed before the child can give up the asthma. In this connection, "parentectomy" (Peshkin, 1963), that is, separation of the child from the parents, as a therapeutic approach in asthma of children, is of interest. In the light of the phenomenon of reverse reciprocity between somatic and psychological manifestations, we can readily understand why the rapidly remitting child will do well when removed from home. The more overtly neurotic child does not have the same kind of malignant relationship which the persistently steroid-dependent child has with his mother, one which resists any external measures and can be modified only in psychotherapeutic work with both the mother and her sick child. Therefore, the more overtly neurotic child will be able to make use of the opportunities for growth and for self-assertion offered in residential treatment, while the more overtly sick child, because of his specific dependence upon the mother, persists in clinging to her. In these cases the inhaler, the medication, and certain rituals become the symbols for the life-sustaining mother to which such a child will cling tenaciously (see chapter 15).

Although, according to Abramson (1963), "40 percent of children with intractable asthma who do not respond to any conventional treatment lose practically all their asthma within a short period after being temporarily separated from their parents," it does not seem to me that physical separation of the asthmatic child from his parents is the answer to the problem of treatment of asthma in children. We have to keep in mind, especially with younger children, that they have to return home and to remain with their parents for many years to come. For that reason alone some work with the parents needs to be done in order to provide a more suitable environment and more suitable parental figures for identification for the child. Even with older children (who can use the progressive instinctual forces available during puberty and adolescence and a more favorable reality which allows for more freedom and independence from, and even rebellion against, the parents) a modification of the parental attitude, especially by the mother, is necessary so that the child will use these forces not in a pathological but in a more healthy way.

It should be obvious by now that I do not regard the treatment of asthma as a simple matter. But then again even the rehabilitation of a neurosis requires expert handling and time. In a psychosomatic disease, such as asthma, the underlying personality disturbances and interrelated family dynamics are of a more severe pathological nature and one should anticipate and be prepared for the magnitude of the task. I am certainly not saying this in order to discourage doctors from treating asthmatic children. On the contrary, I rather hope that a fuller understanding and a more thorough approach by child psychiatrists to the problems involved in childhood asthma could be a stimulating and educational influence on pediatricians, allergists, and all those who see the child early enough to be able to spot the forerunners or earliest stages of asthma, when by proper management the full course of events could still be prevented.

15

A Psychoanalytic Study
of Bronchial Asthma
in Children

Of the early psychosomatic diseases in children, bronchial asthma is one which has attracted the attention of psychologists, psychiatrists and psychoanalysts. Separation anxiety as a precipitating factor has been stressed by most investigators. French and Alexander (1941) regard the conflict between the wish to cling and the impulse to separate from the mother as the basic conflict in asthma, but these authors, rightly, do not consider this as a specific conflict for asthma. Repression of crying from fear or rage is stressed as a significant dynamic factor. The factor of maternal rejection in bronchial asthma in children is emphasized by Gerard (1940) and others. Her studies showed that a constitutional factor of allergic sensitivity was present in these children but was of secondary importance. These children developed a resistance to allergens in treatment, although their allergic sensitivity had remained unchanged.

Maternal rejection plus allergic sensitivity plus inhibition of crying does not necessarily lead to bronchial asthma. In addition, it has been found, in the history of many asthmatic children, that they have been "crybabies," that they were allowed to cry, that they had temper tantrums and manifested aggressive behavior even during their asthma, and also that they had been indulged by their mothers. More recently, investigators focusing on the mother-child relationship in work with asthmatic children have been impressed not so much with maternal rejection as with the existence of a very close relationship between the mother and her asthmatic child. I am referring here particularly to Coolidge (1965), who speaks of asthma as a special type of communication between mother and child, and to the studies on preschool children by Mohr et al. (1961). No definite personality structure specific only for the asthmatic child has been established. The question then, as to why these children, under these circumstances, developed bronchial asthma rather than any other syndrome, remained.

The phenomenon of coexistence of different psychosomatic symptoms in the same child, for instance eczema and asthma, or diarrhea and asthma, or migraine and asthma, and others, and the phenomenon of alternation of different psychosomatic symptoms in the same child, for instance first eczema and then asthma or first asthma and then ulcerative colitis (own observation), or first mucous colitis and then asthma (own observation), or migraine alternating with asthma (own observation), as well as the phenomenon of alternation of asthma with overt neurotic, psychopathic, perverse, or even psychotic behavior should make it obvious that more complex and more specific factors would need to be identified in order to be considered as specific dynamics in bronchial asthma. Fenichel's suggestion (1945) that certain organ neuroses (he specifically mentioned stuttering and bronchial asthma) be differentiated from conversion hysteria as a special group of pregenital conversion neuroses gave the direction for my research.

In this chapter I shall attempt, on the basis of my clinical experience, to define more clearly some of the significant factors found to be operating in the genesis, dynamics, and treatment of certain types of asthma in children, and to compare my findings with those made by other investigators. My experience with asthma in children is derived from three approaches, which permitted me to study this syndrome from various aspects: (1) psychoanalytic treatment of four asthmatic children ages five to eleven, (2) psychoanalytic treatment of two asthmatic children, aged six and seven, and their mothers either concomitantly or with the mother treated first in preparation for treatment of the child (mother then was seen whenever necessary), (3) psychoanalytic treatment of the mother only of one asthmatic child, twelve years old, and one casual observation of the parents of a five-year-old child with asthma in statu nascendi.

In addition, I have treated, for briefer periods of time, four children with asthma and have supervised the treatment by others of four more children.

Psychoanalytic Treatment of the Child: Jim (10½)

Of the first group, ten-and-a-half-year-old Jim is of particular interest because he was an identical twin whose brother, Patrick, also had asthma. Jim had been referred to us, upon his mother's request, by the allergy clinic of the hospital where he had been a patient for the preceding five years, since his first hospitalization there. The referral note in his chart read: "There is an unhealthy family situation which mother feels is contributing to Jim's asthma."

My contact with his mother was limited to three occasions during his entire treatment, which lasted for two years. I saw her for the first interview and twice during critical situations in his treatment. She was seen once a week in casework in the beginning and later on only infrequently.

In my initial interview with the mother, I wondered why she was seeking treatment only for Jim and not for his brother. The mother felt that Jim's asthma was founded entirely on an emotional basis, and she wanted him treated so that he would not grow up to be a neurotic like her husband or herself. She had no such feelings concerning Patrick's asthma. In fact, she was convinced that his was entirely on a physical basis. She felt that, although the boys were identical twins, they had decidedly different personalities. Jim, according to his mother, was a very good boy who listened to her. He was well behaved and got along with other children. She thought that he responded with attacks of asthma to emotional situations arising in the home. Patrick, on the other hand, was an aggressive boy who liked to push the other children around, did not get along in school, and presented some behavior difficulties. These difficulties increased when there was friction in the home.

The mother had always showered Patrick with affection because he was the weaker of the two, and, although Jim now seemed to be weaker, she still felt that Patrick needed her affection more because, when she did not give it to him, he became very difficult to handle. She felt that Jim was keeping his worries to himself and that these were coming out in his asthma. "It's like my arthritis," she said. She considered her arthritis to be a reaction to her marital problems. The marriage was unsatisfactory; the father had left the family for short periods of time on several occasions. It seemed that the mother depended greatly for closeness and affection upon her two sons.

Patrick had developed asthma at the age of three, before Jim, who got it at about age four. Jim's asthmatic attacks had been more frequent and more severe than Patrick's, and, at the age of five, following his father's induction into the Armed Forces, he had such severe asthma that he had to be hospitalized, and his father returned home. As soon as his father arrived, Jim's asthma, which had not responded to medication, subsided.

The statement of the mother that the first three years after the birth of the twins were the happiest in her married life is of interest concerning the time of onset of asthma in Patrick and possibly also in Jim. Her husband had been very proud of the twins and affectionate to her for the first few years following their birth, but then he had resumed his former behavior. The onset of Jim's asthma pretty much coincided with his father's leaving home. At six, when Jim began school, his asthma became much worse.

It was found, very early in his treatment, that Jim was severely phobic and that there existed a close interrelation between his phobia and his asthma. He secretly kept close check on his mother's whereabouts at all times. He often interrupted playing or even the movies to run home with some excuse to look for his mother. Manifest phobic behavior, however, was not accepted readily either by Jim or his mother.

After Jim had been in treatment for several months, he had experienced considerable relief of his asthma. He was allergic to many foods, pollens, dust, and feathers (he slept on a special pillow), and he had been on a strict diet for the preceding five years. By this time, Jim had been taken off all medications, he was not on a diet, and he was coming to the sessions in any weather. In fact, on two occasions he had come in pouring rain, with signs of a cold, but he did not get sick. After leaving my office his cold cleared.

One day he came to his session wheezing pretty badly. He thought he knew why he was wheezing. He was to go on a trip with the Boy Scouts and to stay away for two nights. Although he was looking forward to this trip, he said, he felt apprehensive at the same time, especially when thinking of bedtime. But this time he was determined to go. (Several weeks before, he had had a succession of asthmatic attacks on a similar occasion and had stayed home.)

On this occasion, he told me that nights he would lie in bed thinking that life was too tough and that one has to die anyhow. Then he would start wheezing and coughing. He would sometimes have an attack even before falling asleep but mostly he would be awakened by one. His mother would then get up, come to his bed, attend to him, and give him medicine. His bedroom was not separated from his parents' bedroom by a door, but was actually an extension of their room. There was a deep-seated feeling that life was not worth living.

That these feelings and fears, as in a true phobia, related to a fear of his mother's dying, that is, to a conscious fear which covered up his unconscious death wishes toward her, was brought out in a nightmare: A bomb dropped over his school. Everybody was killed but him. He ran home. His mother was alive. In association to this dream, he revealed that he was continually worried aobut his mother's dying. That he had specific fantasies about the nature of the death was brought out in another nightmare: There was a fire in the neighborhood; a house was burning. He went home. He smelled gas. (They had had a lesson about deadly gases in school that day.) He knocked the windows in to look for his mother. On the whole block gas was escaping. He called for ambulances. Bodies were carried out. His entire family was unconscious from suffocation. On this occasion he told me that he was not particularly sensitive to smell, but that when his mother puts perfume on, he starts wheezing.

Jim had been to camp several times, but he always had reacted with an exacerbation of his asthma and had spent most of his time in the infirmary. Once he had to be sent home. He had been in treatment now for almost nine months, and camp time was approaching. The day his trunk left for camp, Jim had an asthmatic attack. The analysis had been dealing with his fantasy of magical control over life and death, and the fact that this control was expressed by breathing or not breathing. He told me that, often when he felt wheezing coming on, he would think of me and tell himself that I would take care of everything, and I had interpreted to him that he wanted to endow me with the magic that he attributed to his mother and himself and give me the responsibility for his life and breathing. I also had interpreted to him that no one, and certainly not I, could take the responsibility for his asthma, and that only he himself, could stop it if he wanted to.

It was during this phase of his treatment that I saw his mother for the second time in order to interpret to her that her anxiety and her anticipation that Jim would have asthma (as he had always had it) were like a signal for him to *have* asthma, and that he needed her nonverbal permission to leave her and to have a good time without her in camp. She had, on one occasion, said that Jim could not enjoy himself or have a good time without her anywhere.

Jim went to camp and for the first time had a very successful stay, without any incident of asthma and without taking medication, keeping a diet, or sleeping on special pillows. This was a very important experience because it proved to him that he was not at the mercy of his asthma and that he had some control over it and, therefore, responsibility for his illness.

A nightmare in which he dreamed that he had the worst teacher in the new school brought into the analysis his transference feeling and helped explain why his wheezing and asthmatic attacks occurred mainly on weekends. He had had this dream on a Friday night when, in reality, he should have felt relieved at not having to be in school. He mentioned that his mother liked to be away much of the time on weekends, and then casually also said that he did not see me on weekends. He had actually changed schools, and any change was very dangerous to him.

In the analytic situation, there was the particular danger of attaching himself to me. By this time, he had developed a very strong transference neurosis, which culminated in what Jim felt was his most severe asthmatic attack. Becasue this was also his final attack during his treatment, which extended for two years, and during a nine-year follow-up, the analysis of the circumstances leading to the attack will be dealt with more closely.

One Sunday morning, about one year after Jim's treatment started, his mother called me for the first time. She told me that Jim had had a very bad attack of asthma in the night and she had had to call the doctor. Jim received injections, but they did not help him very much. This attack had not quite subsided, but he was already developing another severe attack. She told me that Jim mentioned to her that he had had a very short session with me on Friday. This was also the first time that he had come alone from his session, and he had gotten lost on the way home. I suggested that she bring Jim to my office.

He didn't look well, and he was breathing very heavily. He told me that he hadn't felt well on Friday night. While in bed, he had begun to think of the session and how little time I had spent with him. He coughed and wheezed so badly that his mother had given him medication. He didn't have a good night and didn't feel well the next morning. He was wheezing and coughing badly and stayed in bed all day. He got up in the evening to watch TV, when he suddenly broke out in perspiration and felt nauseous. He vomited. He couldn't catch his breath for quite some time, and everybody was very frightened. The doctor came and gave him an injection and medication. He fell into slumber. He awoke in the middle of the night with a terrible fear that he couldn't breathe and remained awake for some time with the vaporizer. He couldn't get up in the morning, and his mother gave him medication, but, in spite of it, he felt increasingly worse.

Jim knew that this attack had something to do with his feelings about the session on Friday. He told me that he had felt very unhappy on the way home when he had taken the wrong train and had gotten lost. He had been forced to call his mother, who gave him directions how to get home, and he had thought that it had not been worth the trouble of coming for the session. He then remembered that we had talked on Friday about the meaning of his attacks as a method of killing himself by stopping breathing. I interpreted to him his disappointment in me and the fact that he felt he was better off by staying attached to his mother and not making any changes. He said that he had thought I was not interested in him, since I had given him so little time on Friday. To my interpretation that in this attack he was killing me in himself, he said with a broad smile, "This attack was killing more than two people."

This episode is typical of a negative transference reaction occurring during treatment of psychosomatic patients. Jim was afraid to attach himself to me because I was not willing to take the role of the omnipotent mother but expected him to control himself (that it, his asthma).

The second year of his analysis, after the cessation of the asthma proper, was characterized by an increase in dreaming and fantasy material. Jim remembered having had frequent nightmares up to the age of five, the time when his asthma developed fully. He also had suffered from a fear of the dark, and he had had sensations that somebody was grabbing him from behind. He still had this fear. He used to awaken very early in the morning, but he was afraid to get out of bed to go to the bathroom and would wait for his brother to waken so that they could go together. He had not had any nightmares during the five years before he came into analysis.

Correspondingly, with the improvement of his asthma, he developed (or rather had a recurrence of) a sleep disturbance, with frequent nightmares. During his treatment the character of his dreams underwent considerable change, as did his manifest behavior. In most of his dreams, now, he was the aggressor, riding the most beautiful horse, being the best shot. Rivalry with his brother and father now came into the analysis. He was jealous of his brother who, "by two stinky minutes," was the older one and acted like a big shot. He expressed fantasies of killing Patrick. The best thing, Jim said, would be to poison him. He remembered, when he was about four years old, once asking his father for poison for Patrick. He now fought with his brother, and a few days previously he had torn a ligament on his hand when hitting him. We were discussing the connection between temper tantrums and asthmatic attacks, and Jim said that he had always been aware of this and that he would try to tell himself to control his temper. While talking about it, he complained about his hand hurting him. It was the hand on which he had torn the ligament. He smiled when I explained to him that he could not allow himself to hit his brother without hurting himself even more.

He showed apology for his father's behavior by telling me that his father's parents were separated and that his father had had no upbringing. For the first time, Jim talked about the arguments between his parents and said that his father liked to embarrass his mother.

A series of dreams in which men were attacking each other from the back brought into the analysis the homosexual strivings directed toward the father and the brother. These were prominent in the analysis and covered up his very intense, unresolved, positive Oedipus complex. The onset of his asthma during the oedipal phase and the aggravation of it when the father left would seem to be related to his oedipal conflict. He apparently sensed his mother's need for a close relationship with him to substitute for the unreliable father. This increased the intensity of the conflict and the guilt feeling for his father's leaving (his disappearance) which, to Jim, meant that he had killed his father. Jim's asthma subsided when the father returned. Of interest in this connection is an observation reported by the mother: "The farther his father was shipped, the worse Jim's asthma became." His destructive (murderous and suicidal) and forbidden sexual impulses were discharged in the paroxysms of the asthma which, at the same time (through breathing or not breathing), gave him magical control over life and death.

It was also of interest that, as Jim improved, his brother had more frequent asthmatic attacks and became more difficult in general. Gradually, their relationship changed, with Jim becoming the leader. When Jim's treatment terminated he was thirteen and, by this time, had a genuinely positive relationship with his brother, whom he helped in many ways. Patrick continued to have episodic, nonseasonal asthma and experienced increasing difficulties in his scholastic and social performance.

Patrick consulted me, upon Jim's suggestion, during his late adolescence. It was obvious that an unconscious homosexual conflict was a major factor in his difficulties. Some time after I had referred Patrick for treatment, Jim asked to see me. He wanted to know whether he should have further treatment. Obviously, the fact that his brother was now being treated presented a threat to him. Since he did not feel any urgency about it, and since treatment, from a realistic point of view, was not feasible, he decided to wait and to contact me if there should be any urgency.

Psychoanalytic Treatment of Both Mother and Child: John (6)

When his mother began analysis, John was six years old. He had chronic, perennial asthma and many allergies to foods and inhalants. He was on a restricted diet and received medications, but there was little improvement in his asthma. In addition, he was a behavior problem.

The mother had reacted to John's birth with depression. She had found it difficult to care for him; he was a feeding problem and had many colds. She was concerned about his colds, as she had suffered

from colds herself as a child and had had pneumonia from which she
almost died.

John had a tonsillectomy, his mother said, when he was two and a
half years old, and , following this, he developed spells in which he
behaved as if he were dazed. Shortly thereafter he had his first attack
of bronchial asthma.

In the analysis of John's mother, it was found that she unconsciously
identified John with her younger brother, who she felt had displaced
her in her mother's affections. The unresolved rivalry and death
wishes against this brother were unconsciously displaced on John. His
mother had unconscious impulses to choke him, and she would
sometimes grab him and hold him very tightly as if "to squeeze the
breath out of him." At the same time, she also identified herself with
John. She had wanted John to be a girl, and she gave him a girl's name
which she changed only in the second year of her analysis.

John's mother had a very strong unresolved dependency upon her
own mother and still felt that not only her health but actually her life
hinged upon the mother's care of her. She had always felt that she
could get her mother's care only when she was sick.

It was found that John's mother was unconsciously reenacting with
John her relationship with her own mother, playing both parts—that
of the omnipotent mother and, through John, that of the helpless child
who could not live without its mother. It was a fascinating experience
to observe how this rapport between mother and child operated—the
sensitivity with which John perceived and responded to his mother's
needs for him to be sick. Episodes from this phase of the analysis of
John's mother have been reported elsewhere. (M. Sperling, 1949; and
see also chapter 3).

With increasing insight, John's mother was able to recognize and to
control some of the ways in which she signaled her needs to him. She
also abandoned the diet and medication for John. There was a
remarkable improvement in his asthma after the first year of his
mother's analysis.

With the asthmatic attacks decreasing and his general health
improving (he had, prior to his mother's analysis, had only fifty days'
attendance in a school year), the psychopathology underlying John's
asthma became more apparent. The father, who did not accept the
psychosomatic nature of the asthma, nevertheless agreed to have John
treated by me, because of the problems he presented. John behaved in

a very infantile way; he made a nuisance of himself in school, he did not play with other children, and, in spite of his superior endowments, he did not learn. An attempt to have John sleep away from home one night had ended in John's having such severe asthma that his parents had to call for him during the night.

John was seven years old when he began his analysis. It was found that he had a fantasy of having been dead and brought to life again. The origin of this fantasy could be traced back to the tonsillectomy and his reaction to the experience of anesthesia. He was very distrustful of women. He had a fantasy that women wanted to murder boys, specifically him. This fantasy, too, related to the tonsillectomy, which he had interpreted as an attack upon him: the mother getting the doctor (representing his father) to kill him.

Of particular interest, in this connection, was his mother's reaction to his spells which followed the tonsillectomy. She had given him a kind of shock treatment by trying to slap him out of it, or by pouring cold water over his head. She had recognized the withdrawal quality of these attacks and had felt very much threatened by it. She herself had a strong tendency to withdraw from reality. She had difficulty getting up in the morning. She had a waking-up ritual and often, for example before preparing a meal, became so fatigued that she needed hours "to sleep it off." Her migraine headaches also necessitated her withdrawal into bed in a darkened room for hours or days.

It was found that John, unlike his mother who had libidinized sleep, was afraid to sleep because of the close identification in his mind of sleep and death. When John had asthma, his mother was very attentive. She came to his bed and stayed with him and gave him the inhaler and medication, which meant, to him, that she permitted him to breathe, that is, to live.

An important observation in their analyses concerned the phenomenon of corresponding fantasies in John and his mother. (This was noted in a later phase of John's analysis, when he was able to tolerate anxiety consciously and had hardly any nocturnal asthmatic attacks.) They had, in common, a marked intolerance to anxiety. John's mother could not accept any overt display of it in him, because this represented a threat to her own precarious balance. Anxiety attacks would have caused the mother to withdraw from John, whereas the asthma, and especially the frequent nocturnal attacks, brought her closer to him. When he developed, instead, a sleep disturbance with nightmares, they frequently centered around snakes coming into his room. He had a fantasy about a snake winding around his body and constricting his chest.

In the analysis of the mother, it was found that she also was preoccupied with fantasies about snakes. In fact, she had a fantasy in which she was a snake. During one phase of the analysis, this fantasy assumed a hallucinatory quality. With signs of anxiety, she complained about the strange feeling. She believed that her whole body contracted and stiffened. "I have the feeling I am a snake," she told me (1950b). In this connection the mother's habit of grabbing John and squeezing him tightly, "as if to squeeze the breath out of him," is significant also.

John had been found allergic to animal hair; in fact, his asthmatic attacks in school had been attributed to the presence of a hamster. In the course of the analysis, John became the proud owner of a dog. An episode reflecting his father's attitude about the dog and John's asthma is reported in chapter 4.

John would have liked to go horseback riding, but if he merely came near a horse track he began to wheeze and get asthma. After John realized that he was afraid of horses and after we had analyzed the unconscious meaning of the horse as the father who would bite him, that is, castrate him (an anxiety similar to that of Little Hans (Freud 1909) but expressed by John somatically), John, to his father's surprise, went horseback riding and had no allergic reaction

Two other phenomena which I observed in his analysis are important. One occurred in the early part and the other toward the end of his treatment. In the early phases of his analysis, John began to soil himself. He came home with a bowel movement in his pants or soiled himself in situations in which, before, he would have had an asthmatic attack. This soiling was clearly an anal-sadistic attack, which was later replaced by the use of anal and other forbidden (obscene) words. He also, on occasion, urinated on the toilet seat or the bathroom floor. He knew that this angered his mother. When she scolded him, he said: "This is why I get asthma, when you yell at me."

On a few occasions at a later phase in the analysis, when he began to assert himself and dared to argue with his father, he ran out of the house in the evening and stayed away for several hours, walking in the streets alone. Although this was not adequate behavior, it was a more appropriate way of trying to separate himself from the frustrating parents than was the asthma or the soiling.

John's analysis was terminated when he was nine years old, mainly upon his father's wish, who felt that John had improved sufficiently. His analysis was incomplete. It was my impression that there were in John, as had been found in his mother, latent psychotic elements with some disturbance in the sense of reality and of object relationships, which would have required much longer analysis. I maintained contact with the family up to the time when John was sixteen. He had stayed free of asthma and had been doing well. I learned that John went into treatment at nineteen, upon his own wish, with the presenting symptom of insomnia.

Psychoanalytic Treatment of the Mother Only: Hans (12)

This approach is of interest particularly from the standpoint of the effect, upon the asthmatic child, of the modification of maternal attitudes only. (Actually, John, during the first year of his mother's analysis, could be considered as such as case.)

The mother of twelve-year-old Hans came for analysis because of depression and marital difficulties. In the course of her analysis, it was found that she suffered from periodic skin rashes and angiovascular edema. For this and her allergies, she was under the care of an allergist. On this occasion I learned that Hans had suffered from hay fever and asthma since the age of five and was being treated by the same allergist. Neither the mother nor the allergist had ever made any connection between her emotional state and her allergic manifestations. As this connection began to unfold in her analysis, she gradually could give up her diet, the medications, and the treatment by her allergist. Experiencing a heretofore unknown freedom from her allergic symptoms, she began to wonder about her son's asthma. She felt that she had a very good relationship with him. He was very affectionate and attentive. In fact, very often Hans and not her husband would notice her hairdo, her dress, and so on, and comment upon it. He always wanted to be near her, wanted to know where she was going and when she would be home, and, after school, preferred to be with her rather than with other boys.

As the mother's analysis progressed and she became aware of her sexual fears, which had interfered with her relationship to her husband, she began to view her relationship with Hans differently. She realized that she was using him as a (sexually) less dangerous and more eašily controllable substitute for her husband. She also became aware that she, herself, was phobic and actually needed Hans around because she was afraid to be alone in the house.

During the second year of his mother's analysis, Hans decided that he, too, did not need injections and medicine, and he stopped his treatment with the allergist. Although the mother did not oppose this, she was anxious because it was spring and the time when he would get his desensitization to be prepared for the summer and camp. The previous summer Hans had suffered considerably from his hay fever and asthma, although he had been under treatment.

Hans was obviously undergoing some changes. He made more friends and even stayed with them overnight on week-ends. He had had far fewer colds and hardly any wheezing. My patient felt that her husband was changing too. Their relationship was greatly improved, sexually and otherwise.

The incident which is really the primary reason for reporting this case occurred during the summer when I was on vacation and Hans was in camp. One night the camp director called to say that Hans had had an asthmatic attack and that he had refused to let the camp doctor give him an injection. The doctor needed the parents' consent. The mother spoke to Hans and left the decision up to him, indicating that she had confidence in his ability to control his asthma. The asthma promptly subsided without any medical aid. From the standpoint of the mother, we could understand, through ananlysis, the meaning of her behavior. By leaving the decision up to Hans she had, in effect, told him that she was willing to set him free, that she thought he could manage without her, and that it was now up to him.

As far as Hans is concerned, we are left to conjecture, because we really do not know what this meant to him. I can, therefore, report only the facts. Hans is fifteen now, and his mother is still in analysis. Hans had been completely symptom free during the past three years. He went back to camp once more, without any incident and with much more active participation in camp activities. The year following this he declared that he was not going to camp and that he wanted to spend one summer at home. My patient seemed very concerned about this and continually made suggestions to Hans about trips he should take or about going to another camp. She feared that his staying home would interfere with her freedom. My suggestion that she let Hans make his own plans and that she analyze her anxiety was followed by a surprise. Hans changed his mind and signed up with a friend for another camp. Later in her analysis, we found out that the mother had anticipated being saddled with an undesired visitor for the entire summer and that she had unconsciously wished that it would be Hans, instead, who would stay with her.

Whether Hans' decision to stay home that summer was in response to his mother's unconscious wish could not be determined. In cases where I had the opportunity to treat mother and child in concurrent analyses, I could observe in minute nuances the effects and changes of the interplay of the mother's unconscious wishes and the child's unconscious responses (M. Sperling, 1950a, 1959d). On the basis of my experience, I would be inclined to think that a similar rapport operated between Hans and his mother.

There are some similarities between this case and that of Jim, particularly in the mother-child relationship. Without analysis of the child, this is about all we can say. What seemed of interest to me is the fact that a chronic asthmatic condition in a twelve-year-old boy could be decidedly influenced through the analysis of his mother.

Although the improvement in this boy's asthmatic condition was accompanied also by favorable changes in his total personality and actual functioning, I consider that the direct treatment of a child of this age is essential for lasting results and certainly for a cure. Unless the unconscious fantasies underlying the asthma are exposed and devaluated through analysis of the oedipal conflict and the preceding preoedipal relationships are at least partially analyzed and changed, there can be no basic change in the personality which uses the syndrome of asthma, or another somatic syndrome, to deal with these conflicts.

The case of a five-year-old girl with asthma in statu nascendi, where only the parents were seen in consultation, seems of interest because of the very favorable effect upon the child's further development. Patricia's parents consulted me because they feared that she was developing asthma. Since age four she had had a stuffed nose and difficulty in breathing, and now she was beginning to wheeze on occasions.

The mother told me that Patricia was preoccupied with death. She had repeatedly said that she wouldn't want to die. She asked her mother if she would die and said that she wanted to marry her father. She wanted to sleep with him and have a baby. The mother had explained to her about babies when a neighbor had been pregnant and had given birth. One day, when Patricia was sucking on a carrot, the mother became anxious and told her to stop. Patricia asked, "So what could happen? I could choke."

When father administered nose drops, he tickled Patricia with his nose. The parents were in the habit of walking in the nude, and the father took showers with Patricia. When she asked him whether she could marry him, he teasingly told her to ask him when she was older, that he couldn't tell her then. The parents dated the onset of the breathing difficulty to an incident that had occurred when Patricia was four and at the zoo, where she had been bitten by a monkey.

It was quite obvious that the child lived in a highly sexually overstimulating atmosphere and was caught in an intense oedipal conflict. The father, in particular, was quite actively seductive with her. The mother definitely appeared to be jealous of the child's relationship with the father. Whether this had been the father's intention, I could not determine. She seemed to react to Patricia's openly expressed oedipal wishes with anxiety and, as I suspected, with retaliatory death wishes against the child. She was manifestly anxious about Patricia's breathing and had expressed anxiety that Patricia might choke. Since treatment of the child was not feasible and both parents had had psychoanalytic treatment themselves, I explained the situation to the father with particualr emphasis upon the connection between the child's breathing difficulty and the sexual overstimulation and to the mother with the emphasis upon her own anxieties. According to the parents, who have remained in touch with me, Patricia has been doing very well during the past three years.

Separation anxiety as a dynamic factor in asthma has been stressed, particularly by French and Alexander (1941). I wish to emphasize even more the close similarity in the personality structure of the phobic person and that of the patient with asthma. We know that, in a phobia, the phobic clinging to mother or her substitute has the meaning of counteracting the unconscious death wish toward her (M. Sperling, 1961a). In the asthmatic attack this conflict is acted out somatically through the respiratory system as a conflict over breathing: to breathe or not to breathe has the meaning to live or to die, to let live or to kill. The unconscious meaning of the asthmatic attack is revealed as a form of magical control over the life and death of the ambivalenty loved object and of the patient himself.

I should like to start my discussion of the factors which I consider significant in the genesis, dynamics, and treatment of asthma with the case of Jim. His mother obviously sensed his attachment to her and encouraged it as long as it was not overtly phobic. The oedipal phase had been particularly traumatic for him. Asthma set in when the conflicting feelings of oedipal love and hate for the mother reached a climax and the intensity of the unconscious death wishes against the mother urged for immediate fulfillment. For a short time, Jim alternated between sleep disturbance and asthma, but the course of the development into an asthmatic was the most probable under his particular circumstances. We shall follow these circumstances more closely. It was a time of severe marital friction. Jim's father left the family after a fight with the mother, and subsequently was inducted into the Army. To Jim, this was a confirmation of the magical effect of his unconscious death wishes against his father (positive oedipal conflict). He had particularly severe asthma then, which necessitated hospitalization and which subsided with his father's return. The sleep disturbance with nightmares preceding the onset of the asthma was an indication of the severity of the oedipal conflict, as well as of the specific source for this intensification, namely sexual overstimulation. He had a recurrence of the sleep disturbance with nightmares preceding and during the resolution of his asthma.

I have made similar findings in the analyses of other asthmatic patients, and I am inclined to consider this a typical occurrence. These findings would indicate that there is a definite connection betwen asthma and a specific type of infantile neurosis preceding it, namely, a sleep disturbance with nightmares. This particular kind of infantile neurosis I have classified as Type II of pavor nocturnus, and I consider it the traumatic neurosis of childhood from which the later sequelae, such as psychosomatic disease, psychosis, character disturbance, or neurosis, develop (M. Sperling, 1958).

The two important questions which arise here are, (1) Why did, in Jim's case, the traumatic neurosis lead to the development of a psychosomatic disorder and not to a manifest phobia or any other neurotic disturbance, and (2) Why was it asthma and not another psychosomatic disorder?

Those who lean heavily on the constitutional factor might be satisfied with the fact that it was certainly present in Jim's case. Nevertheless, he did not develop asthma before the age of four, although this factor was present from birth, and he did not have asthma after the first year of analysis and during the nine years of follow-up although his allergic sensitivity remained unchanged. The factor of somatic compliance operates also in conversion hysteria, but we know, from the theory of conversion hysteria, that the organ or organ system is chosen not because or only because of organic inferiority but mainly because it lends itself to the somatic expression of specific, unconscious fantasies (H. Deutsch 1929, Fenichel 1953, M. Sperling 1953, 1957, 1960a, 1960b, see also chapter 7).

In connection with our first question, certain behavior of the mother is of interest. Although both of her children had asthma (in fact, Patrick had developed asthma prior to Jim), she was interested in treatment only for Jim. She said that she did not want him to grow up a neurotic. What actually determined the mother to seek treatment for Jim at the time she did was the fact that she felt that Jim was using his asthma as a means of controlling her. On several occasions he had threatened to have an attack if she did not comply with his wishes. Jim had had much more severe asthma when he was five and six years old than at the time he came for treatment. It was quite apparent that the mother reacted much more to his neurotic behavior than to his asthma. She considered Patrick's behavior as much more normal; he was aggressive, more like his father, and, therefore his asthma was "organic." She, herself, felt inhibited—"His asthma is like my arthritis"—and she could not tolerate this in Jim. She could not tolerate the development of an overt phobia in Jim because this would also have meant that he controlled her, while, in the asthma, she controlled him. He could not breathe, that is to say, he could not live without her.

This was particularly well illustrated in the analysis of another child who had had asthma from the age of four. When she went to camp her mother would visit and spend a great part of the time there. She would sit on a bench with a medicine bottle, watching her daughter play. The little girl would be running around, but when she glanced at her mother she would start to wheeze. She would then stop playing and run to her mother. The mother would put a spoonful of medicine into her mouth, and the child would return to her playmates. Through her behavior the child was indicating to her mother: "I am really not having a good time without you. You see, I need you to give me medicine." To the mother, giving her child the medication had the meaning of controlling her. Under this condition she could permit the child to play with the other children.

This aspect of the mother's need for control and its effect upon the child was brought out with great clarity in the analysis of the mothers of John and Hans. Neither woman could accept any overt neurotic manifestations in herself nor, therefore, in the child with whom she identified herself.

Workers in the field have been impressed with the factor of maternal rejection in bronchial asthma of children. My findings regarding the quality of the mother-child relationship differ from those described by others. I have studied, through the method of concurrent psychoanalytic treatment of mother and child, a variety of psychosomatic disorders in children and could observe in operation the fundamental workings of the mother-child relationship. The case of John may serve as an illustration for this relationship in bronchial asthma. What, on surface observation, might appear to be rejection of the child, was found, in the analysis of the mother, to be a cover for keeping the child dependent upon her for the gratification of her own, infantile needs (primarily the maintenance of a fantasy of onmipotent control over life and death). Other infantile (sexual) needs of the mother can be well rationalized by the illness of the child, because it is exptected of a mother to take care, in certain physical ways, even of an older child when he is sick. The mother of the psychosomatically sick child rejects the child when he is healthy and wants to be independent, but she rewards him when he is sick, with a high premium of exclusive attention and preoccupation with his illness. I consider this quality of the mother-child relationship—the psychosomatic type of object relationship (M. Sperling, 1955c)—to be an essential etiologic factor in psychosomatic disease of children.

More recently, research in bronchial asthma in children, focusing particularly on the mother-child relationship, by

Coolidge (1956), Jessner et al. (1955), and Mohr et al. (1961), would seem to confirm my concept of a relationship of special closeness between the mother and her asthmatic child.

Another essential determining factor in the genesis of asthma, as I have found in psychosomatic disease in general, is pregenital fixation. In bronchial asthma this fixation is particularly to the anal phases of the psychosexual development. These findings would seem to confirm Fenichel's assumption (1943, 1945) of the anal basis of bronchial asthma (displacement from below upward). In this connection certain behavior of asthmatic children is of interest. For example, John, during a phase of his treatment when he ceased to have asthmatic attacks, became very noisy and used anal language. Similarly, he would soil himself on occasions. Because the psychosomatic object relationship originates in earliest infancy, although it may remain latent until the anal phases when, with progressive development of motility and strivings for independence, a battle for control between mother and child sets in, there will be a certain degree of oral fixation in every case of bronchial asthma, even if there are no manifest clinical evidences for this in the history of the particular asthmatic child. High intolerance against impulses, with an urge for immediate acting out, is characteristic for the pregenitally fixated patient. The differences in the level of fixation and the differences in the degree of fusion between libidinal and destructive energies will be reflected in the variety and severity of the psychopathology of the asthmatic patient, as well as in the differences in the severity, in the course, and in the outcome of the asthma proper. With this in mind, we can better understand certain phenomena observed in children with bronchial asthma, such as destructive, and particularly self-destructive behavior, even leading to suicide; the connection between perversion and bronchial asthma; and the connection between certain impulse-ridden-character disorders, such as obesity, enuresis, and psychopathy, and bronchial asthma. I should like to make these points clearer with some case illustrations.

From birth, eight-year-old Jeffery had always been a high-strung and difficult child. Feeding difficulties started when he was only a few months old. He had colic and diarrhea, and, because of this, his bowel training was difficult and delayed. At the age of four he developed severe asthma. Preceding the asthma, he had had eczema and allergies for which he had been on a restricted diet. At four years of age, he made his first suicidal attempt. He took a large amount of sleeping tablets. He was unconscious and had to be rushed to the hospital. There was no doubt in his mother's mind that the child knew what he was doing. At seven he attempted suicide by trying to choke himself.

Jeffery was a highly intelligent boy with very good insight. At the time I saw him, he was in the process of developing a very severe obsessive compulsive neurosis. He also had feelings of depression. He sometimes said, "If that's how I am and if I can't be any different, then it doesn't make any sense to live. It isn't worth while." He was preoccupied with death, specifically with his mother's death, as we found in treatment. This preoccupation with death is a typical feature in the asthmatic child, as it is in the phobic child. It relates to similar basic situations in both conditions: intense death wishes coupled with the belief in the magical power of the wish. Jeffery remembered anxiety attacks at the age of four.

The parents' marriage was unsatisfactory, and both parents were highly seductive with the child. At seven, preceding his second suicidal attempt, Jeffery had a severe anxiety attack. It had to do with dying and with his mother; something with her dying, he said.

The severity of the psychopathology seems to be in direct proportion to the severity of the asthma proper. I have found that, in those cases where there is a large admixture of oral and anal sadistic impulses with a more labile fusion of libidinal and destructive energy, the underlying mood is one of depression, with marked self-destructive tendencies (see chapter 8). Jeffery would seem to fit into this category.

In other cases which, clinically and in their development, appeared to be quite similar to that of Jeffery, the dynamic situation was different. To illustrate: Richard, nine years old, also had been a difficult child from birth. He was a restless sleeper and a poor eater. At two and three he often wandered away, and his mother had to pat his head and shoulders for hours at a time to get him to sleep. He came into her bed nightly. He had only mild eczema, but he scratched himself very severely. Even at nine, when he was excited, he scratched himself and rubbed his belly. His mother never observed him masturbating. At three he had a tonsillectomy and adenoidectomy, but continued to have a running nose and disturbed sleep.

When he was four, the mother abruptly stopped the head-and-shoulder patting. Also, shortly afterward, a sister was born. At that time Richard developed attacks of vomiting and complained about bellyaches. He usually first had an attack of vomiting and coughed severely, and then had an asthmatic attack. His attacks occurred mostly at night or early morning. These were the times when he used to wake up and get into bed with his mother. The asthmatic attacks took the place of the sleep disturbance. The mother was still assisting him with dressing, feeding, and bathing, rationalizing that Richard insisted that she wash him around the genitals and that she dry him.

Attempts to send Richard to camp had ended in failure. In spite of daily Adrenalin injections, he had such severe asthma that his mother had to bring him home. He had been found allergic to a great many substances, food and others. He responded poorly to diet and medication.

The true reason for the mother's asking for psychiatric help for Richard at this point (he had been under the continuous care of an allergist) was the fact that his behavior was becoming embarassing to her. He was increasingly impatient and demanding and had temper tantrums. He accused her of lying, and he used anal and obscene language. He often said to his mother, "Go out of my room. I can't breathe. You take the air away from me."

Richard was very distrustful of me. "I don't trust ladies," was his attitude. He was certainly right not to trust his mother, because, as soon as Richard formed a relationship with me, she withdrew him from treatment.

In this case, anal-erotic and anal-sadistic features predominated. Richard's oedipal phase appeared to have been very difficult. At three, he had a tonsillectomy; at four, his sister was born; at five, he had an appendectomy for which he was totally unprepared, the mother having told him that he was going to be x-rayed.

An important factor in his development was the relationship with his father. His father had been absent for a long period of time during Richard's early childhood. The father was a rather kindly person, who liked Richard. Intense oedipal resentment toward the mother and oedipal guilt toward the father prompted regression to the anal phase. The tonsillectomy which, like the appendectomy, he experienced as an attack, may have set the model for breathing to become the function to be taken into the conflictual sphere. In the analysis of John, it was possible to establish the etiologic significance of the tonsillectomy.

It was my impression that Richard's development was leading toward that of a character disorder with latent homosexuality. I should like to illustrate further this connection between asthma and deviate sexual behavior. Dora, five years old, had suffered from asthma since the age of three. She was allergic to various foods, dust, pollen, and so on, and she had been on a restricted diet and slept in an "aseptic" room. She came into treatment because of behavior which concerned her mother. She was lying and stealing, was difficult to handle, and was wetting her bed. No connection between the asthma and this behavior had been made, nor had asthma been the reason for seeking treatment.

With the resolution of the asthma (after I had dispensed with the allergist, medications, and diet and put the child into a room with carpeting), startling behavior was observed in her play sessions. She became wildly excited, screamed, jumped around, used floods of obscenities, and stamped her feet. This, as we found, was Dora's reaction to the primal scene and rage at her parents, particularly her mother. It was found that the mother had been very seductive with Dora; she had an unusually close physical contact with her, consisting of mutual looking, smelling, and touching of certain parts of the body (breasts, genitals, buttocks).

Of interest in this connection is an episode which occured during the treatment (which I supervised) of an eleven-year-old boy with chronic asthma. This happened during the phase in treatment when his asthma had improved considerably and the

therapist was dealing with his anality and homosexuality. He
had told her of the activities between himself and a group of
boys and that they were calling each other girls' names. In one of
his sessions, he reported the following incident: He had had a
bowel movement at school. Since there was no toilet paper, and
he had not known what else to do, he had wiped himself with his
hands and had told his friends about it. Interpretation of this
acting out of his coprophilic impulses led to further exploration
of his anality, which had been greatly intensified by actions of
his father (enemas and touching of his behind) and other
experiences with older men.

We now return to our still-unanswered second question:
Why is it asthma and not another psychosomatic disorder which
these children develop? We have found, as predisposing factors,
pregenital fixation, a specific mother-child relationship (the
psycho-somatic object relationship), and a somatic predisposition operating in these cases. The conflicts are not specific for
asthma. The urge to cling and the wish to separate from
mother, the positive and negative oedipal conflict, are universal
and basic to human development. The somatic predisposition,
although frequently present, is not always demonstrable in
asthmatic children. It is latent and apparently needs to be
activated by certain factors, which can also be extrinsic factors
such as allergens. It has been found that this somatic
predisposition, the allergic sensitivity, although it remains
unchanged, can be inactivated through psychoanalytic treatment. It also has been found that, under certain circumstances,
individuals who do not have an allergic predisposition can
develop conditions which closely resemble, or perhaps even are,
genuine bronchial asthma (Rogerson, et. al., 1935; Weiss, 1923).

What, then, are the specific factors which must be present to
bring about the complex syndrome of asthma? The study of the
structure of the conversion symptom provides the answer. We
know that the conversion symptom is structured like any
neurotic symptom: An unconscious fantasy is fulfilled; fulfillment of the wish (the id aspect) and punishment for the
gratification (the superego aspect) are expressed at the same
time. A conversion symptom can be understood and resolved
only in analysis, which exposes the specific, unconscious

fantasies that have been gratified in the symptom. I have been able to demonstrate in other psychosomatic diseases (ulcerative colitis, ileitis, allergy, migraine, chronic diarrhea) the existence of such specific fantasies. I have suggested considering these conditions as pregenital conversion neuroses.

Let us now examine the case material with this view in mind. Can we discern unconscious fantasies specifically related to the syndrome of asthma? Jim's analysis revealed that he had specific unconscious fantasies concerning death and how it could be brought on. It was always through some form of suffocation, poison, or poisonous gases. The smell of his mother's perfume would cause wheezing or asthma (respiratory introjection described by Fenichel 1953). The analysis of John revealed specific fantasies of death through suffocation, stemming from the experience with anesthesia, and fantasies of suffocation through constriction by a snake. All the children were preoccupied with death brought on through suffocation. Jeffery's suicide attempts were carried out in this way. The unconscious fantasies underlying the asthma and expressed somatically in the paroxysm of the asthmatic attack are specific fantasies for the individual patient and not for asthma in general. There will be certain similarities in the fantasy life and behavior of asthmatic patients, for instance, in those with predominantly anal fixations or in those with predominantly oral fixations.

One of my asthmatic patients, a six-year-old girl, had fantasies of living under water, with a plastic dome, where she could breathe freely. Such water fantasies in asthmatic patients have been described by others (Knapp, et. al., 1960) and are considered as belonging to the group of intra-uterine fantasies. This patient was an enuretic, and it seemed to me that the water fantasies were related to her enuresis and to the urethral fixation in her case. It was found later, in the analysis of her enuresis, that the plastic dome had something to do with the big round wet circle on the sheets when she wet herself at night. Such conditions do coexist with asthma. In this case the asthma responded very quickly to analysis, whereas the enuresis proved to be most persistent and took the place of the asthma. Here, the characterologic and perverse features were predominant.

Of particular interest, in this connection, is the phenomenon of change from one psychosomatic symptom to another in the same patient. I could demonstrate, in several of such cases, that the change in symptom followed the change in unconscious fantasy which had been exposed and devaluated in analysis. I had one such experience with a boy with ulcerative colitis, who had a short-lived episode of asthma at the beginning of the treatment of the ulcerative colitis. At that time (1946) I made reference to this case and to the possible connection between ulcerative colitis and asthma as two different forms of dealing with a similar conflict, namely, the elimination of a sadistically incorporated object (see chapter 7). In the one form there were oral incorporation and anal elimination; in the other, respiratory introjection and expulsion. From this point of view, asthma could be considered as an attempt at a specific somatic solution of this basic conflict.

In the treatment of bronchial asthma in children, the recognition that the basic dynamic structure is the same in asthma as in phobias is of great importance. Phobias are neurotic conditions based on unconscious conflicts in which the fantasy of omnipotence and magical thinking play a predominant role. Phobias respond to environmental manipulation, but such responses are only a surface adjustment. The phobic core remains, with severe crippling effects upon the personality of the child (M. Sperling, 1960a). The same is true for asthma. Asthmatic children, too, respond to environmental manipulation, but the asthmatic core remains, with crippling effects to the child. We know of the beneficial results of hospitalization and residential treatment (Abramson, 1961; Hallowitz, 1954), but these methods of dealing with the child's illness are of limited value, because they do not effect basic changes in the personality of the child. Unless the child is treated and, in many cases, particularly those of young children, unless the parents are also treated, no lasting results will be achieved. With older children, as in the case of Jim, this can be done through direct work with the child and minimum work with the mother. The same is true for phobias. With younger children, however, treatment, if it is to be successful, involves much work with the mother. In some cases of young children who are still at the

developmental phases in which the superego and the mechanisms of defense are not yet firmly established, analytic work
with the mother alone may result in the cure of the child's
condition. This, too, is similar in the case of phobias, where the
mother needs the phobic child for the maintenance of her
fantasy of omnipotence. The healthy child who can become
independent and leave the mother, that is, live without her, is a
threat to the maintenance of this fantasy.

The child's asthma is a reassurance to the mother that she is
indispensable to his life. In the asthmatic attack the child
submits to the mother (or her substitute) in reality. When he
appears most helpless (sick and unable to breathe), in reality,
he has assumed unconsciously via the symptom a magical
control over life and death which, in some cases where the
unexpressed rebellion against this submission is extreme, may
lead to suicide, overt or psychosomatic.

PART 6

TIC DISORDERS

16

Tic Disorders and the Gilles de la Tourette Syndrome

Tics are involuntary movements of voluntary (striated) muscles. We can speak of tics only after full coordination of muscles has been achieved. Jerking movements in infants or young children are frequent but these are not tics. Tics due to organic causes like brain injury are excluded here, and only tics where either a definite emotional etiology or no etiology could be established are considered. We can differentiate between single and multiple tics or tic syndromes and a condition referred to as maladie de tic in which muscle systems of the whole body may be involved. Tics are repetitive, quick movements which, in some cases, can be so violent as to resemble convulsions without loss of consciousness, Tic convulsif (Kovacs, 1925; Wilder, 1946).

The usual onset of tics in children is in early latency. In some cases, an immediate and direct relationship between a traumatic event and the onset of the tics can be established. This is particularly true in cases of single tics. In such a case, the tic may represent the memory of the traumatic incident retained in reaction of the child to this incident, or it may represent the outcome of a conflict between an action which the child would have wanted to carry out but did not in response to the trauma. It may be the result of a conflict aroused by the trauma; for instance, the blinking of the eye in response to an exhibitionistic trauma expresses the conflict between looking and closing one's eyes. Certain tics, like shaking of the arms or the head originate on such a conflictual basis, for example, where the child inhibited the impulse of hitting or fighting off the attacker. Compulsive, repetitive features are common to all tics. While tics occur in children of both sexes, they are more prevalent in boys. Children with hypermotility where environmental restrictions interfere with the child's activity seem to be more predisposed to the development of tics. In fact, lifting of these restrictions and providing suitable outlets such as physical activities, sports, or dancing for discharge of muscular energies are often valuable aids in treating children with tic disorders. Precipitating traumatic events may be surgery, illness, birth of a sibling, sudden stopping of masturbation (due to masturbation threats and fears of consequences) in an environment that is excessively restrictive and overstimulating at the same time. Pediatricians sometimes confuse tics with chorea (St. Vitus disease) and treat these children with rest and confinement to bed, that is, with methods that are responsible for the production of tics, rather than for their dissolution.

A few clinical examples of the less severe tic disorders illustrate some common features in the genesis, dynamics, and course of this syndrome. These will be followed by a presentation of the more severe tic disorders referred to in the literature as maladie des tics and Gilles de la Tourette syndrome.

Freddie (9)

Nine-year-old Freddie was referred to me because of headaches and twitches of the facial muscles and jerky movement of the shoulder. He had developed these tics at six, at which time he had been confined to bed because a diagnosis of chorea had been made. He had been very unhappy about his confinement, and his tics increased in severity. We found that at the time preceding the onset of his tics, his parents had separated. Freddie, who was a very active boy, had lived in the country before the separation where he had an opportunity to release his energies in outdoor activities; he had a good relationship with his father who would take him hiking and who encouraged sports and physical activities. After the separation, his mother moved into a small city apartment and Freddie found himself confined to a small space with a depressed and irritable mother.

On the surface it appeared that the relationship between Freddie and his mother was an affectionate one, but it soon became obvious that Freddie felt hostile and resentful toward her. It appeared that the mother had displaced a great .deal of her resentment and need for revenge from her husband onto Freddie, and he seemed to sense and react to this. He was the middle child sandwiched between two sisters with whom the mother got along well. She had little understanding of Freddie's needs and restricted his activities severely. The father would have liked to resume the marriage under the condition that his wife allow him a certain amount of freedom which she could not do. She had left her husband once when her children were still small and had taken them to live with her mother for one year. The mother could not accept my suggestion that she seek treatment for her depression, and as soon as Freddie's headaches and tics improved, she withdrew him from treatment. During the five months of treatment, we had dealt mainly with the dynamic role of repressed aggression manifested in his headaches and in his tics—both equivalents of temper tantrums. The freeing of aggression had resulted in great symptomatic improvement; however, there was no opportunity to deal with the sexual aspects of his symptoms, and his treatment, although very satisfactory from the symptomatic point of view, has to be considered incomplete. There were, nevertheless, marked changes in his personality. He had become a more assertive, aggressive, and active boy.

Dickie (6)

Dickie was also six when he developed a facial and vocal tic. These tics could be observed in statu nascendi during his treatment. He had been referred to me because of a severe sleep disturbance with nightmares, which was very disturbing to his parents. The content of his nightmares showed that Dickie was in an acute oedipal conflict with sadistic impulses and death wishes directed towards both parents. It was during the dissolution of his sleep disturbance and the nightmares that Dickie developed tics. The vocal tic was a barking sound. Dickie had a puppy which somebody had given him and although he had previously been afraid of dogs, he became very attached to this puppy. His mother, however, did not like dogs, and one day when Dickie came home from school, the dog was gone. His mother had decided to give the dog away without discussing it with him. After working through his anger at his mother, which was manifested in the facial tics and his identification with the lost puppy, especially in the barking sounds, his tics cleared up. Tics sometimes start as grimaces and threatening faces which children make deliberately. In some cases, the child may lose control over these movements which then remain as facial tics. In Dickie's case, these tics represented an inhibited (aggressive and sexual) attack on his mother as a barking and biting dog, but he was not consciously aware of this. In order not to be rejected by his mother, he had to be a "good" boy and repress overt manifestations of aggression.

The relationship with me enabled Dickie now to express his aggressions more openly in his treatment. One episode may illustrate this: One day, Dickie came to his session with a baseball bat which he put down beside him while we played a game of cards. He said that he was determined to win this game. When I asked him why he had brought the bat, he said, "To hit you over the head if I lose." Here, the connection with headaches is of interest. Before, he would get a headache in such a situation. He gradually learned to handle his aggressive and sexual impulses more appropriately, without resorting to headaches, tics, or nightmares.

Miles (9)

Miles was nine when he was referred by his school because of a peculiar tic that was disturbing in the classroom. He was making gasping movements and sounds, like a fish who has difficulty breathing out of water. His treatment revealed that Miles' tic represented an unconscious identification with his mother who was a chronic cardiac patient with severe difficulty in breathing and who was making gasping sounds. She had been hospitalized several times because of her condition, but even when she was at home, Miles had to take over many of her responsibilities, such as the housework and shopping. Since he had to be home after school, he had very little opportunity to play with his friends. Treatment revealed strong unconscious hostility and death wishes against his mother. For these feelings, he overcompensated by being oversolicitous with his mother and by unconsciously identifying with her in the symptom. After this was brought out and worked through in his treatment, the tic disappeared.

Because of the increasing severity of his mother's illness, treatment had to be terminated at this point. After his mother's death, Miles had a serious accident. He was run over by a car on his way home from school and had to stay in the hospital for some time. He was seen afterwards for a short period and helped to work out his guilt feelings about his mother's death. We found that unconscious guilt feelings had played a part in his accident. He made a very good adjustment and remained symptom free during a follow-up of six years.

Myrna (11)

Myrna was eleven when she was seen because of blinking of her eyes for the past five years. Her tics typically increased in intensity whenever she was under tension. We found that the onset of her tic coincided with the birth of her brother. Her unconscious feelings towards her brother were expressed in the blinking of her eyes. The conflict between seeing and denying the existence of a penis and that caused by the existence of her brother, with whom consciously she had a very close, overcompensatory relationship but whom she envied and hated unconsciously, were thus preserved and enacted in her tic. She responded very well to psychoanalytic therapy.

Carol (12½)

A very similar situation was found in the case of twelve-and-a-half-year-old Carol. Carol, too, had developed blinking of her eyes and facial tics four and a half years before, after her brother was born. Both Carol and Myrna had been only children until then. Carol's tics, too, became more intensified in stressful situations and particularly in the presence of her mother, who reacted to Carol's tics with great disturbance. In treatment, it was necessary to bring to the fore and work through with Carol her penis envy and resentment of being a girl and her hostility and resentment against her mother who, she felt, preferred her brother. The mother was unduly disturbed about her daughter's tics and rationalized her feelings with the fact that Carol was a girl and that the tic was spoiling her beauty. The overconcern of the mother, in some cases, points to unresolved conflicts concerning her own femininity. This was true in the case of Carol's mother. Of particular interest in this connection, is the next case, which highlights the mother's psychopathology and its role in the tic disorder of her daughter.

Cases of child tiqueurs, especially younger children, with

more severe psychopathology of the mother, the child, or both are treated best by simultaneous treatment of mother and child. With this method the role of the mother's psychopathology and the child's responses can be observed clearly. I have selected two cases, one of a six-and-a-half-year-old girl whose mother had a latent paranoia and one of a five-year-old boy whose mother suffered from a manic depressive psychosis. I intend to emphasize the connnection between tics and paranoid feelings.

Ellen (6½)

Ellen developed a facial tic with blinking of her eyes and jerking movements of her body when she was six and a half. She, too, had been diagnosed at first as a case of chorea and had been treated with rest and confinement to bed for several weeks. This only made her condition worse. Her mother was inordinately disturbed about Ellen's tics and could barely conceal that she considered the tics an indication and manifestation of severe aberration in her child. Treatment revealed that Ellen's tics had originated in response to a very traumatic experience. Preceding the onset of the tics, Ellen had suddenly become sick with an acute appendicitis. She was taken to the hospital without knowing that she would have surgery and remain in the hospital. Her mother had been afraid of Ellen's reaction and, therefore, had not prepared her for the surgery and separation. Soon after Ellen came back from the hospital, her father had to leave town for several months, an event which also had no precedent in the past. In addition, the mother informed Ellen that she was pregnant. Following this, Ellen also developed vocal tics which consisted of peculiar noises and a repeated four-letter word.

Ellen's mother was a severely disturbed woman. She was afraid of the dark and of being alone and would take Ellen into her bed for comfort whenever her husband was not at home. At the same time, the mother felt guilty for using her as a substitute for her husband.

In addition to the facial tics and blinking of here eyes, Ellen would deliberately make grimaces and peculiar movements with her hands which she knew were very disturbing to her mother. Ellen knew that her mother thought that she was crazy, and the movements with her hand, which she would suddenly hold in a peculiar way in front of her mother's face, especially when it was dark, was intended to scare her mother. Expressed and carried out in this tic was also Ellen's revenge on her mother. "If you think I'm crazy, I'll give you cause to think about it." By her tics she had the power to disturb her mother and *make* her think that she was crazy. This meant that she controlled her mother's feelings and thinking. Heightened narcissism, omnipotence, and masochism are important characteristic features in tiqueurs. For the same reason, she would also make peculiar noises which upset and scared her mother very much. Because of the severe psychopathology of the mother and the intense interplay between them, it was felt that treatment of the child alone could not be successful, and because the mother refused to see anyone else, she and Ellen were treated simultaneously (M. Sperling, 1951).

Ellen's mother was very restrictive and had discouraged physical activities which she considered tomboyish and inappropriate for girls. Her treatment revealed that Ellen unconsciously represented to her a younger sister of whom the mother had been very jealous and towards whom she had also strong guilt feelings. The guilt feelings related mainly to sexual activities with this sister whom she had seduced to mutual masturbation. Once, in the sexual play, the patient had been taking the male role, trying to perform intercourse. Her sister had pushed her off and had avoided sleeping with her after that. The mother had always felt guilty about her own masturbation and about seducing her sister. As treatment progressed, the mother's paranoid psychosis became more apparent but also amenable to therapeutic intervention. She actually considered her own behavior as crazy, but she had projected this to Ellen. Ellen's jerking movements had a sexual meaning to the mother. She connected it with masturbation and this was a continual reminder of her own masturbation and of sex play with her sister. Ellen's tics to the mother were a giveaway of her own sexual crimes. It meant everybody could see what a terrible person she was. She felt uncomfortable taking Ellen places. She never liked to sit next to Ellen in the movies. She said that she had a very peculiar feeling sitting next to her because she was feeling that Ellen was twitching. The guilt feelings about Ellen's tics were not only a displacement from the sister to Ellen but had some justification in reality.

Several months preceding Ellen's hospitalization, the mother had taken Ellen to a pediatrician because of a vaginal discharge. Following the advice of the pediatrician, the mother had administered douches to Ellen for a while. To the mother, giving douches to Ellen had the

·meaning that she was repeating, under the guise of administering legitimate treatment, the seduction of her sister with her daughter. In Ellen's treatment, it was found that she had experienced this treatment as an assault by her mother and also as a punishment for touching her genitals. During the time while this treatment was going on, she was suffering from enuresis diurna and wetting herself at school. This wetting was the indication that Ellen felt sexually overstimulated by her mother's manipulation. I learned from the mother that she had bladder trained Ellen at age two and a half by rubbing Ellen's face with a wet diaper, telling her to smell it. Since then, Ellen had never wet her bed at night. Ellen had shared her parents' bedroom up until age four and after that frequently came into their bedroom at night. The mother had observed Ellen masturbate and had issued many prohibitions against it. She had never been able to answer any questions Ellen raised about babies and where they came from and had treated discussion of sexual matters as a forbidden issue. Ellen had a similar feeling about the anesthesia and surgery later, reacting to them as an assault and as a punishment. Ellen's jerking movements with her hands also represented a pushing away of the mother douching her genitals and of the anesthetist in the hospital.

In the treatment of the mother, we were concerned mainly with clarifying and improving her relationship with Ellen. The mother had definite paranoid trends, she revealed the idea that people were talking about her, especially about her femininity and were observing her. She also claimed that she knew when Ellen was twitching, even though Ellen was in an adjoining room and the door was closed. Ellen, at a time when she only twitched in the presence of her mother, would sometimes turn to her little sister (then two) and, looking at her mother, say, "Ask me what I do and tell me that I am crazy." She was still testing and teasing her mother. It was remarkable that under these rather difficult circumstances with such a disturbed mother, Ellen succeeded in freeing herself of her tics. She also made a very satisfactory development in a five-year follow-up.

In Ellen's case, we could see how the mother's paranoid feelings affected Ellen's condition. With the case of five-year-old Paul, I would like to show that a child's persecutory feelings have a basis in reality.

Paul (5½)

Paul came into treatment at age five, referred by the private school he attended because of bizarre and disruptive behavior. In the course of treatment, we found that Paul suffered also from a tic disorder. Only this aspect of his behavior, which apparently did not concern his parents nor the school as much as his overtly disturbing behavior, will be considered here. Paul had developed, between age three and a half and four, various facial tics, including twitches of the nose with sniffing and peculiar twitches of the mouth. In his treatment, it was possible to explore and to understand the genesis and dynamics of these tics which responded very well to psychoanalytic treatment. It was necessary for various reasons to treat Paul's mother in simultaneous analysis (Sperling, 1950a).

In the analysis of his mother, we could trace back the onset of Paul's tics to an incident which occurred when he was three and a half. The tics consisted of twitching and sniffing of the nose, twitches of the cheek with biting the inside of the cheeks, and of picking and eating the snot from his nose. Except for the nose picking, which greatly irritated his mother, Paul's tics were hardly mentioned by her. Paul had been bowel trained by age two, at which time the mother discharged his nursemaid and took over his care herself. Paul reverted to wetting and soiling. One day, when he was about three and a half, he had defecated on the rug in the living room. The mother was so furious that she stuck his face into his bowel movement. Paul, apparently, got the message that he could not afford to oppose his mother openly and stopped soiling. It was shortly afterwards that the tics appeared. Speaking of this incident, the mother related that the maid, who had been present then, had said to her, "You are not a mother. A mother doesn't do that to her child." In a way, the mother was aware of her ambivalent feelings and attitudes towards Paul. She would often find herself thinking when she spoke nicely to him, "Come into my parlor, said the spider to the fly." She was alternately seductive and sadistic with him. Paul felt that he was being persecuted by a witch and that he had to use the magic powers, which he attributed to the urine, feces, tics, etc., in this struggle.

The mother's analysis revealed that she unconsciously identified Paul with her brother, of whom she had been very envious in childhood. This brother had been killed in an accident. She felt guilty about his death, and Paul was planned as a replacement of the brother to his mother and named after him. In Paul's treatment, we found that some of his facial tics, especially the movements of the mouth and chewing of the inside of his cheeks, were a mirroring of his mother. The mother had not been fully aware of her grimaces and tics. Later on, when both had progressed in their treatment and Paul could express some of his feelings more openly, he would say, referring to his facial twitches, "This is the angry face you make." Still later in the treatment, when Paul had given up his tics, the enuresis, and much of his sadomasochistic behavior and the mother had gained insight into her own unconscious motives and could function more like a mother than like a hateful sister to Paul, they were able to communicate with each other verbally and had frequent conversations.

The preservation of a traumatic experience in the frozen stereotyped form of tic is not an infrequent phenomenon among children. This is true also for the imitational tic. This type of tic indicates how keenly children observe and interpret facial expressions and other body motions of the important people in their environment. I should like to give one brief illustration of the frozen tic retained in a symptom.

Steve (6)

Six-year-old Steve suffered from peculiar tic-like movements of his mouth. He would open his mouth wide and make sucking and smacking movements with his lips. The tic had appeared suddenly several months ago and was increasing in frequency and intensity. Brief psychoanalytic therapy revealed that the tic was the stereotyped repetitive memory and confession of a traumatic experience. Steve had been persuaded by an older boy to perform fellatio. The tic, like a typical conversion symptom, expressed both the gratification and punishment of a forbidden sexual wish.

Tics and Psychosis: Peter (8½)

Tics can be associated with a psychosis or the final outcome of a tic syndrome in a child may be a psychosis. I would like to present a brief abstract of a longitudinal study of such a case. For a fuller presentation see M. Sperling (1954, chapter 20).

Peter initially presented a tic syndrome and later developed a psychosis for which he was hospitalized for more than two years in a psychiatric hospital. In supervising the successful analytic treatment of his psychosis, I had the opportunity to observe him both during the initial phase and later after his discharge from the hospital. This case is interesting also as a longitudinal study with a fifteen-year follow-up during which time the patient has remained well without tics and without psychosis, functioning on a high intellectual level and in a satisfactory marriage.

Peter was eight and a half when he was referred to me because of facial and vocal tics and because he was a withdrawn and rather fearful child. We found that his tics had developed following the birth of his sister when he was nearly six. His mother was depressed at that time and appeared to reject him. She needed much rest, and Peter had to be quiet at all times for her sake in order not to wake the little sister. He was expected to play quietly by himself without bothering anybody. His father was working during the day and busy evenings helping his depressed wife with her chores. The mother was not able to follow through my suggestion for psychotherapy for Peter and for herself.

I learned later that because his tics and his behavior had become unbearable to the mother, Peter had been hospitalized. In the hospital his tics decreased gradually and disappeared, but his behavior became more and more bizarre. He was much in demand as a patient for staff presentations because of his seemingly inexhaustible capacity for producing bizarre fantasies and behavior. He was diagnosed as a case of childhood schizophrenia and he remained in the hospital, attending school there and going home for occasional weekends until he was twelve. At that time, his parents consulted me again. They had to make a decision whether to take him home or transfer him to another hospital since the first hospital kept children only until age twelve. They decided to take him home and to accept my referral for psychoanalytic psychotherapy for Peter.

No account of his treatment, which extended over a period of four years, can be given here. What is of interest to us in this study is the fact that this patient, contrary to the predictions by Gilles de la Tourette and others, did not deteriorate mentally, although he had a manifest psychosis and although his tic syndrome had all the characteristics of that described as Gilles de la Tourette. His vocal tics were really obscene four-letter words which he did not fully articulate (for fear of his mother's reaction) but intonated with hissing sounds.

The muscular twitches, which had spread from his face to his shoulders and arms, were his way of expressing his aggressive and sexual impulses towards his sister and his mother and father in symbolic, exhibitionistic, confessional body actions. This form of communication was then replaced by symbolic, exhibitionistic, and confessional psychotic verbal productions, which gained him the full interest and attention of the hospital staff. The element of scaring and shocking people by sudden grimaces, muscular twitches and vocal emissions was retained in an attenuated way in his psychotic verbalizations. It was as if he had replaced the vocal and the muscular twitches with a kind of "mental" ticking.

In his analytic treatment, we found that he had actually enjoyed his exhibitionistic performces at the conferences and had taken pride in the production of his fantasies. It was necessary for his analyst to interfere with this form of exhibitionism by pointing out to him that he was not on exhibition and that she was neither impressed nor startled by this behavior. The analyst had to continually deal with his need to communicate and to confess his "crimes," through both his tics and his psychosis in a way that should not be understood by himself nor by those to whom it was directed.

In connection with this case, who although he had a psychosis never developed mental deterioration as is claimed for Gilles de la Tourette syndrome, a recent publication by Brunn and Shapiro (1972) is of interest. The authors, after a review of the literature and an intensive six-year study of thirty-four patients with Tourette's syndrome, found that Tourette had failed to differentiate this syndrome from other obscure diseases in his time. They found that although sounds or words eventually appear in all patients, coprolalia is not a necessary component of the syndrome and also, that there is no mental deterioration in these patients. Other investigators (Corbett, 1971) and particularly Ascher (1948) and Eisenberg et al. (1959) have, on the basis of their clinical experience, expressed views similar to my own. They have been impressed with the favorable response to psychotherapy and are optimistic in regard to therapy and final outcome. MacKay and Heimlich (1972) report the successful collaborative treatment of an eleven-year-old boy with Gilles de la Tourette syndrome. Paraverbal treatment (use of percussion instruments and songs) was introduced as an additional therapeutic modality which helped him to use, in a more sublimated way, some of the aggressive and sexual impulses discharged in his twitchings and made him more amenable to psychotherapy. At the same time, intensive work was done with the family. When the patient left the psychiatric hospital at the end of the second year, he had to be placed in a residential setting. Because of the degree of pathology of the parents, he was not able to remain at home. He was symptom free at a follow-up at eighteen.

Tics and Their Relation to Other Psychosomatic Symptoms: Barbara (7)

Tics can be followed or replaced by symptoms other than bizarre behavior, psychosis, or acting out. In the psychoanalytic treatment of a seven-year-old girl, Barbara, who suffered from ulcerative colitis, we found that she had developed facial tics and shaking of her arms at four and a half, shortly after her brother's birth. She had been very angry at her mother then, but her attempts to express this or any overt aggression were met with rejection by her mother. We also found that she had had a tendency to temper tantrums earlier, between two and three, which had been forcibly suppressed by her mother. Barbara obviously realized early in life that she could not afford to have manifest temper tantrums without being rejected by her mother. In her case, the tics at age four and a half could actually be considered as an equivalent for the earlier unacceptable temper tantrums. This relationship with her mother, who could not tolerate any manifest expression of rebellion and assertiveness but demanded complete submission, passivity and dependence, was a major dynamic factor in the genesis of her ulcerative colitis which she developed at age seven (see chapters 6 and 25).

In Barbara's case, we could see that unconscious aggressive and sexual impulses and the rebellion against her mother were expressed in the disguise of "uncontrollable" somatic symptoms which replaced the willfully produced temper tantrums first in the form of "involuntary" twitches of the motoric musculature and then in the form of cramps and explosive diarrhea through the smooth, involuntary musculature of the gastro-intestinal tract. In Barbara's case, it was essential to work simultaneously with the mother because any improvement in the child's condition which led to an increased ability to express herself more openly was met by the mother with rejection of Barbara and an increased resistance to her treatment.

In some cases, especially in the case of mothers with paranoid tendencies, the mother's morbid preoccupation with her child's tics serves to reinforce them. The child correctly senses that this overreaction expresses specific feelings of the mother and that he can affect his mother's feelings by twitching. This then means to the child that he has control over his mother or father or both, as the case may be. It is of interest, however, that in most cases the tics are particularly pronounced in the presence of the mother (for her benefit). In the treatment of mothers of children with tic syndromes, we found that the tics have specific meaning for these mothers, particularly sexual meaning. Ellen's mother felt as if Ellen was ticking for her in response to her sexual needs. The mother externalized her guilt feeling which then turned into anger towards her child for complying with her unconscious needs. A vicious cycle develops whereby the mother's reaction increases the child's needs for ticking, which serves also as a discharge to relieve tension by symbolically permitting gratification of the child's sexual and aggressive needs.

The paranoid feelings of some of the patients suffering from tics are based, to a large extent, on reality experiences in childhood. The child may exaggerate these feelings and use them with little discrimination in other situations and with other people. The development and the basis for this "paranoia" could be seen clearly in the simultaneous analytic treatment of mother and child. Here we could observe that the symptoms originated in response to maternal expectations and needs (Ellen, Michael, and Peter). The parents, in such a case, are actually persecutors who carry out their persecutory activities under the guise of parental care. I have dealt, for many years, intensively with this problem in my work with severely disturbed and psychotic children (M. Sperling, 1974, chapter 22). In this connection, the recent research by Niederland (1959) into the childhood history of the famous Schreber case is most illuminating. Niederland found that underlying the bizarre behavior and psychotic fantasies of Schreber was a childhood reality represented by his physician father. The latter used bizarre physical approaches and instruments on his little son, which could easily have provided a reality basis for the development of Schreber's later illness.

Tics as Masturbatory Equivalents and Identification with Mother: David (6½)

David was six and a half years old when his mother consulted me. He had suffered from multiple tics for the past half year. His mother, while concerned with his tics, obviously used this as an opportunity to seek help for herself. This was a very favorable circumstance for David because he benefited from his mother's treatment indirectly and required only brief direct treatment, since he was still young enough and his tics were of recent origin. In addition, treatment of his mother brought about a considerable improvement in her relationship with David. Her relationship with David has been an essential factor in the genesis and disappearance of his tics.

When David was three and a half, his mother's sister, who lived with the family, had a baby girl, and shortly after this aunt moved, his mother got pregnant and gave birth to a baby sister when David was four and a half. He had shared the parental bedroom until his sister was born and had shown great interest in this event. He had frequently questioned about how babies grow but the mother could not answer these questions. She was very irritable and restrictive and when she observed him masturbating in the toilet, she forbade him to do it. She also restricted his physical activities and did not let him play with other boys. He had to rest a lot, especially since his sleep was disturbed during this period, and he would frequently wake up screaming that his legs hurt him. Medical and orthopedic examination was negative. She did not allow any overt manifestations of aggression. Once when he was angry and pinched her, she not only pinched back but shook him in fury. It was around that time that he began to shake his head and developed facial tics. There was a change in his personality. He began to withdraw. She was ambivalent towards him, mostly angry but she also had profound guilt feelings. She was aware that she did not permit him to discharge any angry or aggressive feelings and that she did not let him be a boy. She felt particularly guilty about a habit David had developed. He would touch his genital region and put his hand to his nose. Discussing this, she confided that she had the same habit until adolescence and sometimes would find herself still doing it now. She also had had tics until adolescence. She was not aware that she was still grimacing and twitching when she felt angry and frustrated, but David was very aware of his mother's facial expressions and mirrored them in his tics.

The mother had had a very traumatic childhood. She suffered from episodic depressions and was frigid in a very unsatisfactory marriage. She hated her father, who she felt had exploited her after her mother's death. She had carried over this hate to her husband and son, both of whom she was trying to emasculate. Her gradual understanding of her problems and relationships in her treatment enabled her to become more tolerant and accepting of her husband and David. David was seen in therapy for about four months, during which time he expressed in play and verbally his hostility and resentment toward his mother and jealousy of his sister at home. We found that his tics developed after he had stopped masturbating rather abruptly, due to his mother's intimidation and threats. He had impulses to hit, kick, and kill his mother and his sister. These impulses had to be repressed because any attempt of expressing, overtly, resentment and aggression towards his mother was met with increased rejection and restriction by her. The changing feelings and attitude of the mother towards David made further direct treatment unnecessary. David's tics had disappeared, and he was allowed to lead the life of an active boy of his age. The mother remained in treatment for two years, during which time the satisfactory development of David could be followed closely.

Tics Persisting into Adulthood

I have selected two clinical examples to illustrate some sequelae of tics persisting into adulthood. Childhood tics may either persist or recur in certain traumatic situations or come out in certain characterological changes.

A Woman (29)

A twenty-nine-year-old single woman came for analysis because of feelings of inadequacy and depression. She had a tic disorder consisting manily of eye and facial twitches from childhood. These tics had started at about six. The patient was the youngest in a family of five girls. At that time, the sister next to her was sick with rheumatic fever and was getting all the attention which the patient had had up to that time as the baby of the family. She had felt that she had been a disappointment to her parents; they had wanted a boy, and she now felt that because of this sister, her whole life was spoiled. Her mother was particularly concerned about the eye twitch and took her frequently to eye doctors but nothing was done. She would be relatively free of tics for some time, but whenever she felt frustrated or under pressure, her tics would recur with full intensity. This was particularly disturbing to her during adolescence because she felt especially uncomfortable with boys and the tics interfered with her dating. At twenty-nine she had the same problem with men. She would twitch badly when on a date or when men paid attention to her.

She was still a virgin at twenty-nine, and she had never had a gynecological examination. She was afraid that the doctor would find out that she was not a woman. She was very interested in hermaphrodites and she had the idea that she was a hermaphrodite herself. A memory from childhood of entering a dark room, seeing her sick sister in bed, and having the thought that her sister was dead, lead to the uncovering of a repressed memory of a primal scene experience, with death wishes against her parents and a wish of being in her father's place and of having a penis. This piece of insight helped to explain another aspect of her behavior related to her tics. Whenever she was successful in her job and close to being promoted to an executive position, her tics would become so unbearable that after a while she had to quit the job. She could not permit herself in reality to be successful because this to her meant taking the place of a man, that is, the place of her father. While symbolically in her tics she exhibitionistically displayed that she was not a woman, or not like other women who did not twitch, this behavior also expressed her doubt of whether she did or did not see a penis on herself. A gynecological examination revealed that she was anatomically a normal female with a somewhat elongated clitoris. She had been practicing clitoral masturbation from childhood.

It is my impression that tics in females are an indication of particularly strong unresolved conflicts about masculinity and that female tiqueurs have particularly intense exhibitionistic needs which find distorted expression and gratification in this syndrome. Boys with tics are often effeminate and have conflicts concerning masculine identification. In addition to the general hyperkinesis, exhibitionistic conflicts seem to play an important dynamic role in the genesis and dynamics of tics.

Sequelae of Tics in Childhood: Jane (21)

Jane, a twenty-one-year-old, single female, came for analysis because she experienced difficulties in her work and in her social relationships, especially with men. She also suffered from bouts of depression and a general dissatisfaction with life. She was an attractive, intelligent girl with an unusually strong exhibitionistic tendency, which got her into trouble. She had an insatiable need to attract attention wherever she was, especially in public places. For that purpose she would behave in a way that would usually embarrass those who were with her. In her analysis, we discovered that this unrestrained exhibitionistic behavior was an alternative or rather a sequelae of a tic disorder from which she had suffered in childhood. In her analysis, she worked through the onset and course of her tic disorder. She remembered that her tics first started when she was seven and in the first year of school. One day, she was sitting on the stoop of her house with her mother who was teaching her how to read. She wanted to play and was very impatient and resentful that her mother kept her and insisted that she take her lessons. They were reading the word *Mother*, which her mother was spelling for her, urging her to pronounce it. Jane pronounced the word in a very mocking tone and her mother got angry and hit her. Jane started to move her hand in a very peculiar fashion which she showed to me explaining that it meant pushing her mother away from her. At first her mother did not notice it and Jane did it voluntarily, but soon she lost control over it and had to do it all the time. It became so intense that she had to be fed because she could not hold a spoon or a glass. Very often, when she was holding a glass, she began to shake in this way with her hands, spilling the milk, which delighted Jane but upset her mother. Soon other tics developed, particularly sounds. She used to give a whistling sound which irritated her mother, and her mother slapped her in the face for it. From then on, she had a whistling tic which she could not stop. Her mother became very upset and began to take her to doctors. One doctor diagnosed her condition as St. Vitus' dance, and she was put to bed in a darkened room for two weeks. It did not help. Another doctor treated her with injections. She did not like the injections, and she hated both her mother and the doctor because she felt that they were both in conspiracy and out to hurt her. She hated her mother violently and went around saying, "Fuck, fuck, fuck." Her mother hit her for it because she would say it in the presence of anybody. So she would say it under her breath, "from my belly," as she explained, and this too became a tic. Finally, one doctor diagnosed it as a nervous condition, and she was referred to a psychiatrist when she was about nine. She had to go five times a week and she resented it terribly. She could not play with her friends because she was never home. She accused her mother of taking her away from her friends. When the children came to her house, her mother would always have fights with Jane in the presence of her friends and humiliate her. Jane accused her that for that reason nobody wanted to come to her house.

Her relationship with the psychiatrist and her understanding which she gained in the treatment she used against her mother, now blaming her for everything with the backing of the psychiatrist.

Later in the treatment, when her mother let her go alone, she would play hooky most of the time, either not showing up for her appointments at all or coming so late that no work could be done. Finally, she declared that she was through and that she would not go anymore. By this time, she had given up her tics "but the silly behavior" had started then. Whenever somebody would come to the house, Jane would put on a spectacle, run and dance around wildly, and behave in a crazy fashion. At times she would sit and stare into the air and act very mysteriously. Then she would suddenly jump up and perform a mirror dance or the like. This behavior she had retained up to now and it was the cause for her unsatisfactory relationships with friends, male and female. When she went out with somebody for more than one time, she would start this behavior and people would become disgusted with her and drop her.

Notes on Treatment

In cases of children with tic syndrome, it is essential to bring about a modification in the environment, but particularly in the maternal feelings and attitudes towards the child; otherwise the results of treatment are undone at home, and treatment in such a case could be very long or be abruptly terminated. With young children, very often environmental manipulation, by providing outlets for motoric release such as sports, dancing, lifting of restrictions and improvement in the mother-child relationship are sufficient to permit a gradual decathexis of the muscular system as the organ for the discharge of emotional tension. Even analytic treatment does not always give good results with tiqueurs, especially in chronic cases, because the psychic content underlying the tics is often so repressed and removed from the patient's consciousness that it is difficult to bring it to the fore. This phenomenon may play a role in the impression of those investigators who consider tics as an organic disorder. On the other hand, tics in children may disappear spontaneously, only to be replaced by some other pathological behavior which may be less obvious and disturbing to the environment and is, therefore, not considered connected with the tics. Tics are most frequently replaced by character disorders with overt acting out behavior, or in some cases, by psychosis or psychosomatic symptoms, such as ulcerative colitis or migraine headaches. Tics, like other neurotic symptoms, do not disappear spontaneously without sequelae, unless the underlying repressed conflicts, wishes and fantasies are at least partially resolved. I am here in disagreement with other investigators, especially those who are not psychoanalytically oriented and whose criterion for assessing normal and abnormal personality and character development include only the manifest behavior. With young children of prelatency or early latency, indirect treatment through modification of the mother's feelings and attitudes toward this child may suffice by allowing a change in the course of the child's further development from the pathological state to a more normal one (Sperling, 1950a).

Mahler (1949) differentiates between organ neurotic, which to her is psychosomatic, and impulsive tiqueurs. Adopting the view of F. Alexander (1948) that psychosomatic means organic and that therefore the psychosomatic symptoms unlike hysterical conversion symptoms have no psychic content, she runs into difficulty reconciling her clinical findings with her theoretical views. Clinically, she found in her organ neurotic tiqueurs unconscious conflicts and fantasy material, as in neurotics, and a more favorable response than in the impulsive tiqueurs, which she considers more difficult to treat because they are "like the delinquents, artful in evading the therapeutic interference by acting out and projective mechanisms." What is most disconcerting is that the impression is conveyed that the so-called organ neurotic tiqueur is not only not responding to psychoanalytic therapy, but that the application of it is dangerous because it breaks down his defense systems. It may be worthwhile to stress again that the tic disorder was one of the three conditions (stuttering and asthma are the other two) which prompted Fenichel (1945) to introduce the concept of pregenital conversion. According to Mahler, the tiqueur with consolidated organ neurotic motor syndrome has a better prognosis." The armor plating of his ego" protects him against the upheaval of puberty while the patient with tic disease, whose defense had been broken down by ineffective deep psychotherapy, did not do well. She concedes, though, that it may be due to faulty techniques where there has been a release of aggression and a liberation of erotic drives through symbolic interpretation without concomitant strengthening of the ego. The impulse-ridden tiqueur, according to her, has an unfavorable prognosis.

Simultaneous Analysis of an Adolescent Boy with Maladie de Tic and His Mother

Michael (14)

Michael was brought for treatment at fourteen, suffering from a severe case of Maladie de Tic. He had multiple tics beginning with the head, face, and eyes and extending to the shoulder, arms, trunk, abdominal muscles and legs. The head shaking and facial tics had begun in early childhood around the age of six. Gradually other tics developed. The multiple body tics and eye tics became more apparent after a stay in camp and following eye surgery when he was twelve and a half. Michael's mother, Mrs. Z, appeared depressed, disturbed, and overly concerned and preoccupied with her son. The father had engineered treatment for Michael while the mother had seemed unduly anxious and threatened by it. In addition, it was obvious that Michael felt forced into treatment. This was his general feeling about everything—a feeling which was, as we found out later, to a large part justified since both parents were overbearing and overcontrolling.

From my previous experiences with such patients, I felt that the chances that Michael would stay in treatment and cooperate without the participation of his mother were very slim. I decided therefore to treat mother and son simultaneously though I would have preferred to treat first the mother and then Michael. This was not possible because Michael was in serious difficulty in school and the parents were very determined that he receive treatment immediately. Mrs. Z related that she had been melancholy after Michael's birth. She had been in the hospital for two weeks and then gone home with a nurse who stayed another two weeks. She could not eat at all, had to be artificially fed, and had lost thirty-five pounds within a month. She could not take care of Michael, and since he had to be shifted from day to night nurses, she decided to go and stay with her mother. After four months she felt better, but up to that time she had been crying all the time. She said that since then she had not had any prolonged depression again but had had depressive episodes espcially when confronted with some task like expecting company, going places, or meeting people. She toilet trained Michael at eight months. He wet his bed until three. In retrospect she said she realized that perhaps Michael was not ready for it so early but when he was eight months her husband wanted to go on a trip for a weekend and since she had to hire a nurse and leave him home with her, she decided to bowel train him first. Her neighbor had told her that Michael had cried the whole time. She sent him to nursery school when he was not quite two and a half years old. When she was pregnant again, she did not prepare him for the baby, nor did she tell him that she would be in a hospital. She found out that Michael had been very disturbed when she was away from home giving birth to her younger son.

Paul, the younger boy, developed allergy at sixteen months. He was still covered with eczema, on restrictive diets, and receiving injections for hay fever and asthma when his mother started treatment with me. At twenty-three months he lost the eczema and also around that time trained himself by simply asking her to take him to the toilet. (She had tried to train him at eight months but he had refused, so she had not forced the issue.) Casually at the end of the session, she mentioned that she was one of nine children, next to the youngest and that her mother was a rather old woman when she gave birth to her.

In her following sessions, she began to talk about her fear of mental illness although nobody in either her or her husband's family was mentally sick. She had married during the war when her husband was in the Army and she wanted to be with him. At first he worked in an office; later, when he was in basic training, he began to complain about pain in his leg. He was hospitalized and eventually discharged. Sometime later when looking through his papers she noticed that the cause for his discharge was psychiatric illness. He had never told her this, nor had she ever spoken to him about it. He would still sometimes complain about his leg, and jokingly she would ask why his leg never hurt when he was playing golf.

She began to complain that now she was getting worse. She was developing a voracious appetite and was gaining weight. This resistance in the mother manifested itself not only in her negative therapeutic reaction but also in an intensification of Michael's resistance. He was still being brought to my office and called for by his father which he resented. Although there was some justification in this arrangement as transportation was rather difficult, I wanted him to assume more responsibility for his treatment and suggested a meeting with his parents to work out a different arrangement. Michael had threatened to stop treatment, and his mother now confirmed that she had been supporting him in this. Now, however, she confessed, she was glad that her husband had taken a firm stand. She became preoccupied with her weight gain, complaining that she was getting fat, in spite of the fact that she was now starving herself. She had refused to consider a European trip her husband had planned because she would only gain weight. As an adolescent she had been plump and unattractive. Boys had ignored her. She started dating at seventeen; but had very few dates. She had achieved a good figure only some eight years ago and men had begun to pay attention to her and tell her how attractive she was. Now she was losing her good figure and attractiveness to men. (It was not interpreted to her at this point that her good figure and Michael represented male symbols to her.)

Mrs. Z now complained that after the last two sessions her face had swelled. The first time she had suffered a similar swelling had been nine months ago when a man, answering an ad for the sale of their home, had bought it on sight in spite of the prohibitive price they had placed on it. While talking to him on the phone she had felt her face getting hot, and when she hung up it was swollen and itchy. The doctor had diagnosed it as angioneurotic edema. For the past five years she had suffered from abdominal cramps which the doctor had diagnosed as allergic. He felt that this symptom might well be allergic too.

She was also suffering the return of an old symptom—the need to urinate several times during the night. The first time she had been told that this was due to a tipped uterus. When this was corrected the condition had disappeared.

Recently she had taken her younger son to the doctor for a sty. Even though a blood test had proven negative, she entertained depressing thoughts about friends who had lost their children and a boy of ten who had died of cancer.

She wondered why she did not feel elated. Now that she had everything, a new house, new furniture and a trip to Europe. Yet she was not enjoying it and did not even feel like taking the trip.

She complained that her eyes were itching; they were slightly red. I interpreted to her that she felt it would not look good if she went around crying; that since she had everything people would wonder why. Having an allergy, however, she could rub and have red eyes "legitimately," she replied. "I used to cry a lot when I was depressed." She then remembered a dream. "It was a very funny dream, in fact the whole thing was very funny." She had dreamt that she was pregnant, and at that moment she and her husband had been awakened by a loud noise. The box with the sanitary napkins in her closet had fallen down. She had very few associations. She was expecting her period. This was usually unpleasant and preceded by a few days where she would feel upset and depressed. (Although it was quite obvious that she was concerned with replacement for Michael and that she was preoccupied with pregnancy wishes and fantasies and discharging and materializing some of her unconscious fantasies in her allergies, no further interpretation was given at this point.)

She was also upset because she was having a dinner party, and although she liked to entertain, she had sleepless nights worrying that everything might not be perfect. She always had to excel and be noticed and admired. Now she had a swollen face and red eyes. This was interpreted in the transference as her feeling that I was not only not helping her but making things worse and exposing her unfavorably. Everybody could see that there was something wrong with her (her swollen face and red eyes). She said that when I had been talking to her before, she had felt like crying. This happened very often to her at home: she just feels like crying without any apparent reason. Her complaints flowed freely: she had to take care of everything and everybody. She never kept them (the men, two sons and a husband) waiting for a meal. She was also very punctual for and never missed a session. The other day when she felt sick and even had a little temperature, she had let her maid go home early because the maid felt sick also. Then she prepared a snack for herself and later made the dinner for the family. Her husband told her that she was OK but that he hated women. He had to deal with them in his business. She was aware that he could not be without her. Last year she was away for one night and he missed her. He would not even let her go with the girls to a milk farm. Why did she feel like crying when she had all this and should be enjoying life? What had she done to deserve all this? After some silence came her confession: when she was six a neighbor had abused her in the barn. She had not known what he was doing, even later when she married, she was very ignorant in sexual matters. She had had no sex education. Her husband could have taken advantage of her, but he was a nice fellow. She then wondered how had this all come up. In all these years she had not thought of this. Why now? She said she had felt guilty about Michael. She had met him in the city the other day and the family went to the movies. He sat next to her. He was twitching terribly. She did not like to sit next to him and certainly not in a dark movie. When a seat became free next to his father, she told him to go and sit there. The next day they were supposed to go to their new house and spend the day at the country club. She felt that she did not want Michael to go with them. She spoke to her husband, expressing feelings to him about hating Michael. That morning Michael was looking at her and asked whether he had to go with them. They looked at each other and she was astonished because she felt that he had read her mind and knew that she did not want him to join them. He stayed home alone. She was ashamed to admit that she had a very pleasant day. She is puzzled by him now, he seems to behave differently.

The other night some people came over and brought their twelve-year-old daughter with them. Michael went upstairs and changed his clothes. He then came into the living room and spent time with the girl. He did not twitch at all that evening. She was flabbergasted. When he was born she had become depressed though she was not depressed later when his younger brother was born. She had wanted a child badly; she had been married then for three years and had even gone to a doctor to find out why she had not conceived yet. After Michael was born she felt she was tied down and had lost her freedom. This did not happen when Paul was born although she then had two small children to care for.

During the three sessions she had tried to release and at the same time hold back her feelings of hate for Michael and men in general. She at the same time developed a rash all over the upper part of her body. She had even thought she had German measles but the doctor found nothing wrong with her. She was taking Cortisone in order to get rid of them in time for an important cocktail party on Sunday. She knew she would not be able to go because she could not wear a cocktail dress, that is, "expose" her decolletage. While talking she was crying and telling me that she cried at home also. I said to her that while the tears were good for the rash (by liquefying it) it would be better to talk about what was really troubling her instead of crying and producing symptoms. She replied, "You would say that I have the rash because I don't want to go to the party." She laughed and said, "I *don't* want to go to the party. I feel tired and depressed and not like going to a party." She cried again and then said that there was a coldness between her and her husband. They were not fighting, it was just a coldness. She then confided that they were having intercourse only every four to six weeks and "I am still a young woman." I interpreted to her that as Michael was showing his feelings in his twitches, she was showing her feelings in a rash and allergies but that there was a sexual basis for these feelings and symptoms for both of them.

Mrs. Z now complained that she was losing her appetite and that she had nausea in the morning. That is how it started before, when she got depressed. She was getting jittery and attributed this to the moving date coming closer and her need to get ready for the trip. She was worried about leaving the children. She had been sending Michael out to eat several times a week. She had never done this before, always preparing meals for him at home. She remarked on how good he was now, too good, it was unnatural. She had noticed that he was controlling his tics and also his temper. The other morning, though, he got angry and dropped a bottle. She said that she was worried leaving him, but she was reluctant to speak about specific fears. She then opened up and revealed her true concern. She knew of a fourteen-and-a-half-year-old boy who had killed his mother and sister. Another fourteen-year-old boy killed his brother. When the doctor they had consluted before they came to me said that Michael should be watched because he might harm himself, she was worried that he might do harm to others.

She can get very angry at him. Once when he was about five years old, she slapped him in the face so hard that she left an imprint of her fingers. She used to have arguments with her husband and afterwards would not talk to him for days. Now, even if they have an argument, her anger does not last. She could not understand what happened: just as she could not stop eating a few weeks ago, she now had to force herself to eat.

It was obvious that she was trying to deny completely her involvement in treatment and her developing dependence on me. Her depressive equivalents were a reaction to the anticipated separation and a reflection of her present state of anxiety. But this was only one aspect of it. Another powerful dynamic factor in precipitating this state of anxiety and depression was her conflict over whether to stay in or to break off her analytic therapy. She knew that if she stayed she would have to confront her infantile sexual (perverse) impulses, especially her very strong voyeuristic, exhibitionistic, and sadomasochistic impulses, which she considered "crazy," as well as her infantile relationship with her husband and Michael, and Paul, whom she realized she was making pathologically dependent upon her.

It was an advantage of the simultaneous treatment that I not only could observe how unconsciously attuned and obliging Michael was to his mother's needs but could also deal effectively with these resistances in their respective analyses. In the beginning of their treatment, Michael had obliged his mother, who felt threatened by it, with an exacerbation of symptoms, thus demonstrating that the treatment did not help him. Now he was obliging his mother by trying to take a flight into health. He was now a very good boy, who controlled his tics and his temper without, like his mother, permitting exposure and analysis of the pathological aspects of his sexuality, aggression, and object relations. When I confronted her with her wish to terminate treatment and also with the fact that her resistance was carried over to Michael, she at first denied having had such thoughts but then said, "It's true, but I did not tell Michael about it." The resolution of this resistance was a major achievement and provided access to the feared and hidden sexual fantasies, fears, and wishes of both the mother and Michael. The mother introduced the subject by wondering why before when the boys went away for a weekend she was relieved and now when they were supposed to be away the next weekend, she wanted them to be home. Laughingly she asked "Am I afraid to stay home alone with my husband?" For the first time, she mentioned that Michael was in the habit of coming into their bedroom to say good night after they had kissed good night before going to bed. A few days ago, she had told him not to do it. He asked, "Why don't you want me to kiss you good night again?" She explained something about privacy, and parents sleeping together having intercourse. He said, "I understand, that's how I am here." For two nights he did not come in, but then he resumed the habit again. In the new house, they will have the bedroom door closed but in the old house it was always open so she could hear the children. Actually she did not hear them. Once Paul had a bellyache during the night and called her. He had to come to her room and wake her. She does not like a closed bedroom door. It makes her feel very uncomfortable. During her depression after Michael's birth, she had the feeling that now that her husband had a son she would lose his affection.

Gradually she began to talk about her feelings about sex. She again recalled the experience when she was eight. The question arose in connection with my remarking that she seemed to be afraid to stay alone in the house. She said that this man had raped her but then corrected herself and said that it happened several times. She would go to his house and sit on his lap and he would tell her "don't look down." She had a similar experience when she was about twelve, when the man who owned the drugstore wanted to seduce her. She always worried what Michael was doing behind closed doors, wondering whether he masturbated. She could not conceive that he could do such a thing. While complaining that her husband was not giving her enough sex, she was telling me that she liked to stay in the bathroom until he fell asleep. She said she had not used the diaphragm for the past year because she had trouble inserting it, and since her husband did not like to use a condom they were at an impass. She thought that she should really have herself fitted, but her doctor had said that she had a tipped womb so that was why she had trouble inserting it.

She did not like her husband's relatives and while talking about this realized that this was because she was envious. She would be reluctant to see her husband's relatives and when with them she would tire, develop heacaches, and usually fall asleep on the way home so she would not have to talk with her husband. While telling me this, she developed a headache which resolved as quickly as it had developed when I interpreted her anger at me.

She said that her eyes were swollen today and that they had been swollen also at her previous session when she had cried a lot. She was expecting guests tonight and tomorrow, and they will see her face and eyes. After a short silence she revealed what had really upset her. That morning she had walked by Michael's open door and he had been on his bed masturbating. She could not understand why she felt that this was such a terrible thing, but that she did and was very upset about it. She then related that she had not been on a subway for many years, since she had seen a man masturbating across the seat from her. In fact, this had happened twice. She said she had always feared Michael might masturbate ever since he was a little boy. The link between Michael's twitching and his mother's feelings about the penis and masturbating were quite clear now. She said that when she gave birth to Michael she was happy he was a boy because of her husband who wanted a son, but then she felt that she had lost her husband's love to Michael and that he loved Michael more than her. Seeing Michael masturbating that morning had provoked a very strong reaction in her. She had felt sick and nauseous and had had to pull over to the curb for a few minutes while driving to my office. Now she consciouarly thought of quitting treatment. She said she was not afraid of sex with her husband. I questioned this and recalled her dragging out the evenings and going to bed after he had fallen asleep. She said that sometime ago he had tried to have "oral intercourse." She was terribly upset but consented to show that she loved her husband. She then wondered if her husband were a sex pervert and maybe Michael inherited it from him. Maybe that was why she did not want to go to bed readily. I pointed out to her that she was overreacting to Michael's masturbation and exhibitionism. Further, she was showing by her swollen eyes and face that there was something wrong with her that she was afraid to know about consciously. She replied that a friend had taken her into her confidence and told her of an affair she was having with her husband's friend. After that she had felt sick and nauseous.

For the first few weeks of his analysis, Michael hardly talked at all but appeared very tense and twitched all over. It was not until his mother had overcome to some extent her fear of and resistance to his treatment that he became more relaxed. He had referred to his twitches as jerking, and I had interpreted them to him as a means of scaring me off and shocking me. I was trying to make a link between his tics and his aggressive and exhibitionistic needs and to encourage him to express his aggression and other impulses more openly. That he under-stood and reacted to this as a threat (rightly) may be illustrated by the incidents which followed.

The other day he had said to his mother that I told him his tics had to do with sex. He was watching for her reaction, expecting her to take him away from somebody who was talking to him about sex, which she surely would have done had we not worked this problem out with her first. It also clearly showed that Michael was aware of his mother's sensitivity to the dangerous subject of sex. Then Michael proceeded to show me (and his mother) that I was a bad influence on him and caused him to lose his temper. One evening he had been doing his work for school, and because he could not find something, he spilled ink all over his hands. He was overtly angry but suddenly became sleepy and tired and went to bed at ten o'clock which was unusual for him. He had obviously been frightened by his temper and escaped into sleep. The mother reported that the next morning she heard him curse and use obscene language. He threw his pants to the floor and there was ink all over. Her reaction to this behavior was most revealing and also showed that Michael was clearly aware of her sensitivity to "mental illness," or more precisely, that she thought of him as "crazy." She had a quick pain in her chest. She worried what he might do and had thought that he could kill or harm himself. She realized that was why the doctor had told her to be around him all the time and not to leave him alone at all. I pointed out that she was afraid of her own feelings and temper and what she might do. She said that she used to have a terrific temper; when the children were small, her husband would say, "stay away from Mommy, Mommy's dangerous." But her temper changed and she developed allergies. I interpreted to her that she, as well as her children, expressed themselves in physical symptoms, rather than in overt behavior, because that would mean to her that they were "crazy." Michael had tics and Paul had allergies. She said that to her mental illness was the worst of all evils. When she had been pregnant, she was preoccupied with worry that the baby would be born with a mental abnormality. She had two miscarriages four years after the birth of her younger son. The second time it was a three month fetus, and the doctor had told her not to get pregnant anymore because the fetus showed abnormalities.

Selected Fragments from Michael's Analysis

While these feelings were being worked through in the mother's analysis, Michael was loosening up considerably in his treatment. The fact that I was neither scared by his tics nor his temper and was confident that he could be aware of his feelings and impulses and express them in more appropriate ways, was obviously reassuring to him. He confided to me an experience that was very disturbing to him, about which he had spoken neither to any of the doctors he had seen nor to his parents. He had experienced déjà vu on two occasions and taken this as an indication that there was really something wrong with his brain. He was greatly relieved to find out that these phenomena were expressions of unconscious wishes and memories and were not a sign of insanity. Since the analysis of these déjà vu experiences would take up much time and space and has no direct bearing on his tic disorder except that it opened up for analysis his strong feminine wishes and homosexual feelings toward his father, it will be omitted here. (M.Sperling, 1964a, see also chapter 20).

The analysis also mobilized early childhood memories, and he began to bring some memories and dreams into his analysis. These memories were mostly unpleasant, and many were outright traumatic. He said that he remembered having his tonsils taken out when he was two or three. He also remembered his eye doctor who prescribed eyeglasses for him when he was four or five. When he was not quite six and in the country with his parents, he once stepped into a beehive and was stung by seven bees. After the age of six, he was always sent off to camp and was never with his parents during the summer. Something happened at eight. He thought for a while, "Oh yes," his best friend had an operation (hernia). He then said that he too had an operation nearly two years ago. It was an eye operation for his muscles. Although he was only a few days in the hospital, it was very unpleasant, he was nauseous and could not eat. At eleven he had a tooth extraction under gas. He remembered dreaming "he was at a parade." During the analysis he had recurrent dreams about being at a parade. These dreams expressed his exhibitionistic masturbatory impulses and the punishment for it. Illness and surgery were a punishment for his forbidden and dangerous impulses. We found later in his analysis that he had experienced the eye operation as a castration. He was in a panic and feared that he would be blind but did not verbalize his feelings. He abruptly stopped masturbating and suffered a severe exacerbation and spread of his tics. He remembered the first day of school, he told me. His mother had brought him there. There was no particular feeling attached to this memory. In this connection, his mother's version of his early childhood and her feelings are significant.

She had sent Michael to nursery school when he was two and a half so she wouldn't have him around. When Paul was born, her husband would take Michael in the morning and bring him home at five o'clock. At four and a half he went to kindergarten alone. Although it was three blocks away, she let him go alone because there was no crossing. She took him there the first morning. She had to take the baby with her and that was too much for her. When he was two he had TB. He had to be in bed several weeks and had x-rays every month, then every three months, then every half a year until he was eight. She thought that he contracted it from a sleep-in maid so her husband did not want her to have any sleep-in help. He had a tonsillectomy at two and a half with bleeding afterwards. They couldn't find a doctor so the dentist in the building gave him first aid. She used to lose her temper very quickly when he was younger. Once she grabbed him by his head and shoulders and shook him. Shortly afterwards the headshaking and shoulder twitches developed. She would feel guilty afterwards and be very affectionate with him and hug him and kiss him.

During the phase when his mother was working out her resistances and becoming more aware of her sexual problems, Michael was beginning to bring dreams into the analysis. He reported two dreams which he said were typical and recurrent, both had to do with falling. He had such dreams frequently. In one, he was on a window ledge and falling and in the other he was falling out of a boat on a lake. His bisexual orientation and feminine wishes were brought out more clearly in a dream in which he lost his Bermuda shorts and went to buy a replacement. He associated Bermuda shorts as something both boys and girls wear. In the dream everything was turned around. Left was right and vice verse. He was on the left side, in reality the store was on the right side. Left to him meant something wrong. Another dream brought his conflict between hetero- and homosexuality into full analytic focus. In this dream, he was in a car with a girl. There was another boy his age who got into the car and took over the wheel. They fought. The boy wanted to go in another direction, opposite to where he was going. This dream quite accurately depicted his emotional state, his conflict of being pulled in opposite directions. His fear of sexual and aggressive impulses and of losing control over himself was coming more to the surface. He said his tics were much worse when there were people close to him as in a car with other people, or especially with his mother. He wished to push them off or out of the car but was not consciously aware of his wish to exhibit himself and to commit a sexual attack. His conflict about his exhibitionism was particularly intense and, as will be seen later, led to some acting out of his exhibitionistic tendencies, particularly in relation to his mother. His mother was perceived by him as a temptress and stood for lack of control. His father, although feared and hated, was a superego symbol. During this phase of analysis, his sleep was disturbed and he had frequent anxiety dreams. In one dream he was in a restaurant with another boy. It was dimly lit. It was about nine o'clock. He left and said that he would be back at twelve. He had actually been in a restaurant the previous night with his best friend and a girl and he had left around nine o'clock because he had work to do. This friend, he told me, had changed very much since his father died. He was speaking loudly and using obscene language. Michael was embarassed by and felt sorry for his friend. The girl with them in the restaurant was another boy's girlfriend. A related thought to this dream was, Would he be better off with his father alive or dead? The next dream, also an anxiety dream, showed that he thought he would be better off with his father alive and that he needed him as a means for control. In this dream he was in a car. At first he could not start and then he could not stop it; the brakes failed. The car was starting to roll into the street where there was a lot of traffic. He wanted to pull the emergency brake. His father woke him. This dream initiated a discussion of his problem of starting and stopping, of losing control, of the dangers of traffic, of intercourse, and of using his penis. He could even get killed for it, and he needed to have his father wake him to prevent him from doing such dangerous things. His ambivalence about his father—looking at him as a savior and wishing him dead at the same time—and his doubts about whether he had a chance in his treatment to be cured came out in a dream in which his father woke him too late. In the dream, he was late for school but when he looked at the clock he realized that it was one hour fast so he really was not late. That meant that he still had a chance. Actually he was very compulsive and had never been late for school, and actually his father was the one who would usually wake him for school.

The following material is from the second year of Michael's analysis. The mother reported that she and her husband came into Michael's room and her husband noticed that Michael's fly was open. Before she would have been so aware of it, but now she had not even seen it. Michael said to his father, "Haven't you seen a fly open?" Later when he opened his pants so they came practically down, she said, "Have you eaten so much that your pants are too tight?" She was surprised at herself. She would have been uncomfortable before. Instead of twitches he was now showing her the real thing.

Did she now have to worry that her son was a pervert, she asked. After a while she said that she was thinking of a boy in her class when she was eleven. He was twitching and fidgeting and exposing himself. Why didn't she tell the teacher? She could have changed her seat. Was it curiosity, fear, ignorance? When I reminded her of her not wanting to sit next to Michael in the movies because he was fidgeting, she said, "I have the exact same feeling with Michael as I did with that boy." She did not want to sit next to a man in the movies. She had never thought of this boy and her feelings, what if this had never come up? She apparently realized the significance of this material in relation to her feelings about Michael and his tics, but also that she was giving up her "secrets." She talked about her fascination with the genital region of a man. In the past she would look only at that, but now she was no longer so interested in it.

The other day Michael had come into her room to show her that his pants were too tight. She said he should put on some of his new ones. He then called her into his room to show her that the new ones did not fit either. He stood there with his penis sticking out, the pants half down. She was very upset, but she did not say anything because Paul and her husband were in the next room and the door was open. The next morning she passed Michael's room. The door was open and he was dressing. She said to him that he should close his door and he said that was useless because his father came in every minute. She told him,

"Your father will learn to knock on your door." In one of the following sessions, she complained that her chest was heavy, that she was not getting anywhere. She had yelled at her younger son for no reason, only because she was angry at Michael. The day before she had to drive him to his session because he had practice and she had promised him that if he couldn't get a cab, she would drive him. This was to have been her free afternoon, she was crying. I asked her why she was so furious at me. She said, probably because of the "rocking in the car." Michael had an erection, he was wiggling and was very restless, looking at her to see if she had noticed. Now her chest felt freer. She had said before, it would have been better if she had not started here at all. Before treatment Michael would twitch fiercely when in the car alone with her and she saw no connection with sex and perversion. Now it was all out in the open, and she could no longer pretend not to see or to know what was going on. She could no longer deny to herself that she actually stimulated him and looked for this behavior. Now she was finding out what was covered up by his tics and her allergies. She was preoccupied with the idea that he could do something to a girl with his penis. "How do children get such feelings? What do children know about sex?" she asked. "How do they become like that?" It was inconceivable to her that he could be so stimulated sexually. She was still holding on to her infantile ideas about rape and sexual violence.

This was the second year of analysis for both Michael and his mother. Michael's tics had improved considerably. He was now able to make connections between his tics and precipitating events or situations. He had hardly any tics in school now, but he noticed that he was twitching a lot in one particular class. Talking about it, he said that he liked this particular teacher, who seemed to be understanding and sympathetic and that he felt drawn to him. Realizing the sexual implications, Michael said "I hope he doesn't understand what I am communicating to him with my tics." The uncovering of the unconscious conflicts, fantasies, wishes, impulses, and affects underlying his tics presented some problems in his analysis. It was the aim of the psychoanalytic treatment to strengthen the ego and to modify the superego thus enabling the patient to acquire more adequate impulse control and a more sublimated use of his sexual and aggressive energies. With such patients until this is achieved, some degree of acting out of impulses during the phases of treatment when the repressed energies are freed from the symptoms is unavoidable (M. Sperling, 1967c). Michael's acting out was limited to his home and was directed primarily towards his mother and the analyst. His exhibitionistic behavior, especially in the presence of his mother, was meant to test her by her reactions to see whether she really accepted him as a male or thought that he was "crazy" and preferred him to have tics rather than a functioning penis. Michael was quite aware of his mother's sensitivity in this matter, and his exhibitionistic behavior barely disguised as "sloppiness" was intended to upset her and to show her that the analyst was transforming him into a pervert. It was a plea to take him out of treatment. As with any acting out, Michael's was also a resistance to treatment, intended to intimidate the analyst and to show that treatment was not helping. There were good reasons for this resistance now, because we were nearing the analysis of his positive and negative oedipal wishes and his murderous impulses toward his parents.

Having the mother in treatment proved to be a great advantage. She did not respond to Michael in the way she used to and he expected her to. Here are some illustrations of how she now handled Michael in situations.

One evening they were sitting at the TV, Michael was in his pajamas with his fly open and penis sticking out. She said that before she would have experienced nausea, the hot and cold feelings, and would have been sick. She felt nothing of the sort but calmly told him to button up because his penis was showing. For the first time in her life, she got her period without premenstrual tension. She hardly knew she had it. Her husband upon seeing a napkin was surprised and asked "How come you didn't have the stay-away-from-me signal?" I interpreted to her that now she could accept that Michael had a penis so apparently she could accept that she had a menstrual period. She said that her complaints about her husband not making enough love to her were really not warranted and that he was actually very attentive to her. She also said that she felt differently about her sons, referring to her previous feelings, when she could not accept that boys, especially her boys, have a sex life. They had a conference with Michael's guidance counselor. She remembered before, when she used to answer all the questions, the dirty look the principal had given her when she registered with Michael. This time she let Michael speak for himself. She even poked her husband under the table not to mix in. The dean suggested to Michael not to take five majors, but Michael without a twitch insisted that he could manage five majors and convinced the dean.

In Michael's analysis, his fear of his impulses and losing control was a major issue. During this period of analysis, his sleep was disturbed and he had frequent nightmares. A series of anxiety dreams helped bring into analytic focus and resolve some of his basic problems. Feelings that he could not grow up to be a man and have a "normal" sex life as long as his parents were alive came to the fore. In recurrent dreams his parents were killed or died, and he was casually talking about it to his friends and people. But this was not the solution because he felt he needed his parents, especially his father, who was still functioning as an "external" superego for Michael, demanding and enforcing controls. In one dream, Michael had been sent on an errand by his father and when he returned his father told him that his mother had slipped and hit her throat against the sink and died. He remembered that when he was nine his mother had an operation for goiter. She was quite sick then and was in the hospital for several weeks. He thought then that she might die. Masturbation and any sexual activity was dangerous because of the violence attached to it. This concept had been reinforced by the mother's feelings about these matters.

The nature of his unconscious masturbatory fantasies and his homosexual tendencies were brought out in his dreams and associations. For example, in one dream he was playing baseball with a bat. (We had discussed previously on various occasions the symbolic meaning of ball=testicle and of playing=masturbating.) He knew there was a strangler around who had strangled three people, his parents and his brother. Michael went into the men's room. He could not find the right door out. He kept opening the wrong doors and could not get out. Then he was playing again and saw a man coming down the hill. This was the strangler. He ran to hide in the men's room.

When he played golf the next day and used the men's room, he really had difficulty in getting out. He could not find the right door. In association to this, he remembered an experience which he reluctantly related. He had gone to the movies one night with his friend. He had an argument and the friend left. He hitched a ride; it was a nice man but when he was in the car, the man put his hand on Michael's penis. Michael pushed his hand away and wanted to get out, but the door was broken and he couldn't open it. He was very frightened but finally opened it. The man said, "But this is not where you wanted to get off." He hid until a cab came.

In another dream he was throwing cigarettes in the room and thought if these were girl cigarettes it would be better. He did not know what to make of it because there are no special brands for girls. He was silent for a while and then said that he had thought of something which really had nothing to do with the dream. He thought of another dream which he had told me some time ago about playing baseball. This dream had to do with a homosexual experience. He then realized that the two dreams were related and expressed perverse wishes. "But why girl cigarettes?" he asked. "Cigarettes are really not for throwing around, but for smoking and taking into one's mouth." He was smoking and his parents didn't think he should. The wish for fellatio was defended against by not having the cigarette in his mouth and by a wish that it should be a female (nipples) rather than the male genital.

Michael was in analysis for four years. He then attended an out-of-town college and chose a career different from that of his father, so that he established himself completely on his own. He made a very satisfactory heterosexual adjustment. He is married, has a family, and is functioning very well. He has a rather good relationship with his parents now that he is successful and a father himself.

The analysis of Michael's mother was terminated after two and a half years. We felt she had gained sufficient insight and maturity to function adequately as a mother and wife. Her treatment was particularly helpful to her younger son, Paul, who suffered from allergies and asthma and had been on restricted diets all his life. Realizing how she was fostering his dependence and rewarding him for his illness by the special care and attention, she began to disengage herself from this relationship and to encourage him to become more independent. She gradually discontinued the diet and other special attentions with the result that Paul "outgrew" his allergies and asthma.

Considering the fact that both Michael and his mother were in rather precarious mental states when they began treatment, the results are most satisfactory. It is my impression that the allergies and the depressive equivalents were failing in their defensive function and that the mother was close to a psychotic break. Michael too had a very difficult time; his tics were becoming increasingly worse and he was in the process of withdrawing more and more from reality. In this connection a case reported by H. Bruch and Lawrence C. Thum (1970) is of interest. The mother's psychosis erupted during intake when she was questioned about her own background and her attitude toward her son. From birth on she had considered him the incarnation of her own evil and aggressive impulses and had made control of his impulses the aim of her life. The authors, like the mother, want to deny or ignore the existence of sexuality and its role in the patient's and his mother's behavior and symptoms. The mother was especially disturbed about the vocal tic of her son which consisted of three letters. When the psychiatrist at the intake interview pronounced them as the four-letter word, the mother became extremely disturbed and this signalled the onset of her psychosis. The authors seem to consider the onset of psychosis in the mother as a fortunate event for the patient. The mother in the psychotic episode went through a kind of catharsis, verbalizing some of her feelings and impulses. The change of the pattern of interaction between her and her son was helpful to the boy's further development.

From my psychoanalytic experience with similar cases, my interpretation of this case would be somewhat different from that of the authors. In my opinion this mother, like Michael's, had projected her own "wild," or perverse, crazy sexual impulses onto her child and tried to control them in the child instead of dealing with them in herself. When the psychiatrist took over and she felt threatened not only with loss of control over her son, which meant loss of control over herself, but also with being found out in her sexual impulses and feelings about her son, she broke down, and made a confession, "I am crazy, I have crazy impulses." Her son was saved, he did not have to have the psychosis for her, she had it herself.

In the case of Michael and his mother, psychoanalytic treatment succeeded not only in preventing psychotic episodes of the mother and/or son but also in achieving a considerable integration of personality with sufficient ego growth and superego modification to make symptoms unnecessary for both.

The role of sexual factors and the relationship with the mother has also been noted by Aarons (1958) in a case of Maladie de Tics in an adolescent boy. Wilhelm Reich had already, in 1925, considered the psychogenic tic as a masturbatory equivalent. In the case of Michael, the tics were a form of sexual communication between him and his mother, permitting the acting out and gratification of mutual perverse needs, especially exhibitionistic and voyeuristic impulses. Studying both partners of this relationship psychoanalytically provided unusual insight into the interrelated dynamics and, in fact, made treatment of Michael possible. At the present, there seems to be a trend among psychiatrists to turn away from psychoanalytic methods and to ignore the role of infantile sexuality and early experiences, and fall back on organicity and organic treatment. In view of this, the presentation of the treatment and favorable outcome of this case seems particularly indicated.

PART 7

MIGRAINE

18

Migraine and
Psychogenic Headache

The problem of migraine and psychogenic headache has attracted considerable psychiatric attention. A number of psychiatric investigators in their studies of the psychological aspects of this syndrome have noted a definite relation between the frequency and intensity of the migraine attacks and such factors as anger, resentment, disappointment, criticism, and frustration in work. Selinsky (1939) stresses anxiety and resentment as the prominent emotional forces in migraine and considers attacks of headache as a "physical expression of inhibited protest carried out in a morbid manner." In a psychoanalytic approach to this subject, Frieda Fromm-Reichmann (1937) concludes that migraine is an expression of deeply repressed hostility against a beloved person, occurring in patients with an unresolved ambivalence conflict. Various authors (Knopf, 1935; Touraine and Draper, 1934; Trowbridge et al., 1943; Wolff, 1937; and Moersch, 1924) in personality studies of migraine patients have described a variety of neurotic features such as rigidity, tenseness, sensitivity, ambition, submissiveness, and domineering behavior.

These features are not pathognomic for migraine sufferers. They apply to sufferers from a variety of psychosomatic disorders. All, however, have one basic denominator in common: a pregenital character structure, i.e., oral and anal fixations with low tension tolerance and an urge for immediate discharge of oral and anal sadistic impulses. Because of their character structure, and primarily because of their type of object relationship, which I have called the psychosomatic type of object relationship, these patients do not carry out these impulses in reality and in manifest behavior (Sperling, 1955c, 1957, 1960b, 1960a). In fact, they are not consciously aware of having such impulses, nor do they experience consciously the affects associated with them, in contrast to the psychotic, the psychopath, and the pervert, who are aware of their impulses and act them out in reality. The psychosomatic patient, like the other neurotics, represses objectionable and dangerous impulses and internalizes his conflicts and objects. Therefore, he is not manifestly in conflict with his real objects, his environment, or with society at large. The psychosomatic patient discharges these repressed impulses in the form of somatic symptoms.

But why does one patient produce migraine and another with a similar psychosomatic disposition and in a similar life situation produce ulcers, asthma, or colitis, to name only a few symptoms? The subject of specificity has remained problematic and is a relatively unexplored area in psychosomatic research. While it cannot be fully discussed here, one of the most important misconceptions will have to be dealt with. It would seem to me that much of the confusion in this area is related to the misleading concept of personality profiles, put forward by Dunbar (1947) and Alexander (1950). Certain observations reported by myself and others (Engel, 1955; Mohr et al., 1963; Monsour, 1960; Sperling, 1955c) would seem to invalidate such a concept. I refer particularly to the phenomenon of alternating psychosomatic symptoms—for example, the same patient may alternate between attacks of migraine and ulcerative colitis. My own observations include alternations between asthma and skin disorders, between ulcerative colitis and ulcers of the leg, between rheumatoid arthritis and ulcerative colitis and metrorrhagia, ileitis and spasm of the eye, ulcerative colitis and headache, and petit mal and headache. In these cases there was a shift in symptoms whereby one symptom was given up in favor of another. Such a shift in symptoms during treatment usually indicates a progressive development and occurs when the unconscious fantasies underlying the first symptom have been exposed, but the basic conflict and the quality of the object relationship have not yet been altered. Patients may also switch spontaneously from one symptom to another, going to and fro, for example, between ulcerative colitis and migraine (Engel, 1955; Monsour, 1960).

What are the specific factors which need to be present in a patient with a psychosomatic predisposition to determine which specific psychosomatic symptom he will produce? The study of the structure of conversion symptoms might enhance our understanding. In the conversion symptom, as in any neurotic symptom, there is fulfilment of a wish (the id aspect), while, at the same time, the punishment for the gratification of this forbidden and dangerous wish (the superego aspect) is also present in the symptom (Freud, 1915). A conversion symptom can be understood and resolved only in analysis which exposes the wish and the specific unconscious fantasies which it expressed and which have been gratified in the symptom. I have demonstrated, in the study of a variety of psychosomatic diseases, that the somatic symptoms represent the expression and fulfilment of specific fantasies and impulses of a pregenital nature (oral and anal sadistic). I have suggested that these conditions be considered pregenital conversion neuroses (M. Sperling, 1973).

Because the conflicts in the psychosomatic patient are internalized, the struggle with the frustrating object is carried on internally; in this case, in the head. What specific forms the fantasies will take may depend also on chance experiences. These fantasies are different for each individual, and it is the task of analysis to bring them to the fore and make them conscious so that they lose their pathogenicity. There is a certain similarity, however, in the nature of these fantasies for each psychosomatic symptom. In migraine, the basic similarity in them is that they deal in various ways with attacks on the head. The situation which precipitates a migraine attack represents to the patient a situation of complete helplessness. In the psychosomatic patient, such a situation leads to an instant, transitory regression to the level of primary narcissism. On this regressed level, he deals with the traumatic situation omnipotently. The psychosomatic patient establishes omnipotent control by mobilizing the somatic channels for instant fulfillment and for the discharge of rage. The accompanying manifestations of nausea, vomiting, and diarrhea represent his attempts to rid himself of his destructive impulses somatically as the only possible, immediate mode of discharge (emergency devices in a crisis). The destructive wish is fulfilled and the object and the patient saved from immediate destruction. My interpretation is that each migraine attack represents a repetitive unconscious killing of the frustrating object. There is no conscious awareness of this, no guilt feeling, and no depression. As in a true psychosomatic symptom, these are replaced by the physical pain and suffering the patient inflicts on himself in the symptom.

The majority of the adult patients come for treatment not because of the migraine, although this is a prominent symptom of long standing, but because they suffer from depression. Subsequent work with migraine patients, who came for analysis with migraine as the presenting symptom, has provided additional material and a fuller understanding of the interrelated dynamics and has enabled me to study the relation between migraine and depression on the one hand, and between migraine and states of withdrawal, petit mal, and epilepsy on the other. Before presenting case material and my conclusions based on it, I find it necessary to differentiate, from the dynamic point of view, between migraine proper and other forms of psychogenic headaches. In some cases of psychogenic headaches, the head may unconsciously symbolize the penis, and the pain and other sensations experienced there, such as fullness, enlargement, shrinking, splitting, bursting, or explosive pain, are sensations belonging to erection, ejaculation, and orgasm displaced from the genitals to the head. In these cases, castration anxiety is the main dynamic force, and the conflicts belong to the oedipal and phallic phases. Headaches of these types may be considered classical conversion symptoms. Specific fantasies of a phallic nature together with an overcathexis of the head are the determining factors in the symptom formation in these cases (castration via the head—

often also a form of intellectual castration). The head lends itself particularly well to the expression of bisexual conflicts and can represent both the female and male genitals. Birth fantasies, especially in men, may be expressed through the head, and the sensations and pain are the equivalents of labor pain. In Greek mythology, Pallas Athene sprang from the head of Zeus. The "brainchild" and "laboring" over intellectual problems are indications of such thinking in everyday life. Monsour (1960) considered as the dynamics of migraine in his patients the displacement from the female organs to the head of an unconscious intent to abort or give birth. In some females, the onset of headaches at menarche and premenstrually may be a form of painful "masculine" protest, indicating a conflict about accepting the female role. The narcissistic overevaluation of the head has been considered a dynamic factor in migraine by other investigators (Fromm-Reichmann, 1937).

My second remark concerns the incidence of migraine. Migraine is still believed to be more prevalent among intellectuals. Statistics show, however, that the migraine syndrome is not restricted to groupings on the basis of age, sex, intelligence, or social position, and that it is much more common among the population at large than is usually recognized (Jelliffe, 1933).

A further remark concerns the treatment of migraine patients. In the thirteen to sixteen years of follow-up of the twenty-three patients (fourteen adults and nine children), I found that their treatment was a complete success. There has been no recurrence of the migraine headache in any of these cases to date. So far as I am aware, such results have not been obtained with any other method of treatment. In psychoanalytic treatment, the pregenital character structure of these patients has to be exposed and changed. They have to be enabled to become conscious of their oral and anal sadistic impulses and learn to tolerate psychic tension without immediate discharge of it somatically or by acting out in reality in destructive behavior (rages directed against others or the patient himself). In this connection, the onset of migraine in certain types of personalities in a certain life situation is especially instructive. It occurs in a situation which provokes intense rage and at the same time does not permit the discharge of this rage in overt behavior.

Paula (6½)

Paula was six and a half when she was referred for treatment because of behavior and sleep disturbances. She was very aggressive toward her mother and younger brother, but timid and inhibited in school and with other children. She was very controlling of her mother, who had to sleep with her and to whom she clung in a phobic manner.

Paula had been treated ineffectively for her headaches, thought to be of an allergic nature by an allergy clinic for about two years. In the course of her analysis, I learned of these severe headaches and that she often awoke from a nightmare during the night and in the morning with a headache. Her nightmares were of a claustrophobic character. In them, Paula would find herself imprisoned in a cell or closet, unable to escape and fearful of suffocation. Witches wanted to choke her. Wild animals wanted to eat her up. These nightmares revealed Paula's very strong oral sadistic impulses which had been reactivated and intensified by the birth of her brother when she was four. They also revealed her murderous impulses toward this little brother of whom she was very jealous and envious. These impulses were turned against herself in the typical mechanism of nightmares. She often complained that she could not stand her brother's loud voice and his crying and that it was this that caused her headaches.

In the course of the analysis, with Paula's understanding of her repressed hostility toward her mother, whom she wanted to take away from her little brother and from her father, and with her understanding, too, of her murderous impulses toward her brother, she lost her sleep disturbance and her headaches. She had developed increased confidence in her ability to control her impulses, manifested also in an improved relationship at home and in the ability to play and socialize with other children.

Young children who had not developed rigid defensive attitudes as yet often express their feelings in their treatment in a most instructive manner. One day, Paula told me: "Don't think he's [brother] not bothering me anymore. I can't stand him when he is noisy and teases me. I feel like choking him. But now I know that I won't do it."

A Boy (12)

In a twelve-year-old boy referred for treatment because of the sudden onset of peculiar behavior conspicuous of schizophrenia, one outstanding complaint was that of severe headache. He had suffered from headaches as far back as he could remember and had received dietary treatment, medication, and injections with hardly any experience of relief. Together with the onset of the peculiar behavior, which included his acting and talking like a baby and refusing to go to bed for fear of death in his sleep, his headaches had become more severe.

In the analytic treatment, his immediately acute disturbance could be understood as a reaction to an operation which his mother had undergone. This had served to reactivate an unsolved traumatic experience of his fourth year when his mother also was in the hospital, giving birth to his younger brother. It was at this time, also, that his headaches first began. In his case, the analysis of his nightmares proved particularly interesting. In these nightmares, terrible things always happened to him and he barely managed to awaken before being killed. The way in which he was to be killed was consistently by an attack upon the head; most frequently a rock was to fall on his head, or he was to be shot in the head, or someone was to throw a stone at his head. With awareness of his very strong repressed hostility against his younger brother and of his wish to harm him, there occurred a significant change in the character of his dreams. While previously he had been the victim, now he allowed himself, at least in his dreams, to be the successful attacker. Prior to the treatment, his mother had twice found him trying to gag his brother, "in play," as he explained to her. Becoming conscious of these impulses against his brother enabled him to express his hostility in a more appropriate manner and made the headache unnecessary.

I should like to add here that some favorable changes took place in his environment. His mother's attitude was much different; she overcame to some extent her rejection of him, which had been covered up by an overprotective attitude, and even allowed him to own a dog, in spite of his brother's allergy to dogs.

He also liked his new schoolteacher, while he disliked his previous one intensely. This was mainly due to his very much improved relationship with his mother. And for the first time in his life, he went to camp for the summer.

A Girl (15)

A fifteen-year-old girl had suffered from severe migraine headaches since the age of ten. Her attacks were so severe that she would be sick for two to three days at a time, had to stay in bed in a dark room, and could not tolerate any noise.

Around the age of ten, in a fight with her brother, she hit his head against the stairs and almost killed him. She was very frightened about this loss of control, and it was shortly after that she developed the migraine headaches. There were other noticeable changes in her behavior at that time. She became markedly inhibited and developed many compulsions and rituals. All these, her analysis showed, were mechanisms designed to help her keep in check her destructive impulses. Shortly after her brother was born, when she was four, she "accidentally" set herself on fire and nearly burned to death. This patient also, both prior to and during part of her analysis, had a number of serious accidents, in particular, "falling" accidents.

Certain visual phenomena initiating and concomitant with migraine attacks are common and well known. This patient would see yellow lights before developing a migraine attack. The color yellow had for her a specific unconscious significance which she brought to light in her analysis. Her mother had had jaundice during the latter part of her pregnancy. Her brother had been very sick as a baby. The patient remembered him lying in the crib and looking very yellow. Apparently he too was jaundiced, and he was hospitalized for some time. The patient remembered that one late afternoon at dusk (this particular time of day and its light have remained of significance to her) when she looked into his crib, he was not there. Apparently he had been taken to the hospital. To the patient, the fact that he had gone meant that he was dead, and she did not expect him to return home alive. The material which demonstrates these connections more clearly cannot be cited here; it would require the detailed presentation of the associations, fantasies, and dreams of many sessions, which led to the reconstruction of these events and her reactions to them at that time. In her analysis it was found that her migraine represented the equivalent of an acute attack of depression with suicidal impulses, resulting from her attitude toward brother and death wishes against her mother. She was extremely attached to and dependent upon her mother and could not conceive of being able to live without her.

This case lends itself to discussion of several aspects of the migraine syndrome. To begin with the role of the constitutional element: the mother of this patient also suffered from migraine. She also had had attacks of syncope which the patient had witnessed on at least one or two occasions. The mother, a compulsive, rigid woman, was hostile to psychiatry, and I had seen her only once, in the initial interview. She had reluctantly agreed to treatment for her daughter because medical treatment had been ineffective, and because a highly regarded, psychoanalytically oriented member of the family had insisted upon it. It is frequently found in the history of migraine patients that some other member of their family also suffers from migraine. This factor would seem to support the concept that the constitutional element is very important, but what follows may indicate that this is a misleading concept. The above patient, whom I treated at the age of fifteen, consulted me again when twenty-eight because of marital problems. She was frigid, and also had some difficulties with her two children. I then learned that she had had no recurrence of the migraine through all these years, in spite of some difficult emotional situations, while her mother had remained a severe migraine sufferer. I do not seek to prove or to disprove the existence of a constitutional factor in migraine, but this case, as is true of all my other cases, proves that this factor is irrelevant and that its role has to be played down and devaluated in the treatment of such a patient. In this case, I did so to impress the patient with the fact that she did not have to be a lifelong migraine sufferer like her mother.

Discussion

Psychodynamically, migraine sufferers are orally fixated individuals and closely related to the two main oral types: the depressive and the impulse-ridden character. We can now understand from a dynamic point of view the frequent association of migraine with depression and other oral character manifestations. In these cases, very strong dependence upon the mother or mother substitutes (Johnson, 1946) is often overcompensated by exaggerated independence, self-sufficiency, and domineering behavior. The oral fixation also can be seen in the sexual behavior of the migraine and headache patient.

The very strongly developed anal sadism in these cases is coped with by reaction formations and not by true sublimations. This explains the rigidity and tenseness so often found in these patients. Occasionally there is a breakthrough of these sadistic impulses.

The personality of the patient with migraine and chronic headache is characterized by an extreme inability to tolerate injury to his narcissism. The hypersensitivity of the headache patient noted by most observers (Weber, 1932) is one way in which their highly narcissistic orientation manifests itself. Any such injury to the patient's narcissism—sometimes so insignificant that it is completely overlooked by the environment—provokes an intense rage reaction with an urge for immediate discharge. To be fully conscious of this rage is considered dangerous by the patient, who fears that he cannot resist the urge for destruction of the frustrating object or of himself. Repression of this rage and of the impulse to kill serves to protect both the object in the outer world and the patient himself. At the same time, the gratification of the impulse is achieved unconsciously in the symptom. Every successive headache in the migrainous patient is such a repetitive unconscious killing of the frustrating object. There is no guilt feeling, the punishment being inflicted by the patient upon himself in the physical pain and suffering. The choice of the specific symptom, headache, is determined by the specific impulse to kill the object by an attack upon the head as an expedient and primitive way of killing, whether this be by choking, bashing in of the head, or shooting through or crushing the head. The accompanying manifestations of nausea, vomiting, and diarrhea represent the patient's attempts to rid himself of his destructive impulses somatically.

In the treatment, the underlying pregenital neurosis has to be exposed and the patient enabled to become conscious of his oral and anal sadistic impulses and to learn to tolerate a certain amount of psychic tension. This is the basis for control over and true sublimation of such impulses.

I should, perhaps, mention here that I do not use any medication. In fact, treatment is aimed at helping the patient to wean himself very early from whatever medication he may have used previously. The emotional factors which trigger off the mechanisms, psychological and physiological, which lead to the migraine attack are those which have to be dealt with. Once these factors are exposed and resolved through treatment, the migraine attacks cease. There is a phase during the treatment when the patient learns to abort attacks. This occurs at the time when he has not yet given up the urge to gratify destructive impulses immediately and still needs to assure himself by a short-lived attack that he is in omnipotent control. I will illustrate this with one example from that phase of the treatment of a thirty-two-year-old woman with severe migraine. Before having a migraine, she felt its onset; she saw lights and colors before her eyes and pinwheels like zigzags. This time, she said to herself, "I don't have to kill him [her husband], even if I'm very furious." She was very angry with him. He had been very short and cross with her and the children. She thought of a remark I had made when she told me about a migraine headache she had begun to develop on her way to the session but which had stopped suddenly. I had said, "So you decided to let me live." She had another migraine headache. She saw red, white, and blue, like blood pulsating, filling, and receding. She felt very uncomfortable, and it made her feel dizzy. Then the pinwheel grew bigger and bigger, and she could not see things clearly. It was as if pieces were missing. She saw only half of the chair, and then it was like a blank. She lay down and decided to take a pill, but, by that time, she could not even see or read the label on the bottle. She lay still for a few minutes, but did not develop a migraine. She thought of the two other times when she also had stopped it at the onset.

This behavior is similar to that of patients with other psychosomatic syndromes. In this connection, I am thinking also of a phenomenon observed particularly in asthma and in patients with petit mal and epilepsy. It has been found that psychoanalytic treatment does not alter the allergic sensitivities of the asthma patient, although it cures him of his asthma (Gerard,1946; see also chapter 15).The same holds true for petit mal and epilepsy. Abnormalities in the electroencephalogram are retained by these patients after successful psychoanalytic treatment, yet they no longer react with the characteristic attacks to precipitating events.

With regard to the interrelated dynamics of migraine and depression, I wish to draw attention to the similarity in personality structure. Fixation to pregenital (particularly to oral sadistic) levels of instinctual development, a highly narcissistic orientation with extreme vulnerability to the slightest injury, and the persistence of magical thinking are characteristic for both depression and migraine, especially in those types who alternate between the two.

The change from the somatic symptom (migraine) to manifest depression or hypomania is of particular interest. Why does the same patient at one time suffer from depression or hypomanic state, and at another time migraine? What does this mean dynamically? This phenomenon of alternating psychosomatic and overt neurotic or psychotic behavior has also been observed in other psychosomatic diseases. I have been able to relate the occurrence of this phenomenon to sudden changes in object relationship. In the case of the psychosomatic patient, there is an increase in object cathexis in the situation of loss or threatened loss of the object. This loss can be real or imagined, coming from the object or the patient himself (giving up the object in rage). Not only is the object retained in reality by the psychosomatic patient, but the tie is strengthened by the illness. The giving up of the object (destructively) occurs symbolically through the symptom.

In the case of depression, there is a decrease in object cathexis and withdrawal from the external object. The struggle goes on with the internalized object within the ego and superego. With the increase in object cathexis and the turning toward the external object, there is repression of destructive and objectionable impulses directed toward the object and the self. In this relationship, the psychosomatic type of object relationship, it pays to be sick, particularly since the destructive impulses are gratified in reality. By the very fact that he is sick, he can indulge himself and be indulged by others. In depression, there is an overt accusation and exposure of the frustrating object and a giving up of the real object, which is lost to the patient by real or fantasied destruction—a killing off of the object in fantasy and mourning for its loss. The factors which bring about and determine these fluctuations in object cathexis in these patients with very ambivalent object relationships have to do with narcissitic injuries and disappointments suffered in reality or in fantasy.

The Relation of Migraine Headaches to States of Withdrawal, Petit Mal, and Epilepsy

Certain sensations experienced by some migraine patients immediately preceding the onset of the migraine attack, as well as their behavior during the attack, indicate that they are under the influence of strong tendencies to withdraw from reality. I have in mind here particularly those who, as a prodromal symptom, experience dizziness, often so intense that they have to hold on to some external object to prevent themselves from falling. Their migraine is usually so severe that they have to stop whatever they are doing and withdraw to bed in a darkened room. Some of them are extremely sensitive to noises and any external stimuli and find relief only in sleep. Some patients actually suffer brief lapses of consciousness preceding the onset of a migraine attack.

Migraine attacks can be triggered off by stimuli specific to the patient because of their association with his unconscious fantasies. These may be visual, olfactory, or auditory stimuli, very similar to those which trigger off petit mal or attacks of epilepsy. In Paula's case, migraine attacks were precipitated by certain noises which unconsciously reminded her of the crying of the hated sibling whom she would have wanted to kill by choking or hitting over the head, or, as in one instance, by stuffing something into the baby's mouth and putting a pillow over its head. Some migraine patients also have an aura similar to that in petit mal and epileptic patients. To differentiate between these prodromal symptoms in certain migraine patients and petit mal may at times be difficult. I believe that there are transitions between these conditions and some basic similarities in their dynamics (Cesio, 1954; Engel et al., 1953; Garma, 1959; Sperling, see chapter 20). I have found as a regular occurrence in petit mal that, during the phase of treatment when the patients no longer have petit mal attacks, they develop headaches of a very characteristic type. Most patients describe them as a sensation of being tapped on the head. One patient, who had suffered from petit mal and grand mal and who developed migraine headaches during the transitory phase, had the sensation, especially when walking upstairs, that somebody was pushing her on the head. She had twice fallen down a flight of stairs. She had a remarkable facility for falling during this phase of treatment when she was fully conscious and without any obstacles in her way (epilepsy = falling sickness). At times, this was really a kind of deliberate throwing herself to the floor.

I interpret this change in symptom from petit mal and epilepsy to headaches as an indication of progress in treatment. It represents a different mode of dealing with the same conflicts and impulses which before had led to the attacks of petit mal or epilepsy, and signifies an increase in ego strength. In petit mal there is an instant cutting off from functioning of those parts of the mind which serve the perception and execution of certain stimuli from within and without, instead of a lapse into complete unconsciousness and discharging of these impulses in convulsions as in the epileptic attack. In the migraine attack, the patient remains conscious and in full contact with reality. The mechanism is now acute repression of the dangerous impulses and partial discharge and gratification in the headaches. Whenever a specific experience mobilizes these repressed destructive impulses and a breakthrough into consciousness is imminent, the patient develops headaches. Together with this change in the course of treatment from the symptom of petit mal and epilepsy to the symptom of migraine, there is a decrease in the intensity and urgency of the destructive impulses owing to the fact that the patient is now able to accept the existence of such impulses consciously and has developed a feeling that he does not have to carry them out instantly when met with frustration. I consider that this interrelation between migraine headaches and epilepsy and petit mal is not based primarily upon a common inherited somatic constitution, but rather upon a specific and early acquired attitude of the patient toward dealing with overwhelmingly strong destructive impulses. In this connection, the environmental factors, particularly the interrelated dynamics of the parental attitudes and the child's responses, are great importance.

I have not concerned myself here with the physiological mechanisms and vascular phenomena characteristic of the migraine attack, nor with the physiological mechanisms operative in petit mal and epilepsy. As a psychoanalyst, I have been concerned solely with the study of psychic mechanisms and of unconscious conflicts, fantasies and impulses.

PART 8

EPILEPSY

19

Epilepsy, Psychodynamics and Therapy

In many cases of epilepsy there is a latent tendency to perversion and criminality. These tendencies may be covered up by a sweet or even saintly manifest attitude, so they are not apparent to others. Because these tendencies are not acceptable to the conscious personality, the epileptic patient tries to exclude them from consciousness and to gratify them in unconscious daydreams and in petit mal and grand mal attacks with retrograde amnesia. The epileptic attack is a kind of self-protection from acting out such tendencies in reality and thus protects the environment from the asocial impulses of such a person. The attack also expresses guilt feelings and serves as punishment for the forbidden deeds. Finally, the attack symbolizes death and rebirth.

The nature and intensity of the attack depend on the degree of regression and can range from fainting spells or a fit of rage or migraine headaches to petit mal and grand mal attacks and even to status epilepticus. In these attacks the patient may live out a more recent trauma or a trauma from childhood or regress to the trauma of birth or to a prenatal, that is, an intrauterine, existence. In the attack, the patient may experience his own death or commit a forbidden sexual or criminal act such as vampirism, cannibalism, necrophilia, or murder. In the epileptic furor, the protective function of the attack fails. The patient does not fall unconscious to the floor but may commit some of these criminal acts in reality. For example, Olga, in a fit of rage, would break mirrors and brushes and have accidents. William used to hit his head with his fists or knock it against the wall before he developed attacks. On three occasions he had what he referred to as "live attacks." These were psychotic states. In one of these "attacks" he nearly jumped off the roof. Ann would wake up with headaches; the thought that she would have to get out of bed and go to work was intolerable. She would then have an attack and afterwards feel very tired and need a lot of sleep. She would also have many petit mal attacks but this would not prevent her from having a grand mal attack. William could have several attacks in succession. Olga could remember the content of the petit mal spells which she had in my office. It had to do with a man cutting something which she thought was a human body in half. These fantasies of cutting and dismembering bodies, especially of cutting off the head and limbs, were basic fantasies which had originated in early childhood and which were dynamic forces in her epilepsy. They ultimately went back to her concept of birth and of the cutting of the umbilical cord, which she connected with having had head surgery during the first year of life. Ann was reenacting in her attacks an early childhood trauma of the primal scene where she had played dead. She wanted her copulating parents to stop and not to move. Since she could not achieve this, she became motionless herself. She thought that her parents had turned into wolves and would eat her up if she moved or made any noise. Olga in her petit mal spells where she suddenly stopped whatever she was doing was also reenacting a similar early trauma. She felt that if she wanted something to stop and it would not, that she could not tolerate it and would go crazy. This was her reaction to the primal scene.

In most cases of epilepsy, there are neurotic compulsion mechanisms operative leading to overcompensation and giving the personality of the epileptic the characteristic mixture of religiosity and criminality, "devil or saint." However, compulsion neurotic defense mechanisms are not sufficient to protect the epileptic from having attacks while for the compulsion neurotic they are effective.

The epileptic, like the infant, has a great need for sleep. He cannot tolerate being awakened prematurely and reacts to this with irritability. There is also an inappropriate relationship between the stimulus and the reaction which contributes to the misimpression that the epileptic attack is not initiated by an external event. The event may be so innocuous to the environment as not to be noticed, but it has meaning to the epileptic patient and explains the reaction.

The epileptic suffers from a hypertrophic fantasy life and a wish for withdrawal from reality into sleep and dreams. In the dream and fantasy world, he can indulge in the forbidden wishes and fantasies, and if this is not sufficient, he acts them out in petit mal or grand mal attacks. Amnesia is a protection against remembering the dream and fantasy life and against being aware of them consciously. The frequency, intensity, and quality of daydreams are a very important factor in epilepsy. This aspect could be studied very clearly in Ann. She had long daydreams already at the age of four and intensive dreams and nightmares in early childhood. She had unusually intense daydreaming in puberty and adolescence which at times was of a hallucinatory quality. Petit mal began in early adolescence, and grand mal followed in later adolescence. There is a progressive character in many cases of epilepsy with intensification of introversion and need for sleep.

Important implications for therapy can be derived from the need for withdrawal and sleep. Curtailment of sleep and of the use of sedatives and narcotics is essential in the treatment of epileptics. One of the reasons why sedatives are effective in minimizing or eliminating attacks is that these drugs support amnesia and deepen sleep so the objectionable tendencies and sadistic impulses can be lived out in a drug sleep without memory. The patient has to be encouraged to work in spite of the attacks. Although sudden withdrawal of medication can be very dangerous, medication, because it increases the introversion and daydreaming and makes sleep deeper, should be slowly reduced. In this connection a case reported by Clark (1931) is of particular interest. The patient was a twenty-six year old man who had had grand mal attacks for at least fifteen years. After being diagnosed as hopelessly demented in the state hospital, he was admitted to Craig Colony and had seizures almost every day. Upon Clark's suggestion, the amount of sedatives was reduced considerably. In four months the patient ceased having attacks. He was forced to go to work which he hated. He also was weaned away from his mother, who tried to coddle him all the time. His first spontaneous interest was reading. After trying a variety of activities, he learned the trade of printing and earned his living for eighteen years without the return of symptoms.

Clark, who worked with epileptics in an educational way in the early twenties, considered the epileptic attack a regression to fetal movements. He emphasized the pleasure principle and the libidinal aspects. He did not consider the epileptic capable of adjusting to the environment and recommended that the environment be adapted to the needs of the epileptic patient. There are three basic mistakes in this kind of thinking: (1) epilepsy is regarded as a fate which is inherited; (2) all attacks are based on womb fantasies; and (3) there is no consideration given to the role of aggression and perversion, nor to the importance of infantile traumata and experiences and the repetition of such traumata in the epileptic attack.

According to Freud (1928), every individual is capable of having an epileptic reaction, and orgasm is the prototype of such a reaction. The epileptic attack is a pathological reaction of the brain which can be brought on in various ways, by stimulation, injury, intoxication, and other damage to the brain. Jelliffe and White (1915, p. 28) explained epileptic seizures as a discharge of accumulated chemical energy. Steckel (1924) stressed hate and criminal tendencies as important dynamic factors in epilepsy, as did Wittels (1940). Bandler et al. (1958) concerned themselves with the role of sexuality in epilepsy. On the basis of a combined psychiatric and physiological study of thirty women over three years, these authors concluded that the nuclear conflict is a sexual one. They believe that aggression and other conflicts play only a minor part. According to these authors, attacks occur in relationship to current sexual conflicts and to sexual transference, and past seizures occurred in relationship to past sexual conflicts similar to the current one.

Sexuality is certainly a very important precipitating factor in epileptic attacks. For a long period during his treatment, William would masturbate in the bathroom before coming into the office. During sessions he would ostensibly work himself up sexually by looking at my legs and breasts and by watching every movement. If I interfered or interpreted, he threatened with and on several occasions had epileptic attacks in my office. Thus he "attacked me" sexually without raping or killing me in reality.

To single out sexuality as the nuclear conflict seems to me a one-sided position. The epileptic attack, like every neurotic or psychosomatic symptom, is highly overdetermined. Certainly the quality of the sexual impulses in epileptics has to be considered. We are dealing mainly with pregenital perverse oral and anal destructive impulses. Oedipal genital sexual impulses in these cases are forbidden too, because of their incestuous and murderous nature.

For the connection between sexuality and epilepsy, it is important to consider two kinds of masturbation—(a) with acceptable conscious fantasies and (b) with forbidden unconscious, perverse fantasies. The latter fantasies are acted out in petit mal and grand mal attacks. In the attack, both active and passive sexual tendencies are gratified, including death, birth, and rebirth fantasies. Ann is a particularly instructive case. She was man and woman, attacker and victim; orgasm and death were equated. Because of this equation there is a lust in dying. This information is usually difficult to obtain from the epileptic patient. In her fantasies, Ann was embracing the Angel of Death and experienceing a climax. After the attack, she felt tired and sleepy. In this case, sexual impulses prevailed in the precipitation of the attack. When criminal impulses predominate, the patient experiences guilt and misery after the attack.

Freedman and Adatto (1968) report observations of eight ictal episodes in an adolescent boy. In each instance it was possible to demonstrate that the attack occurred when he wished and feared an attack by the analyst. They consider as the critical factor, which may be applicable to other cases, a situation where

290 Psychosomatic Disorders in Childhood

there is no other available resolution to intense, mutually incompatible feelings.

Gottschalk's patient (1956) often seemed to induce attacks by staring at screens with checkered patterns. He would stare up and to the left. This act was found to relate and to repeat a primal scene observation. This was the way he could look from his bed into his parents' bedroom which had a checkered pattern. Under stress conditions he would actively seek out a seizure. Gottschalk also mentioned that Dostoevsky reported intense pleasure in association with his attacks. Here the observations of Stekel (1924) and Graven (1924) that patients can willfully bring on attacks are of interest. Stekel mentions the case of the catatonic woman who developed grand mal seizures for the first time when she was told that she wanted to kill her father. This woman had been in a catatonic state for thiry years following a rape assault by her father.

The case reported by Menninger (1926) is similar to that of one of my patients, whose epileptic attacks were found to be a reaction to her husband's behavior toward her. Her condition improved when she was away from her husband. In this case it was hate and murderous impulses against her husband by whom she felt continually humiliated. These feelings were major dynamic factors in her attacks. In Menninger's case, the epilepsy began with her engagement, became aggravated with her marriage, and was most severe during her pregnancy. Whenever she visited her husband, there was an increase in attacks. According to Menninger, improvement was due to a combination of factors, among them transference, catharsis, and environmental alteration.

Kardiner (1932) mentions the case of a man who felt that he changed into a woman after attacks. My patient, who fantasied being the creator of the world all by herself, was not only taking the place of God, but was enacting a bisexual fantasy of being both female and male in one. On the conscious level this meant that she was a hermaphrodite. On the unconscious level in her grand mal attacks, she was portraying the cohabitating parents who by their violent movements and noises had shocked her into a motionless state when she was two.

According to Scott (1969), the Apostle Paul, Buddha,

Alexander the Great, Julius Caesar, Mohammed, Pascal, Flaubert, Paganini, Byron, Napoleon, Swinburne, van Gogh, and Pope Pius IX were epileptics. Van Gogh's convulsions, however, were obviously due to intoxication with absinthe and were a kind of poisoning of the brain. He became delirious and hallucinated after drinking absinthe in excess. Scott is not dynamically oriented and does not understand that epilepsy had a protective function, protecting the epileptic from becoming a criminal or pervert in reality. These tendencies are released in the epileptic attack without conscious awareness.

The fact that epilespy occurs in the body should not mislead us into thinking that it is purely a body function. Urination and defecation also occur in the body and Freud has shown that in human beings these functions have instinctual social meanings such as self-assertion, sexuality, or revenge. So is it with epilepsy. Although it can be brought on in animals and in human beings at will by chemical or electric stimulation, when it occurs in human beings spontaneously, it has meaning.

Some of my readers who are used to thinking of epilepsy as an organic disease and of the epileptic amnesia as an unfailing accompaniment of the grand mal and psychomotor attacks might take exception to my attributing meaning to the epileptic amnesia. May I remind them that epileptic amnesia can be lifted by hypnosis, as has been proven by Muralt, (1902), Ricklin (1905), Oberholzer (1914) and Schilder (1928). Anything hypnosis is able to do, psychoanalysis should also be able to do, and more. In addition, with the Ebbinghaus method, it is possible to find vestiges of the experiences during the psychomotor attack regardless of whether it appeared dream-like, confused, or pseudonormal (Schilder, 1928). The term *psychomotor attack* itself is discouraging to the psychoanalyst, since it emphasizes the organic character of the symptom. It should rather be regarded as a short-lived psychosis which should be analyzed. In a case of Noyes and Kolb (1958), a clouded state lasted for several months.

John (9)

John was referred to me at age nine for a short attempt at psychotherapy because of attacks of unconsciousness and convulsions once every two to four weeks. These had developed after encephalitis at age five. Since then, there had also been a progressive mental deterioration from an IQ of 115 to an IQ of 85. I saw him in the hospital where he had stayed because of a leg fracture incurred by falling off a staircase during a seizure.

His attacks had been observed during several stays in the hospital. They involved clonic movements, sometimes of the right arm and leg, sometimes of the left leg, sometimes only of the right corner of his mouth, sometimes grand mal attacks, the head and eyes deviating to the left. The convulsions were followed by vomiting and sleep, but there was no loss of sphincter tone nor biting of the tongue. Several electroencephalograms showed diffusely distributed abnormality. The last one was grossly abnormal. On physical examination, he showed physical awkwardness and ataxia of station and gait. He was dull and exhibited a frequent silly grin. His speech was distinct but slow. He had been regularly taking dilantin, mesantoin, phenobarb, and more recently, phenurone.

When he came for his first session, he knew me already. He seemed to be pleased to see me. When he wanted to hug me, I gave him a doll and a pillow to act out his feelings on, to do with as he would have liked to do with me and with other people. He then said, "I would like to knock the children over the head so they would fall unconscious."

I explained to him that I was interested in what he was thinking and dreaming. He was obviously very eager to please and at his next session related the following "dream": He fell into a hole. He wanted to get some gold but the fat cop didn't let him and put him into jail for ten years. By mistake somebody put the key in and he put his hand through the bars but he got caught. Once the bars broke, and he got out after five years. Somebody asked him about the man who escaped from jail.

This was obviously a condensation of many fantasies and feelings in which he felt caught and tried to escape. The gold and the fat cop pointed to his father; he had already in our first meeting at the hospital told me that his father was a big man and had a lot of money. After finishing the story, which he referred to as a dream, he proceeded to tell me that he would get his father's business when his father died and then he would be the boss. He would then get married when he grew up, although a boy in his class had said he would never get married.

A few sessions later, he spoke frequently about "little John" who wanted him to go back into the belly of his mother. Just that day during recreation in school, he said "little John" had told him he wanted to be back in his mother's tummy and he told him, nothing doing. He carried him out of the school and locked him up. This story reveals his unsuccessful way of dealing with his infantile wishes by trying to lock them up and then feeling locked up himself. I suggested that "little John" might not like that and he replied, "Just too bad, he's still crying." He then continued to talk about his little sister and her name. His present exacerbation had occurred right after the birth of this sister. He became visibly excited as he was speaking about her, especially about her name. She had two names, the last one being Joy. I asked "Who is Joy?" and he said, looking at me, "Little John wants me to slap you in the face." I interpreted to him that he was angry at me for not preventing his mother from having a baby. This interpretation calmed him down considerably.

John was in the habit of falling frequently in school and at home without having attacks. The other day he told me about his grandmother tripping over his legs. (His father later filled in this story telling me that John had actually pulled his grandmother down.) John then continued to tell me with glee in his eyes that he could observe how she turned over. He got up and helped her up. He had blood on his hands. He looked to see where it came from. With a loud laugh, he said, "It came from my grandmother's nose. She will get insurance money anyway," he said, and then suddenly with loud laughter, "If that had been my mother, good-bye baby." This is what he really would have wanted to do, to push his pregnant mother down the staircase. This incident occurred before the birth of the baby when his mother was in her ninth month.

When his mother was in the hospital giving birth to the baby, John hadn't mentioned this fact to me at all. Only after I asked him who had brought him for his session and where his mother was, did he tell me in a very casual tone, "Oh, she had a girl. She's in the hospital. She'll have a boy the next time." He didn't want to talk about it any further. He wanted to play.

In one of his next sessions, he seemed very tired, sleepy and sluggish, speaking slowly and stretching a lot. He spoke about the light in the room bothering him and said something about its being dangerous and blowing me away. Only casually, he had mentioned that his mother had come home the day before with the baby and then added that she had a pain in her belly and that every mother gets that. "They get so excited over the baby." He spoke about the boys in school teasing him and said he had a bad dream: Somebody was under his cot pushing him up in the air, then shooting at him. He was falling down on the man on the floor, then he was taking a gun out of his pocket and shooting the man. He said he had a lot of silly dreams, mainly flying dreams, and he always was falling down. He obviously did not want to talk about the baby. He said that his mother went to the hospital and then the nurse brought her the baby. He refused to recognize the real situation, and a marked change in his behavior impressed me as if he were preparing himself for an attack.

In the session before, he had complained about the maid giving him burned food, burned eggs and cereal. He also said that she did not like boys, did not like him and his father but that she gave good food to his older sister. He said that he would play a trick on her the next time and throw the eggs in her face. Then he told the following story from the time he was in the hospital when he was five years old. It was after visiting hours and he was supposed to go home that day. He fell asleep and then it was night and Dr. K. was on his bed. His parents came to take him home, although they had not expected to. His older sister kicked him down the stairs in the hospital and his brain became infected. It had started with his saying she was dumb and had a brain like a horse and that if he hit her over the head, no brain would be left because she had only two or four brains. When his brain was tested, the man said that he had wood in his head. Then he had to stay in the hospital another week. When his parents came to take him home, his sister kicked him up to the ceiling, broke the light and broke his head, and he had to stay in the hospital a month. When he came home, his sister was in bed so he kicked her down the stairs. Her brain became infected. Then he kicked her up to the ceiling but he didn't break the light, nor her head because that wouldn't be nice. He only cracked her head, but the ceiling started to come down. Telling this story he became more and more excited and said to me, "Take your glasses off. I will show you. You are my sister." He hit the pillow several times, punched it again and then threw it up. He wanted to kiss me when he left and said, "My head is all cleared up now." His older sister, the one who supposedly had kicked him down the stairs, is four years older than John.

It should be stated here that in this seemingly senseless way, John was telling the story of his illness. He had been a healthy child of superior intelligence up to age five. At that time he came to the hospital in a state of unconsciousness and moderate fever. He had several attacks of Jacksonian epilepsy and after thorough examination the diagnosis of encephalitis of unknown origin was made.

The following treatment sessions were taken up with many involved dreams, mostly "bad" ones where he was shot or nearly shot or caught with a rope around his neck and choked. He told me that whenever he felt frustrated with something or somebody he would hit himself on the head and I interpreted to him that this is what he would like to do to those who frustrate him; that he would get angry and want to fight but that he really wasn't allowed to fight. He laughed, relieved.

I had also interpreted this in the transference, that when I said something he didn't like he wanted to hit me over the head too. In the following session, when I said something he did not like, he came at my head with a board. When I reminded him of my interpretation, he stopped and laughed. Later he said that he could anticipate the spells and described the onset of an aura. It was like the ticking of a clock in his stomach. When this happened, he would prepare to fall so that he wouldn't hurt himself. Then he would lose consciousness.

The treatment of these children in their home environment presents some special difficulties. The parents accept as good behavior submission on the part of the child. During the process of freeing aggression from symptoms, the child may meet with rejection from his parents. John too threatened to run away and twice he actually took his hat and coat but returned after a short time. If the child meets with constant disapproval and rejection from his parents, then his conflicts are only intensified. On the other hand, there is no transformation of instinctual energy possible unless this energy is freed from repression. The handling of this transitional phase in the treatment of such children is a difficult technical problem. It is necessary to impress the child with the need to control such impulses, at least in school, because there he runs the risk of being expelled by the school. This actually happened to John. It is essential to get the cooperation of the parents so that they will provide suitable motor outlets for the child, such as hard play or construction work. John had wanted a bike, and we worked out in the therapeutic sessions the dangers involved in falling off and crossing the streets. He pleaded and assured me that nothing would happen and he wanted to "make a deal." The father himself had noted that John did rather well on the occasions when he was allowed to ride his sister's bike, but John told me that he as a big boy resented very much riding a girl's bike. We had agreed that his father would get him a workbench in the basement so that he could work with tools and wood, but somehow this did not materialize. John and his father couldn't agree. John didn't want a very small workbench which his father had offered him. He had been very disappointed in his father. His father, in talking to me about this later, said that he had not understood the boy's needs and felt guilty for the way in which he had treated John, very harsh and rejecting.

The day before this quarrel he had a major attack. John had gone to the doctor for a treatment. The doctor took off the cast without assistance. The entire handling of the fracture was very poor. Nobody was allowed into the hospital. John had three readjustments, two under anesthesia. The cast had an unconscious meaning. In reality, it had given him an exceptional position. He felt stronger with it. In the hospital, he had refused to take any medications. He spit them out. I learned from the parents that after the removal of the cast, an attack had recurred that evening.

The morning after the quarrel with his father, John had a severe epileptic fit from which he did not seem to recover and the parents had called me. When I saw him at his house, he was in a semistupor, lying on the bed with his eyes closed. He seemed to recognize my voice, although he did not seem to be aware of the environment. It was possible for me to arouse him out of this stupor temporarily and to interpret to him what he was doing. He seemed to hear me and to understand although he appeared to be very weak and drowsy. He called me by my name and said something about his father falling down two flights of stairs. He seemed to be concerned about his father. He calmed down and appeared to be quiet but sleepy. John's father told me that they had quarreled and he felt that John must have been very disappointed in him.

This example shows how cause and purpose combine in the motivation of the epileptic attack. The causes: the accumulated angers about the hospital, the handling of the fracture and the taking off the cast, several lumbopunctures, pneumoencephalograms, and anger about the father. The purpose: to protect John's father from his anger (as expressed in concern for his father falling down two flights of stairs).

Bob (17)

Bob was referred for treatment at seventeen. He had had his first attack a year before on the morning after his sister's engagement. He had been free of attacks for nearly a year and had his second attack coming home from a visit to her. She was now married and lived in a different community. He had a third attack, two months later while shopping with his father for a gift for her. He had his fourth attack on the day that she arrived for a visit at his home. He had not seen her yet, since he had left for school in the morning. He had this attack coming home from school on the subway and was brought to the hospital by ambulance. He had his fifth attack, after which he was referred for treatment, on a Sunday morning just a few days after his fourth attack. His sister was still staying at his house at that time. He was shopping at the bakery and fell and injured his scalp. He was brought to the hospital and had to have stitches. On this Sunday, he and his parents were supposed to go to the wedding of his sister's friend. It was for this purpose that his sister had come to the city but because of his attack his parents and he did not go.

At his first interview, he was obviously concerned with making a good impression and being a cooperative patient. We had talked about childhood memories and dreams. At his second session, he said that he remembered early childhood dreams in which falling was the outstanding feeling. In some of these dreams he would be standing on a ridge and falling off. Coming in for his third session, he was humming the song "Secret Love" and then another song "La Mer" or as he said "The Sea." He further explained that this meant "The Mother."

Pointing to the patch on his head where he had the stitches, he said that it had done him good; he had had no attacks since. I asked whether he had to knock himself on the head like that in order not to have attacks. To this he replied, "Do you know how it happened that I fell in the bakery? There was a little old lady who pushed herself ahead of the line in the bakery store. Now, what I could have done to her." While having these thoughts, he explained, he had had the attack.

He always like to twiddle and play with things while talking, but his mother did not like him to do that. In the fourth session he related his first dream. He said that it was a recurrent dream and that he had been dreaming it for about the last ten years. He had it in different versions hundreds of times. This is the dream: the marines are there (this takes place during the war). He is standing on a cliff, falling.

He said that these were his typical dreams, falling dreams, often without content, just the sensation of falling. In his next session, he said that he had had a bloody dream. In this dream someone was all bloody but he didn't know who it was. He then talked about his sister, who had returned to her home, and told me that she was pregnant and due to have a baby soon, and that his mother was concerned about this event and planned to stay with his sister during childbirth.

A few days later he had an attack on the way to school and afterwards slept five hours and missed his appointment. At his next session, he said that he thought maybe the fact that he was going to get a report card on that day had something to do with the attack, which he referred to as "my fainting spell."

His parents had not told him that his attacks had been diagnosed as epilepsy, and I had to explain this to him. He had been humming a song like "What am I going to do about you?" He then corrected his humming to "What am I going to do without you?" "Down by the riverside," "A boy asked for a kiss," "One of a roving kind." This was apparently how he was announcing to me that he was leaving me. His parents had decided to move to the city where his sister lived.

William (13)

William was referred for psychoanalytic psychotherapy at thirteen with the diagnosis of psychomotor epilepsy. At four, when he had an upper respiratory infection with high fever, he had a convulsion and two years later developed brief choking spells. His throat felt as if there were something stuck there; he had to swallow and spit a lot. He also had strange sensations in his hands, especially in the left one, as if they were shrinking or he was losing them. A neurological examination, including EEG, was negative then. At ten he again had a complete neurological checkup. The EEG and everything else were found normal. He was diagnosed as having psychomotor epilepsy and put on phenobarbital. At seven he had psychotherapy for half of a year because of his hand and throat symptoms, but it had little effect. His IQ at that time was 131. At eight he had a tonsillectomy. This only increased his choking sensation and was a very traumatic experience, as will be seen later. When he was nine, his father was hospitalized for several months.

He had been bladder-trained at two but became enuretic at three when he shared a room with his older sister who was enuretic and very seductive with him. There was excessive sex play between them and also with an older boy who seduced William to masturbate him and to perform fellation. The latter William did not remember, but it was repeated in his attacks, especially in the sucking in of his cheeks and of mucus and spitting afterwards. He used to pick his nose and eat the snot. He had conscious coprophagic impulses and was quite self-destructive.

Between three and four, he swallowed orange-flavored aspirin (this color and taste later became a trigger in some of his attacks), and his stomach had to be pumped. He also cut himself with a razor blade and later on used to hit his head with his fist or against the wall. The identification with his sister was a major factor in his wish to be a female and in her place and also in his bed-wetting, which proved to be very resistant to treatment, as was his nail-biting. He would repeatedly tell me that he would continue to wet until he was married. He knew that this was an important outlet for his perverse impulses. When he stopped wetting for several nights during treatment, he complained that he was having nightmares and that I was responsible for it. Here the similarity in the dynamic and economic function of the wetting and the epileptic attack should be noted. At thirteen when he could not relieve his impulses in the wetting he had nightmares. At eighteen when he could not discharge his fantasies and wishes in the epileptic attack, he had psychotic episodes.

This observation has important implications for treatment. It shows why such a patient cannot be treated with psychotherapy and medication at the same time. Psychotherapy is aimed at uncovering the fantasies and bringing them to the fore so the patient can deal with them on a conscious level. The medication deepens the sleep and clouds the memory. Therefore, no fantasies and no dreams are available when the patient is taking sedatives. Retrograde amnesia also functions to protect the patient from the awareness and memory of his impulses. Such a patient will always feel threatened by a breakthrough of his impulses, since there is no impulse control possible without conscious awareness. William was rather carefully protective of himself, considering how often he could have injured himself seriously. When he burned himself, he really did it deliberately. He knew that he was going to do it because he was so furious at his mother. He really let himself go into the attack. Stekel (1924) and his co-workers have drawn attention to this phenomenon of the epileptic patient willfully bringing on an attack.

William once gave the following description of his spells. First he feels slight nausea in his throat and paresthesia in his hand, usually right after masturbating. At the same time he feels guilty. The feeling in his throat reminds him of coffee. Sometimes he has that feeling after drinking coffee. Also certain smells can cause this feeling—for example, the smell of an orange-colored powder which his mother used when he was little. This smell was associated with play dough. This in turn makes him think of the things which he used to do with his sister and with other children—licking her breast, touching and smelling the genitals, touching the boy's penis or showing his penis. The smell also reminds him of children's aspirin, and he thinks of the aspirin which he swallowed when he was little and had to be taken to the hospital. As a small child, he played with razors and cut his hands. He then talked about his oboe teacher, who suffered from epilepsy, took medication, and had settled with it as a way of life. During a lesson, when this teacher, in an epileptic fit, cut his arm on a broken lamp and was bleeding, William could not control himself from laughing. It was a relief that it happened to the teacher and not to him and that it was the arm which was cut and not the penis.

While he was sitting in the waiting room, he had a fantasy about taking off his clothes so that when I came out I would see him in the nude breaking the furniture and smashing the pictures. He said he was aware that he was constantly preoccupied with sexual thoughts. Everything became a sexual symbol to him. He nearly had a spell in the orchestra when he was blowing on the oboe and working it with his hands. This meant to him that he had the breast-penis in his mouth and simultaneously fondled and stroked it with his hands. To top if off, this was exhibitionistic. Something about the oboe stimulated a sexual fantasy. Another sensation which might precede his spells was the following: He would see the air filled with particles but these particles didn't look like dust but rather like little drops. He called it a streak; it came close to being an enormous ejaculation, as if the air were filled with sperm.

In the second year of treatment, William understood that his bed-wetting had a sexual meaning. It was a gift of love from his mother and was a form of communication between them. He also remembered that when he was nine and his father was in the hospital, he had told his mother that he wanted to marry her. One day at the beginning of the session, he said "I have decided to stop wetting." But then he had the following fantasy: He would drop a match and put the couch on fire; the ceiling would cave in and the apartment below would catch fire. The psychoanalyst couldn't escape and would be burned alive. "You'd better have your drapes made of fireproof material so you can hang onto them." He saw me dangling from the drapes and then there was nothing left but a hook. The whole office was burned out. Then he had a fantasy about blood dripping; he was the attacker. He feared that he could go crazy and do something but he wouldn't cut hs throat. "You probably think this has something to do with the feelings in my throat." He had some fantasies about choking. While talking about them, he got some sensations in his fingers. Later he brought up exhibitionistic fantasies which were very embarrassing to him, fantasies that he would go on the street with only a transparent diaper.

Around this time I found out that he would frequently masturbate in my bathroom before entering my office. When I interpreted that in this way he discharged sexual and aggressive impulses towards me, he belittled this interpretation. But following this, he would experience frightening fantasies in my waiting room. At first it was an intruder who was hiding in the waiting room. They fought and shot at each other until the room was in shambles. After that the fantasies changed and more clearly depicted someone who wanted to sexually assault and kill the analyst. It was possible to more deeply analyze his oedipal complex and the mother transference.

William's treatment can be divided into three parts extending over a period of more than seven years (from thirteen to twenty-one). The first three years of treatment brought marked improvement in his general behavior and symptoms. The feelings in his throat and hands were highly overdetermined but yielded to psychoanalytic interpretation. The wish to bite off and swallow his father's penis was a major determinant but there were also impulses to choke others and himself as punishment. He would frequently stick his finger into his throat to pull out phlegm, as his mother had once done when a piece of meat got stuck in his throat.

The symptom in his hands related to masturbation and punishment for it. It was also a displacement of the anticipated castration. It was his hand and not his penis which fell off and disappeared. The tonsillectomy at eight had been experienced as a castration. The fact that the doctor had turned him over before surgery and had given him a shot in the buttocks reinforced his feminine identification. His wish to be both a boy and a girl was clearly expressed in the way he masturbated and in his homosexual practices.

At that time of treatment he was doing well in school, was able to make friends, and had nearly stopped the enuresis. After an initial slow withdrawal, he was no longer on medication. He had infrequent spells which he correctly attributed to the guilt feelings related to his incestuous and perverse masturbation fantasies. Had I terminated the treatment after the first three years, it could have been regarded as a big success.

But toward the end of his third year of treatment, William struck up a friendship with an overtly perverse boy who introduced him to various homosexual practices including fellatio and anal intercourse. This became a very difficult time in his treatment and extended to the period when he was to enter college. His resistance was supported by his friend, who wanted him to stop treatment. I was in a most unfavorable position. While he spent little time in treatment (three sessions a week), he was with his friend almost constantly. In his treatment he got interpretations which he didn't like. I was the one who tried to interfere with his perverse gratifications while his friend was the one who gratified him in reality. In addition, I had spoiled things for him at home. His parents now expected him to control himself and to perform. He was getting older, he would have to graduate, go to college, and assume responsibility for himself. It was preferable and easier to blame his parents for his epilepsy and to show that the treatment was a failure and that I was a fake. Had I prohibited his friendship or terminated treatment, I would have confirmed his wishes.

The fact that he was now gratifying his perverse impulses in reality created a major obstacle to treatment. What brings such a patient to treatment and keeps him there is suffering (mental or physical or both). William now experienced an increase in the frequency of the brief spells and in addition began to have grand mal attacks. He attributed this to his excessive masturbation. He was trying to deny what we had discussed on many occasions, namely, that it was not the manual act of masturbation but the guilt feelings related to his incestuous, perverse, and destructive fantasies which were an essential dynamic factor in his epileptic attacks. At this point, the treatment was an interference; he wanted the gratification of his perverse needs and was accepting the attacks as a just punishment, which from the standpoint of the superego they were. From the standpoint of the id, the attacks were also a gratification of his most forbidden impulses. It was like paying the price and getting what he wanted. He considered terminating the treatment but he could not quit; it would have been an admission that he was giving up. Also his parents wanted him in treatment. They expected better performance and more and more self-control from him now that they had seen that he was capable of it. The only way to get out of treatment was to get me to terminate and this, apparently, he was setting out to do.

He was also at a turning point now; graduation was approaching, he was to enter college which meant growing up, leaving home, assuming responsibility for himself and planning for the future. He didn't want any of this. He began to act out in the treatment and with others. He now began to have spells and on three occasions grand mal attacks in my office during the session. He talked to whomever would listen, telling them about the kind of treatment he was getting. Everyone responded the way he had expected, telling him to quit. In order to justify his behavior he was accusing and blaming his parents and, in the transference, the analyst. It was all their fault. Later he realized that by trying to expose me and ruin my reputation, he had actually been damaging, and exposing himself. In this behavior he acted out a mother transference.

The narcissism, ambivalence and illusions of omnipotence of these patients cannot be stressed enough. In the three psychotic episodes which William referred to as "live attacks," a number of common elements were present, the most outstanding being the need for omnipotent control. All these attacks followed an experience where he felt humiliated and not in control of the situation. While it would appear that a single experience triggered off the attack, careful analysis showed that a series of related traumatic events preceded it. It is significant that the attacks occurred during or just before the summer vacation. This was a time when treatment was interrupted and also when William had to prepare for a summer job which he hated.

The first "live attack" occurred exactly on the day I left for my summer vacation. While the preceding events may be of some interest, the main factor was that he could not stop me from going, that is to say, that this was my, and not his, decision. As he had already analyzed for himself and then later with me when he resumed treatment in the fall, this attack was his way of killing me by replacing me with other doctors and medication.

Preceding the onset of the feeling that he was controlling everybody and everything, he had gone to his cousin's home but was ignored there, which only increased his resentment. Why should he control himself, go to work, and forgo the gratification of his impulses when I had left him and nobody else really wanted him?

A number of preceding traumatic events were involved in the second psychotic episode. He had been beaten up by a younger boy and felt terribly humiliated. He later told me that even if another boy had not helped he could not have fought with the boy who beat him up. At the wedding of his counselor, he felt rejected and in addition it was summer vacation and I was away. The full-blown attack developed at the end of a performance at a summer theater. He wanted to get home and the cars outside didn't move or moved very slowly. This meant he was not in control. His reaction was that he thought he could become the one who controlled everything and felt that with only the slightest motion of his left arm he could make everyone and everything move or stop. He overcompensated for his helplessness by a kind of megalomania.

The third psychotic episode was the most interesting one because it brought out clearly the sexual factors which were involved. The fact that the draft board might consider him for reevaluation was a tremendous threat to him. At that time in the treatment, we were working on his homosexuality and some paranoid misinterpretations connected with it. I was working to get him well, to be a man, to finish school, to hold a job, to be a responsible person. He, on the other hand, did not want to be responsible. Getting well meant being drafted. I was a danger to him and therefore he treated me as such. In this psychotic episode, he attempted to jump off the roof. Later he said that this was a mock attempt intended to scare his parents so they would not reprimand him and not expect him to perform (he was doing very poorly in school at that time).

He had missed an appointment, which was most unusual for him. As I later found out, he had been to the draft board but had not mentioned it in his session, which was also quite unusual for him. I then learned that he had had several grand mal attacks after he had left the draft board. I called his mother to alert her and to see what was going on. His parents went to his dormitory. They found him in his room in bed in a stuporlike state. He didn't talk. According to his mother, he started to but couldn't get a word out. While she was telephoning, he took the receiver and said, "What suggestions do you have for me? What to do?" His mother was surprised that he had talked. He then tried to go out by the window. His room was on the fifth floor. His father pulled him in. They took him home and there he said that he had sensations in his arm and spine like urinating. His father suggested that perhaps he needed to urinate. At that he ran upstairs to the bedroom and said to his mother, "I love you." He also said that he was Jesus Christ and that he wanted to have intercourse with his analyst. William's friend told his parents that William was miserable because of finals. At his first visit after this episode, his mother drove him. He looked forlorn and pulled away from me when I came into the waiting room. He walked toward the window instead of toward the door. He looked and acted psychotic. I said to him that if he didn't come in with me to the office I would call it quits. He looked at me, then at his mother, and then followed me into the office. He started to tell me that he was Jesus Christ and that he wanted to have intercourse with me. I interpreted to him that he had panicked about the possibility of being taken into the service. His behavior would put him into a psychiatric hospital in order to escape the responsibility of reality, the Army and school. He agreed and said that there was nothing for him in life, that he didn't want to work, or study, or do anything. In his next session, he told me that he had called to make sure about the time. My husband answered the telephone and this was a sign that he had "set me back in time." When I didn't answer, this meant I had disappeared and he didn't have to come.

He had a dream. His father gave him money. William was a homosexual. Then he went on to talk about mother, mother earth. He said that he wanted to have intercourse with his mother, that the "light was following him." When he stood before the window in my office looking at the sun repeating that he was Jesus Christ, I told him that he was trying to get himself into an attack by hypnosis—looking into the light, gazing at an object, flipping fingers, and holding his breath. He was running away from his feelings and thoughts and would prefer medication and somebody to make the decisions for him.

He said it was true that he was giving himself spinning sensations and all kinds of body sensations. This was his last psychotic episode. In spite of frequent grand mal attacks, sometimes three in a day, his EEG remained normal.

In the third stage of the treatment, homosexual activities were replaced by heterosexuality. First he experimented with heterosexuality without emotional involvement but finally he had a real love affair. His spells were provoked by homosexual ideas. His sister became a center of resistance. He told her everything that went on in his analysis and used her as a substitute analyst when I was on vacation. On the other hand, he had most of his attacks when he was in her company. She was against psychoanalysis. Perhaps she was afraid "that her role as a seducer would be revealed."

On several occasions, when he was talking to me, he had the feeling that he might have a grand mal attack, but he was able to stop it. He compared this feeling with the sensations he had when masturbating. He had a very similar feeling without masturbating before a spell. It was like a mild warning. When he had it, he knew that the spell was still far off and he was not very scared. The second stage in masturbating, he explained to me, was characterized by a feeling that unless he stopped he would have an orgasm. At this point he could still stop without an orgasm. This feeling corresponded to a feeling preceding the spell when he felt that he was very close to having a spell, but he could still get away without having one. This was a very uncomfortable feeling accompanied by sensations in his throat. What he called the third stage in masturbating was characterized by a feeling that he could no longer stop it and that he had to have an orgasm. This feeling corresponded to a very similar sensation preceding a spell when he had very scary sensations in his throat. He also had these in the first two stages, but in a milder degree. The sensation was that there was something stuck in his throat. When he had this feeling, then he knew the spell was coming. The therapeutic success proved that the interception of the attack in the early stages was not an illusion.

This description is very similar to the one which a patient with mucous colitis gave of the aura which she had preceding an attack. When she had the feeling in her "upper stomach," then she knew that she could still control it, but when she had the sensation in the "lower stomach," then it was followed immediately by an explosive attack of colitis.

We had discussed on previous occasions, and I reminded William again, that these sensations had something to do with fantasies about incestuous objects and were a form of mental masturbation. To this he replied that he was thinking of his father and that the feeling in his throat was like sucking on something. He had a fantasy of grabbing his father's penis. He also thought of the boy with whom he had had homosexual play and of his oboe teacher. He thought of his mother, of her breasts. He wondered how she could have nursed him. He said that he really never saw his mother's breasts. He couldn't understand, when he was fourteen, why I had made such a fuss about his masturbating in my bathroom. But now he realized that this was an attack on me. He also realized that talking so freely about his treatment, especially to the psychiatrist at his college, was an attempt to expose me.

He still felt different from other people. He worried about "the God within me." "Maybe I was God or the Devil (a sort of Anti-God)." But his grand mal attacks were reduced without medication to one in one to two months, psychotic episodes did not recur, and he continued his college education. In general he became more able to enjoy life and less vulnerable. In this situation, when he was twenty-one, we came to the agreement that he should continue his treatment with a male analyst, which he did. There were several reasons for this decision, not the least one being my own increasing infirmity.

20

Psychodynamics and Treatment of Petit Mal in Children

This chapter describes how the psychoanalytic insight gained in the analyses of seven patients with epilepsy (and/or petit mal) was applied to the treatment of children with petit mal in a clinic. To indicate the technique and therapeutic results of my method, and particularly for the purpose of demonstrating some of the psychodynamic phenomenon which I observed in these cases, I shall use the case of a seven and a half year old boy who suffered from petit mal from the age of four and a half years.

Stephen (7½)

Stephen started treatment with me when he was seven and a half. According to the mother, he had been suffering from dizzy spells with brief lapses of unconsciousness since four and a half. These attacks had increased in frequency and intensity—occurring from four to six times a day—over a period of months. There had been intervals of several weeks, but then the attacks would recur with the same frequency. During these attacks, he would remain unresponsive for about a minute. He could tell when they were coming on, and would try to hold on to something in order to avoid hurting himself should he fall. During one such attack he fell and struck his head; his arms and legs had also been shaking. This had prompted his mother to take him to a clinic, which recommended hospitalization for diagnostic purposes.

In the hospital Stephen underwent a series of tests and examinations, all essentially negative. The x-ray of the skull was normal; a neurological examination revealed no findings; the spinal tap was negative; the EEG showed "electrical abnormalities diffusely represented and spasmodic in character." Diagnosis of petit mal was made, and Stephen was referred for treatment to the convulsion clinic. After several months of attendance there, during which his condition had become progressively worse, he was referred to me for treatment.

Stephen's early childhood had been uneventful, according to his mother. Pregnancy and delivery had been normal. He weighed eight and a half pounds at birth, and was bottle-fed up to one year of age, at which time he gave up the bottle voluntarily. Toilet training began at one year and was completed when he was only one and a half. According to his mother, he had never wet or soiled since then. He had a tonsil and adenectomy when he was three and some of the usual childhood diseases. He was always a poor eater and a restless sleeper. He did very well at school. His mother described him as an exceptionally good child. He has a brother five years his senior, with whom the mother is very pleased because he is an obedient and quiet boy. There is no history of epilepsy, migraine, asthma, or allergy in the family.

Stephen's father was a heavy drinker, who left the family upon the mother's insistence shortly after Stephen was born. The mother thought that Stephen's attacks were brought on by overexertion, fatigue, and irritation. She was very restrictive, and did not allow him to play outside because she felt the neighborhood was a bad one. She did not allow him to fight with other children, even with his brother. Because he had been a very active child who never walked but always jumped, she had a difficult time teaching him to be more careful. She would yell and threaten him frequently, and often hit him—especially between the ages of three and four—because he was so 'wild.' She would also spank him when he did not eat. About the age of four she noticed a change in his behavior. He became a quieter boy, but there was something in the look of his eyes that bothered her. The onset of his "spells" dates back to this time.

Stephen was a nice-looking, somewhat slender, friendly child, who established rapport with me readily. In his first interview he told me he remembered the circumstances under which he had experienced his first "spell." He told me that one day he was crossing the street with his mother and saw a truck coming toward him. He got dizzy and felt that if he did not hold on to his mother he would fall to the ground. While he was telling me about this, he let himself playfully fall to the floor several times. Upon entering my office, he had run through the door so rapidly that he fell, and he repeated this falling entrance several times. When he came to see me the second time, he told me that he had had a spell on his way to the clinic and he wondered whether this might have had something to do with his working hard in school. His mother, he said, was very ambitious and wanted him to have 100's in his tests. That day he had two tests and had a hundred on both of them. Again he threw himself on the floor and pretended he was dead. After a while he began to play a shooting game with clay balls. At first he shot at objects in the room, accompanying each shot with ack-ack noises. Then he began to shoot the clay balls at his own head, letting himself fall to the floor each time he shot himself, pretending he was dead. When I walked toward him while he was lying on the floor, he suddenly began to yell in an excited voice, "The truck is coming, the truck is coming." I interpreted to him that he identified me with the truck and that he wanted, but at the same time was afraid, to be run over (by me). He then turned off the lights and began to scare me in the dark by suddenly starting to yell or sneaking up on me. In this session he also mentioned that he was in the habit of getting up at least once each night to go to the bathroom. He told me that on such occasions his mother would often call him to come into bed with her and that he would stay for the rest of the night "just to keep her company." Only the night before he had been in bed with her. He liked to snuggle up close to her because she was so warm and he could feel her body. He mentioned that he had wet the bed on several occasions after sleeping with his mother.

During a two-week vacation from the clinic Stephen had no attacks. On the way to his next appointment after the vacation he had two spells, which he himself related to his coming to see me. He thought this was because he did not like to tell me about sleeping with his mother and other things, yet on the other hand he felt that he should tell me about it because it bothered him. On this occasion he told me about masturbating, for which he felt very guilty. He did it infrequently, he said, because his mother had told him that it was a very bad thing to do. Reluctantly he began to talk about his nightmares. He was particularly bothered by one recurring dream. In this dream a murderer came into the house. Stephen did not know whom the murderer wanted to kill, but he was very frightened and had to have a light on during the night. He also kept his tinker toy under his cover to use as a weapon of defense. The discussion of this nightmare brought to the fore Stephen's jealousy and hostility against his brother. "I could kill him any time when I am mad, but I know I don't have the guts to do it," he told me. He liked to fantasy methods of killing him. "I could use a knife. That would be the quickest way." His resentment against his mother was also beginning to emerge. At first he made joking remarks about her as if testing himself and my reaction. "I should have a scale to weigh my mother and see how heavy she is and see if I can lift her and throw her out of the window," he said laughingly. His mother is quite a heavy woman. She is also the truck which he is afraid of being run over by and yet at the same time wishes it. It became apparent that he was very much afraid of his resentment toward his mother—even more than he was afraid of her in reality. His conflict over whether to submit in complete passivity to his mother or to free himself by overcoming her or leaving her was beginning to crystallize, together with the realization that this conflict was an insoluble one in reality because either outcome was associated with death, his own or that of his mother, or of both.

Stephen liked to play with a shotgun during the sessions while we talked, and occasionally tried to shoot in the direction where I was sitting. I had discussed with him his fear of knowing his impulses because, to him, knowing his impulses meant carrying them out instantly. I had told him that this was not so at all, in fact that it was just the opposite. I had explained to him that to know his impulses would help him to control them, and that because he did not know them he was having the fears at night and the spells by day. In the sessions following this discussion he playfully came close to me with his shotgun loaded with darts and said, "I'll shoot it right through your glasses into your eye." I interpreted to him that by threatening to shoot at my eyes he wanted to scare me and induce me to feel as he did, that his impulses were stronger than he. We discussed his fear of being overwhelmed and having to yield to his impulses further. It was possible to link up the incident in which he crossed the street with his mother and experienced the sensation of falling with his unconscious suicidal impulses and to show him that the spell was the result of and the defense against his wish to fall and be run over by the truck. That these explanations—to the effect that he could know of his impulses and not give into them but learn to control them—had a reassuring effect upon him was borne out by the way in which he played during the sessions. While there was a tremendous release of aggressive impulses with a lot of shouting, shooting, running about, and falling, I was rarely made the target of it.

After Stephen had been under treatment for three months on a weekly basis, the mother reported a very marked improvement in the petit mal. The spells now occurred infrequently and were shorter in duration. But at the same time there was a change in Stephen's behavior which disturbed the mother greatly. He was becoming more aggressive at home and with other children and to the mother's consternation had temper tantrums on occasions and used dirty language when he got angry. This she particularly resented. She was greatly concerned with the neighbors' and others' opinions of her and felt that her children's behavior was a reflection upon herself. She had a need to prove to people how well she had brought up her children without a husband.

It was necessary to work with the mother to help her to accept the child's liberated aggression without again restricting him too severely. This work with the mother was done through our psychiatric social worker, who had had regular weekly or biweekly contacts with the mother since Stephen had begun treatment with me. Although the mother had a good relationship with the social worker and myself and was eager to cooperate, it was very difficult for her to permit Stephen any freedom or separation from her. During this phase of Stephen's treatment, the mother herself developed a variety of psychosomatic complaints, particularly muscle and joint pains for which no organic basis could be found. Her symptoms were obviously related to the repression of rage impulses toward Stephen and were taken by me as an indication of her inability to cope adequately on a conscious level with aggressive impulses.

Stephen continued to play out his aggression in shooting and attacking the enemy and then letting himself drop, pretending that he had been killed. He was bringing out intense feelings of resentment against his brother and his mother. He blamed his mother for chasing his father out of the house. There was some reality in this accusation. The father had come back and wanted to make things up with the mother, who did not let him into the house. This incident had occurred about a year before Stephen had started treatment with me, and Stephen had been at home when it happened. Because Stephen never spoke to his mother about the father, she thought that he had forgotten the incident and that he did not care to have a father in the house.

Stephen continued to have nightmares. There was now a new version of the killer dream. The scene was a dark street. There were no lights at all. The killer killed a whole family—father, mother, and the children. The destructive impulses were gratified now, at least in the dream. The danger of the night and of the darkness, conducive to murderous impulses, is well dramatized in this dream. There was also an element of reality in it, inasmuch as Stephen had now been sleeping without lights in his room or in the foyer.

He would now often draw pictures of devils on the blackboard while he was playing in his sessions, and say, "The devil is dead. I have killed him and now he does not bother me any more." He became much more outspoken in his complaints about his mother, telling me that she would not let him play in the street with other children. "When I am only out a few minutes, she yells at me and wants me to come back to the house. I wish I could live somewhere else," he told me. Prior to his treatment he would sit in the house and have spells. Now he was able to express his feelings and the desire to get away from his mother. This could be taken as an indication that he had conquered his strong suicidal impulses and that death was not the only way out of his situation. He reported that the character of his spells seemed to have changed. Now it was only as if somebody tapped him lightly on the head and the whole thing passed very quickly. He could continue with whatever he was doing during the spell. The other day in school he knew that he had a spell while he was putting clay away in the classroom and then found himself sitting in his place. Although he did not remember how he got back to his place, he knew that he had continued to act properly during the spell so that nobody had noticed it except himself.

I felt that it would be desirable for Stephen to spend some time away from his mother during the summer, and arrangements were made for him to go to camp. He seemed to be eager to go, especially because his older brother would also be going; yet at the same time it was obvious that he was apprehensive about leaving his mother. He had then been under treatment for six months. Shortly before he was supposed to leave for camp he fell and this time fractured his lower tibia. Instead of going to camp, Stephen went to the hospital, where he remained for several weeks because a cyst in the tibia was discovered and removed. I continued to see him in the clinic, where he was brought down for his session in a wheelchair. He himself linked up his accident with going to camp, and said: "I think I'll be ready for it next year."

In play, in associations and in dreams, Stephen's sexual wishes and fantasies began to emerge. Two dream fragments may serve as illustrations (age nine to nine and a half):

1. The dream about planting flowers: He asked his mother whether he could plant some grass and flowers in her pot. He awakened from his dream wanting to go to the bathroom and found that he had wet the bed. This had not happened to him for quite some time.

The last spell, which took place several weeks before the above dream was reported, occurred at home when he picked up some tool. The tool was a garden pick, a long thing like a hammer, he explained, which could be used for digging. He brought out fantasies of stabbing and sticking something into "something," he did not know into what.

2. The dream about fire: There was a fire in the school and then at home. He was speaking to a fireman who had a hose. Stephen too had a hose, which he was holding in his hands. Then there was something about his being trapped in the fire. Again he awoke to find that he had wet the bed. The symbolic sexual meaning of the dream is obvious. The frequent connection between sexual excitement, bed-wetting, and petit mal was clearly brought out here. His bed-wetting was a transient symptom which occurred infrequently. In my opinion it represented a petit mal equivalent.

The character of his nightmares had changed completely. He now had a recurrent dream about opening doors and seeing an ugly face which scared him terribly. In discussing this dream with me, he said, "I know what you are thinking." And after I remained silent, he said, "I know it is a woman's vagina and it does scare me."

As if he were a living illustration of the psychoanalytic concepts of the psychosexual development of the child, his homosexual impulses, which were mobilized in defense against his intense castration anxiety, began to appear. Again the dream material was more instructive. The bike dream may serve as an illustration.

3. He and his brother are riding on bikes. (Stephen has not got a bike in reality, but wants one very badly.) In the dream he is riding his brother's bike. The scene changes, he is going upstairs and is being chased by a monster which is behind him trying to grab him from the rear. (This monster reminded him of a colored boy at school whose name is also Stephen. This boy has a very ugly face, which holds a peculiar attraction for Stephen. He symbolizes for him forbidden homosexual temptations. These are represented in the dream by the monster.) The homosexual desires are elaborated further in a third fragment of the dream which takes place in Sunday school. The caretaker of the school wanted to hit Stephen over the head with a hammer and missed him because Stephen ducked quickly. The caretaker is a man who is very interested in Stephen's brother, because, as Stephen explained to me, his brother reminds the man of his own son who was killed in the war. While the caretaker actually gave Stephen's brother a bike and in many ways treated him like a son, he does not get along well with Stephen. Stephen's resentment, his jealousy, and his wish to be treated like his brother by this man were brought out, and he began to realize that he had actually been provoking the man because of these feelings and also because to be loved by the man had to Stephen the meaning of passive submission to him. He had similar feelings in relation to his brother, by whom he wanted to be loved and whom at the same time he was provoking. He was in competition with his brother for both this man's and his mother's love.

Again the conflict could be seen as one between passive submission and aggressive (sexual) attack now directed toward this man who clearly represents a father substitute. Stephen now seemed to be able to cope with these impulses without having to resort to petit mal attacks. While he obviously did not now feel so completely helpless in the face of his impulses that in defense against them he had to suspend perception of all mental activity and lapse into unconsciousness, he still evidenced inability to cope with them adequately, that is, at a conscious level. Such impulses and wishes, which represent danger and to which the superego objects, were now repressed by him and released in disguised form. This came out in his behavior, in his dreams, and in a new symptom.

Stephen did not now have any spells, but instead of the petit mal attacks he had headaches which he described as follows: "It is like a dizzy spell, it is like a spinning of the head, but it lasts only for a split second and it comes like in waves." He had no sensation of falling and no loss of consciousness.

In chapter 18, I discuss the connection between petit mal attacks and headaches. In this study, I found as the specific underlying dynamic force in the symptom formation the unconscious impulse to kill the frustrating object in the outside world by an attack on the head. Immediate repression of this rage and of the impulse to kill serves to protect both the object in the outer world and the patient from destruction. These repressed impulses are gratified and released in the symptom of the headache which at the same time serves as a punishment.

I had the opportunity to study in concomitant analyses two children with epilepsy and petit mal and their mothers who both suffered from migraine of long standing. My findings in the analyses of these two pairs seemed to me particularly relevant to the question of the psychogenesis of migraine and petit mal. Although I cannot report these findings here, I should like to state that it is my impression that a definite interrelation exists between the psychogenic headache and petit mal and epilepsy. In my opinion this interrelation is not based primarily upon an inherited somatic constitution but upon a specific early acquired attitude of the patient toward dealing with overwhelmingly strong, destructive impulses. Psychoanalytically speaking, this means that this attitude is the result of specific defense mechanisms which such an individual has adopted against instinctual impulses.

Stephen's headaches could be understood on this basis as a different expression of the same conflict which had formerly led to the petit mal attacks. It indicated a change in attitude toward his unconscious and a consequent change of his main mechanisms of defense against dangerous and objectionable impulses. Instead of blocking out the psyche altogether, as he had done in the petit mal attack, he was now blocking out only the dangerous impulses. Whenever accumulated frustration led to an increase in repressed destructive impulses and a breakthrough of them was imminent, he now developed headaches. This change from the symptom of petit mal to the symptom of headaches in the course of the treatment I would attribute mainly to decrease in suicidal impulses and to the fact that he had been able to accept the existence of such impulses consciously and to develop the feeling that he did not have to kill himself instantly when he met with frustration. By this time Stephen had been in treatment for one year with a total of thirty-one sessions. He was now able to face and handle his feelings much more realistically; for instance he could talk with me about his feeling of not having a father and tell me that he had made up a story for the boys that his father was working out of town and visited them occasionally. The fact that he had not a father was still difficult to accept, but he did not resort to petit mal attacks. His mother still gets very angry, he told me. She yells a lot and hits him, but he does not fear her as much as he used to do. Formerly he had been afraid that she might kill him when she got so angry. He knows now that that is what he feared, he said.

I should like to emphasize and illustrate the significance of such a feeling with a fragment from the treatment of another case. This child was in psychoanalysis with me for petit mal and grand mal between the ages of ten and twelve with complete success. I saw her again for a brief period when she was seventeen, in order to help her arrive at a decision regarding her college education. At that time she told me the following:

Up to fifteen years of age her mother still used to hit her. Even now her mother got very excited and yelled. We knew from the previous analysis that this patient was particularly sensitive to yelling. She could not stand it. It did something to her. As a child she used to be happy when her parents went away for a weekend and she was left with the maid because the house would be quiet. Now she was no longer afraid and told me that she could even sometimes yell back at her mother. She felt that her relationship with her mother was very much better now. Yet an episode that occurred two years ago frightened her terribly. In her own words, "I shall never forget it as long as I live." One afternoon she was in her coat, ready to leave the house, when for some reason, some small matter which she did not remember any more, her mother suddenly became very angry and began to yell. Her mother became so excited that she went to grab her and started to claw at her. It was horrible. She thought that her mother had gone crazy, but she did not tell her so. She ran out of the house. That was the kind of temper her mother had.

Stephen now understood that his spells were related to feelings of unhappiness and helplessness, and that they served to remove him instantly from a painful and threatening external situation or an equally painful and threatening feeling from within. "You know," he once said, "at the time when I got my first spells, I must have wanted to cross the street by myself very badly, but my mother would never let me. She would never let me do things by myself."

He went to camp the following summer. He was then nine. He enjoyed the experience and participated in all the activities. After his return I saw him biweekly or once a month. He still had occasional headaches.

Stephen is now eleven years old and a well-functioning youngster. He has not had any spells during the past two years, and for the past year and a half he has not had any headaches. I continue to see him on an infrequent basis in order to follow up his further development. It is my impression that psychoanalytic psychotherapy has not only helped to free him from his petit mal but that it prevented him from developing grand mal attacks, for which he was seemingly heading.

Stephen's case demonstrates the importance of exposing and managing unconscious destructive impulses and of the unconscious conflict in the treatment of his condition.

The basic conflict in petit mal is seen as one between extreme passivity and extreme aggresivity. While this conflict in itself is not considered specific for petit mal, the attitude of the patient toward this conflict, in which either outcome is associated with death, seems to be a specific dynamic factor in this condition. The mechanisms of defense which the patient adopts against these dangerous unconscious impulses and also against a threatening reality are considered the specific dynamic factor. According to this concept petit mal is interpreted as an instant cutting off from functioning of those parts of the mind which serve the perception and execution of stimuli from within and without, because perceptions of certain stimuli would lead to an explosive reaction endangering the life of the patient and that of people in the environment.

The significance of environmental factors, particularly of the interrelated dynamics of the maternal attitudes and the child's responses, was demonstrated in the hope that a full recognition of the importance of changing such attitudes through therapy may prove an essential factor in the prevention of petit mal.

21

The Vicissitudes of
Basic Fantasies
in a Case of
Petit Mal and Epilepsy

Fragments from the analysis and follow-up study of a patient with petit mal are presented with the main focus on two aspects: (1) to study the dynamic role of basic fantasies in symptom choice and to follow their vicissitudes in the life of this patient who was under observation for twenty-five years and (2) to contribute to a fuller understanding of the dynamics and treatment of petit mal.

Olga(11)

Olga began her analysis at eleven because of progressive petit mal attacks. In the second month of treatment she had her only grand mal seizure. There was no repetition during or after her analysis. Her petit mal attacks had been noticed during her stay at a summer camp when she was not quite nine. According to Olga, the first spell had occurred several months prior, at the time when her mother, because of illness, had left her to take an extended vacation. Olga had been seen by several leading neurologists and had undergone various examinations including electroencephalography and skull x-rays. She had been diagnosed as an organic case of petit mal epilepsy and given a poor prognosis with the prediction that she would develop grand mal epilepsy in adolescence. She had been on large doses of dilantin and glutamic acid for the two years preceding her analysis. There had been no improvement in her condition; in fact, she was becoming progressively worse.

The psychological tests at ten and a half revealed Olga to be a girl of superior intelligence but functioning much below her capacity and with considerable irregularity. The examining psychologist had attributed this to an organic disorder. A marked disparity between mental and emotional development was noted which interfered with Olga's emotional control and stability. The examiner felt that this was due to an organic disturbance. Features such as obstinacy, excessive irritability, and excitability considered characteristic for "epileptic personality" were stressed in this report. She was doing poorly in school, she had difficulty in concentrating, and in spite of the large doses of medication, she had up to twenty petit mal spells a day.

Olga appeared to be somewhat withdrawn, but not unfriendly. In her first interview, she spoke of her experiences with the various doctors she had seen because of her illness. The frequent petit mal attacks in school made her feel inadequate. She had difficulty in her work and she was comparing herself unfavorably to the other children. For purposes of establishing contact with her more readily, she was seen—in spite of her age—for some time in the play room. She displayed some difficulty in handling scissors; taking them into her hand she said, "I could cut my fingers off." She said that she had such a feeling whenever she saw knives. She had one petit mal attack during a session in the play room early in the analysis. This was the first and only time this occurred in a session during the entire time of her treatment. I succeeded in getting her to lift the retrograde amnesia characteristic of petit mal and to remember the content of the spell. I knew from my experiences with other patients with petit mal that this was possible. She told me that she had seen a round power saw and her father cutting something into halves. Her father actually owned such a power saw, which she used for cutting wooden logs.

Much later in her analysis, when she no longer had petit mal nor the severe headaches which had followed the cessation of the petit mal attacks, it was possible to bring to the fore the fantasies and repressed affects which had been a major dynamic force in the production of both the petit mal attacks and the headaches. During that phase of her analysis when these fantasies began to emerge into consciousness, Olga was suffering from a severe sleep disturbance with nightmares.

The sleep disturbance with nightmares which had followed the cessation of the petit mal attacks is a phenomenon which in some cases of petit mal and grand mal epilepsy is found to precede the onset of the illness (M. Sperling, 1949, 1958, 1969). This sleep disturbance is an indication of the severity of the conflicts and of the patient's struggle with dangerous impulses, which threaten to break through and to overwhelm the individual during the state of sleep, when ego controls are relaxed.

Olga's nightmares dealt with a recurrent theme worked over in many different versions. This theme was one of mutilations and savage acts like cutting off limbs and cutting up people committed in cold blood by an insane person. Many years later when Olga was married and had children, her doodlings still dealt with this theme of mutilation. She would often find herself doodling cut off fingers and toes. This observation is of interest in connection with the subject of the vicissitudes of basic fantasies throughout life in patients who had undergone analysis.

During the time when Olga suffered from the sleep disturbance with nightmares, she was also interested in reading about people with mutilations. She would look in the newspapers for stories and pictures of people who had been cut up, especially of people who had inflicted such injuries upon themselves deliberately and not by accident. She had a dream, in which she could see how this cutting up was done. A round saw was turning, a person was cut in half; she could see the upper part, the red flesh and entrails. It was cut clean, like a butcher would do it. The lower half was also cut and there was one leg or one arm missing. The skin was white and soft. It reminded her of her own skin. This dream, which was reminiscent of the content of the petit mal spell she had in my play room early in her treatment, occurred when Olga was sixteen and had been free of petit mal for four years.

She had stopped having petit mal attacks after the first six months of analysis. She had been off all medication after the third month of treatment. She never had a recurrence of the petit mal during her entire treatment nor during the follow-up. Olga's treatment actually consisted of three parts and with interruptions extended over a period of more than ten years. The first part of treatment, which began when she was eleven, terminated after two and a half years with cessation of the petit mal and with great improvement in all areas of functioning. Olga returned for more treatment at fifteen when she was in high school and experienced some difficulties scholastically and socially.

The main reason for returning for treatment, however, was the fact that she had developed a new symptom—severe headaches. She described these headaches as painful sensations in her head which she experienced especially when walking up stairs, something she had to do daily at school. She said that she felt a pressure on the top of her head extending to the forehead and at the same time severe pain around her eyes. It was like blinding and like something or somebody pushing her down. She would get panicky and hold on to the bannister. She would experience this sensation sometimes on the subway stairs and in other places but seldom at home. She had suffered many "accidental" falls from stairs, especially at school. The feeling connected with the headaches reminded her of the feeling she used to have with the petit mal attacks. It was a feeling as if she were not quite there and things seemed to be distant.

Following a phase of analysis which dealt mainly with the dynamics of her headaches, Olga developed a sleep disturbance with night-mares. She had many, mostly recurrent dreams. Some of her basic fantasies which had found an outlet first in the petit mal and then in the headaches, in both instances without conscious awareness nor recall, were now emerging in her dreams and daydreams, which she could remember and which could be analyzed. In one dream she saw three people walking out from a hospital where they had been "mended." They came out one after the other, first a woman who was middle-aged with a hat and coat, in a wheel chair. She wheeled herself. Then came the man, and then some other person. The day residue for this dream came from a visit to the hospital she had made that afternoon, to see a boy whom she knew and who had had a severe motorcycle accident, with a broken arm, jaw, and legs. While she was there she also saw a man who had one leg amputated. While she was talking about the dream she was visibly disturbed and was covering her face with both hands. To the three people in the dream she associated her parents and herself.

In another dream of people being cut up she was not an onlooker but a would-be victim. It took place in her house. A woman was to cut up three people and Olga was to be one of them. The woman was doing this with a hatchet as an insane person would do it. She was just going about it in a matter of fact way without feeling or reason. Olga knew, although she did not see it, that the two people were stretched out on boards. This woman had cut them in three places, but first she had cut their heads off. She wondered why in her dreams the people had been lying down on the table or board and let themselves be tied down or cut up. The mad woman was yelling and reaching for her while she was fumbling at the lock. The boards were oak. Her parents' house is furnished in oak; their beds are oak. The feeling in this dream was like that in a dream about snakes, where she had felt paralyzed when she should have been running. The dream about snakes to which she was referring was a recurrent dream from earlier childhood, when she was about six. This dream had made a lasting impression upon her and she referred to it frequently in her analysis. In the dream she was standing in a garden surrounded by snakes. She was petrified and unable to move. In the petit mal attacks, she would suddenly stop what she was doing and remain motionless and unaware of her surroundings.

A week prior to the hospital visit to the boy who had had the accident, Olga herself had fallen off her bike. She was still very accident prone although there had been some decrease during the three and a half years of her analysis. She was to some extent aware now of her self-destructive impulses. She sometimes had the impulse to jump on the track of the subway. She would then have to walk back and hold on to something. In the butcher shop she liked to watch the butcher cutting the meat. She would like to do this herself, she said. When the butcher used the hatchet she often had the feeling that he would cut off his fingers. She also liked to watch fishermen clean fish and would experience the same sensation.

She had seen a picture about a car crash in the newspaper. The man pinned behind the wheel was receiving the last rites. The girl had been thrown through the windshield. She had read about a boy who had fallen into a crevice, with a detailed description of how he died. After reading it, she became very depressed, thinking that such things actually did happen. She had heard of a girl who had been thrown through the windshield and who had been decapitated. She had terrible fears of losing a part of her body, especially a finger, toe, or leg. She was also afraid of cancer because this would lead to amputation. In this connection, she thought of the movie "Gone With the Wind," which she had seen when she was seven or eight. She thought of the scene where the man's leg is being cut off without anesthesia and Scarlett O'Hara runs out of the room. She saw this movie again some years later. She knew where the scene of amputation came and at that point she covered her ears and face.

The picture brought back many feelings from her childhood. She thought of the time when she cut up her mother's music book. "I must have told you about this," she said, and was surprised that she never had. When she was about four years old she once quietly cut up all her mother's music. She wondered how she could have done it, since she was so afraid of punishment and she knew how much her mother treasured her music book.

She could not stand her mother's yelling. Her mother used to get very angry and hit her but does not do it anymore. She had the thought at times, that she could kill her mother; sometimes when she had a knife in her hand she had the thought that she could kill both her parents but mainly her mother. She had always thought that she was afraid that her mother might lose control when she would get so angry and kill her, but now she realized that she was afraid of losing control herself and killing mother. When she would get very angry and was alone in the house she would break things; once she smashed a mirror and a window. She would break her brushes, smashing them against the sink. She bites herself and grinds her teeth. "It's dangerous to be so angry," she said. She was a very stubborn, severe nail biter. This symptom persisted for many years, long after she had given up all other symptoms. Could she really harm herself when she feels so enraged? she would often ask.

In discussing her headaches in connection with the killing impulse, she spoke of the pervading feeling of sadness, that there was no purpose in living; particularly when she would get the pain in her head, she felt this futility. This feeling led her back to earlier feelings before the age of eight when she lived in the country without her parents, only with a maid. Olga's feelings of being rejected and of being exiled were to some extent justified. The mother had used Olga's frequent illnesses as a rationalization for sending her to live in the country. The mother had been aware of her own ambivalence and uncontrollable temper outbursts and had felt that it was safer for them not to live together at that particular time.

Olga used to daydream a great deal while she lived away from home. A favorite daydream was the "pump-house fantasy." In this fantasy she lived in a pump-house near her house in the country. It was filled with the stuffed animals and rag dolls her mother had given her. In the pump-house there was just enough room for her to fit in without being able to move. She was sitting in it with her favorite little doll on her lap. From this period of her life, she also remembered that she nearly drowned in a lake. Somebody pulled her out by the neck. It was in general an unhappy time in her life.

Olga wrote stories about a girl Mary which were indicative of her self-destructive impulses. In one particular story Mary, while crossing the street, was debating whether or not to let herself be run over by a car.

Olga's main preoccupation was about injury to her head. This was evident from her dreams and fantasies. In one dream somebody was swinging a meat cleaver at her head, inflicting a dent from the top of her head through the forehead. This is where she used to have her most severe headaches. In association to the dream, she remembered an incident from her childhood when she was between four and five. It occurred in her country home while two cousins who were visiting were sleeping. Olga, who never napped in the afternoon, took her little baseball bat and hit them over the head. She remembered that there was a big commotion afterwards and everybody was saying that she could have killed them. While talking about this, she experienced a pain on the top of her head. She thought of a recent dream about her kitten that had fallen out of a window. She got visibly anxious and putting her hands over her eyes, she said, "Oh my God, now I know I am afraid that I might jump out of the window." In her mind this meant that she would be falling on the head.

This was followed by material which dealt with "the crazy way" she was handling things in the kitchen, especially sharp knives. The other day she had picked up a few things from the kitchen table and since she had her hands full, she had put a sharp, big kitchen knife between her left shoulder and head. Any awkward move and she would have cut herself. She pointed to the neck "where I have my scar." She meant the scar which she had from a mastoidectomy when she was eight months old. She remembered a photograph from the baby album which her mother kept. In this photograph her head was all bandaged up. Her mother had told her that she had been so sick as a baby that she was not expected to live. In this connection the information given by her mother at the initial intake interview is of interest. Her mother had told me that she had had difficulty in holding Olga as a baby. She was afraid she would drop her and actually did drop her once and Olga fell on her head. Olga was always a sick child, had many colds and pneumonia, and for this reason had been sent at age four to live in the country with a nursemaid.

Further analysis of her fantasies about cutting and falling on the head led to a connection with birth and womb fantasies. These fantasies obviously had played a part in Olga's petit mal and in the single grand mal attack which she had had at the beginning of her treatment, when she was still on large doses of anticonvulsive medication. In the second month of treatment, Olga went by car with her father to visit her mother at a resort where her mother was recuperating after an illness. During this trip Olga had had the grand mal seizure. Her father said that he had left Olga in a restaurant for a short time and when he returned, he was told that she had had a grand mal attack. He found her resting and looking tired. She did not remember what happened. When I confronted Olga upon her return with this information, she knew that she had had an attack and where it had happened, although her father had not told her about it. She remembered that on the trip they had stopped at a place to visit a tourist attraction, some famous caverns, and that she had felt very peculiar, as if she had been there before. In reality she had never been there before. This was one of the few déjà vu experiences which occurred during Olga's analysis. She said that after lunch that day her father had left her at the restaurant for a short time while he went to look after his car, which needed some repair. She remembered that she had felt panicky and lost after her father left.

It was during the second part of her analysis, when she was nearly eighteen, that Olga openly expressed feelings of revulsion at the thought that she had been born from her mother's womb. She had had these feelings for a long time. She was revolted by the thought of female genitals and particularly by the smell of the vaginal excretions. As a child she had been told that God makes the baby and that he needs an angel. When at eleven she found out how babies were really made, she could not accept this. She thought that the baby gets cut out from the belly or that it came out from the pee hole.

The theme of pregnancy and birth continued into the third part of her analysis when Olga was married and pregnant with her first child. In discussing her feelings about pregnancy she recalled her visit to the cavern on the trip when she had the grand mal seizure. She remembered that her mother had once told her that she had been visiting these same caverns at the time when she was pregnant with Olga. To Olga the womb was still a mysterious place and she was also concerned about anesthesia and about not being able to watch the birth process. For this reason, she was thinking of natural childbirth, so that she would be able to see that the baby was really coming out from her womb. Pregnancy was frightening to her also because it meant that there was something growing inside her over which she had no control and which would be taken from her. The worst thing about birth to her was the cutting and severing of the umbilical cord and separating the baby from the mother. To her this meant to inflict irreparable damage to the baby and specifically to its head. She thought of a picture she had seen of a woman with the umbilical cord hanging out from the vagina. To her this looked like a snake and it brought back the terrifying feelings about snakes. She remembered a snake dream in which she had the feeling that she could be eaten alive by the snake. This made her think of tapeworms and the fact that unless the head of the tapeworm was removed, it would continue to grow and renew itself by feeding on its host. This made her think of sensations she had frequently experienced in her bladder when she felt an uncontrollable urgency and need to run to the toilet without being able to urinate. The feeling was that she had to squeeze something out of her bladder but was unable to. We had dealt with this sensation in connection with the analysis of her intense penis envy and wish to produce a penis and to urinate like a man. She had been free of these sensations now for some time. The link with underlying urinary birth fantasies, obvious already then, could now be more fully explored. Olga would have wanted to deny the existence of a womb, as well as of secondary sex characteristics. The onset of the petit mal occurred in early puberty and increased in severity with the progressive psychosexual development. Menarche at ten and a half was a traumatic experience, and her mutilation fears and fantasies expressed also her feelings about menstruation. She felt repulsed by the secretion and smell from her genitalia. She was also preoccupied with the size of her breasts. From puberty on, she had a problem with bras and hiding her breasts. In connection with her feelings about her breasts, something from her early childhood came to light which made her feel depressed. It happened between two and three because after three she had been sent with a nursemaid to live in the country. She used to come in the morning into her parents' bedroom and into her mother's bed and grab her mother's breast, wanting to suck it. As a child she wanted to be like her mother, but during adolescence Olga became very concerned about the size of her breasts. She thought they were too big and she tried very hard to conceal them.

At this time in her analysis, Olga was preoccupied with thoughts about nursing. Her breasts were her most sensuous area, the feelings in her breasts were more important to her than genital feelings. The fondling of her breasts would get her very excited, to the point of having an orgasm, while vaginally she was frigid. The nipple to her was a "sexual organ" and "sucking it" was a "sexual act" reserved for her husband.

In a dream somebody took her down a crevice. It was like a labyrinth but also like a toilet; it was dirty, she was exploring it. The smells were disgusting. The dream reflected not only her feelings about her genitals and being a woman, but also her confusion between the vagina and the anus. Associating to this dream, she thought of the caverns where she had had the epileptic attack at age eleven and a half years. She recalled the panicky feeling after her father left her in a strange place and felt that her attack there was related in some way to her having been with her father in the same caverns that her mother had been with him, when she was pregnant with Olga.

The déjà vu experience in the caverns which preceded the epileptic attack, and one other déjà vu experience in a dream at a time when Olga was concerned with getting pregnant, indicated a connection between the epileptic attack and fantasies concerning intrauterine life, birth, separation, and death. Ferenczi (1955) in particular stressed this factor as well as the sensitivity to smell which he related to the smell of the mother's body and particularly the vagina, in déjà vu. Freud (1914) ascribed the déjà vu phenomenon to the recollection of an unconscious fantasy, and Arlow (1959) emphasized the disturbance of a specific ego function in response to a situation which both symbolized and stimulated revival of an anxiety producing memory, wish, or fantasy. All these dynamics applied to Olga's déjà vu experience and were dealt with in her analysis.

Expression of her fears and fantasies enabled Olga to overcome her anxieties associated with pregnancy, birth, and anesthesia. Because of a breach position, she had to have a Caesarian and anesthesia, which she took very well. She gave birth to a healthy baby girl whom she was able to breast feed and to care for in a genuinely motherly way. It was during the phase of analysis following childbirth that Olga was able to work out some feelings about her early childhood. She had been frequently sick during the first three years of life. She could not recall specific experiences, but there was a feeling of sadness connected with this period of her life. She had one visual image which made her feel extremely sad. She saw herself lying on a high table, looking at a green wall. This particular green color provoked a very strong feeling of sadness in her. She had the feeling that this must have taken place in a doctor's office and that she must have been very small at the time. She questioned whether it was possible to remember something that had happened at eight months. She was referring to her mastoidectomy, which had occurred at that age. This early traumatization and anxiety would seem to me to have been an important factor in the structuring of Olga's fantasy life, her personality development, and in the choice of her symptoms (Greenacre, 1941). A contributing factor to this prevailing sadness which Olga associated with her childhood is the fact that her mother had been depressed following Olga's birth and was not able to care properly for her. Encouraged by the success of Olga's analysis, the mother sought treatment for herself. This was not only very beneficial for the mother, but also was helpful to Olga's analysis.

This chapter focused primarily on the role of basic fantasies and their vicissitudes in a patient with petit mal epilepsy. Although the material presented here was selected with this particular view in mind, it also supports and expands some of the concepts and conclusions arrived at in earlier work with petit mal (see chapter 20). The main mechanism in petit mal was described as an instant cutting off from functioning of those parts of the mind which serve the perception and execution of certain stimuli from within and without because perception of these stimuli would lead to an explosive reaction endangering the life of the patient and that of people in the environment. I have also pointed out the interrelation between petit mal and psychogenic headaches, and expressed the opinion that this interrelation was not based primarily upon an inherited somatic constitution, but upon a specific early acquired attitude of the patient toward dealing with overwhelmingly strong destructive impulses. That is to say that both the petit mal and the psychogenic headaches are the result of specific defense mechanisms which such an individual adopts in dealing with instinctual impulses (M. Sperling, 1969b; see also chapters 6 and 18).

When Olga no longer had headaches, nor the intense and almost perpetual daydreaming which had followed it and which had interfered with her working ability, she could still in certain situations suddenly "go off in a dream" while talking to people. For instance, once her supervisor was criticizing her for some unfinished work. While he was talking, she felt herself going off, cutting him and his voice out of her perceptual sphere. She pulled herself back instantly with "a click in the head." "It was like tuning in again." She explained that she was aware of what she was doing and of the meaning of this behavior, and she remembered everything that happened. Referring to the incident with the supervisor, she said, "I just wanted to erase him. I couldn't stand the criticism."

Olga, like other patients with petit mal, also had a conflict between extreme passivity and extreme activity. The model for the petit mal attack was the immobilization experienced and expressed in the snake dream. The feeling was that if she moved, she would be destroyed. The immobilization was a defense against dangerous activity that would end in destruction and at the same time symbolized the masochistic submission to it and to the aggressor. The genesis and dynamics of the petit mal were rooted in Olga's reaction to the primal scene. Olga's parents were quite exhibitionistic and she was exposed to nudity, open bedroom doors, and parental intercourse. Olga suffered from a feeling that if she could not stop something that she wanted to stop instantly, she would feel extremely helpless and that if she allowed this activity to continue she would go crazy.

We had been able to trace this feeling to her reaction to the primal scene and her wishing her parents to stop but instead becoming petrified and motionless herself. In the spells, she would become motionless and stop everything for a split second. In the dream in which the "crazy woman" was about to kill Olga with a hatchet, Olga instead of running away became paralyzed and unable to move. This dream took place in the bedroom of her parents and two people (her parents) were strapped to the bed with their heads cut off. It is of interest in this connection that Olga, during the early part of her marriage, at times when she was very angry at her husband, would move herself into another room during the night when her husband was fast asleep to protect him from her murderous rage. She was also aware of the temptation to identify with her mother and to have outbursts of rage toward her children. But she was able to deal with these impulses successfully and did a remarkable job in sublimating her destructiveness into creative work.

Falling (experienced by Olga mostly as falling on the head) and cutting and mutilation fantasies were the basic fantasies through which Olga's wishes, conflicts and fears from all levels of development were expressed. Falling fantasies are frequent phenomena in petit mal, and in grand mal epilepsy (also called the "falling sickness"), these fantasies are executed in reality. It is of interest that Olga always knew even in her "involuntary" falls a split second before that she was going to fall. These fantasies express also the submissive needs and the masochistic aspects of the feminine identification of these patients. On a deeper level they are symbolic representations of death and of birth. Olga had strong wishes to jump on the track of the subway, to jump out the window, or to fall off the stairs. These expressions of masochistic submission and of suicidal impulses were at the same time attempts to transform the passively suffered trauma over which she had no control, such as the mastoidectomy and the primal scene experience, into an active experience of jumping on the track and being run over and falling on the head. The injury to the head in infancy had become linked with the trauma of birth and with the castration complex, for all of which she held her mother responsible. In this connection her reaction to her children's birth by Caesarian operation is of interest. She was delighted that in this way any pressure or injury to their heads had been avoided.

When Olga no longer suffered from "involuntary" falls and accidents, she once confided that she had deliberately fallen, or rather thrown herself to the ground. It was a rainy day and she had been shopping for a coat. Her mother did not buy her the coat she wanted. As soon as they left the store, Olga "fell" in the street and got her new coat all messed up and smeared with mud. This need for falling also appeared in her dreams. In one dream, the connection between falling, spells, and birth was particularly clear. In this dream she was on the roof with children. She was falling off the roof. When she came to a split second later, this reminded her in the dream of the spells. In the dream she experienced a click in her head, like the sensation she used to have when coming out of the spell. This click, she said, was like becoming aware again of her environment and coming back to reality.

The basic fantasies of falling, of cutting and mutilation which had first been discharged in the petit mal and then in the headaches without conscious awareness and without recollection, came to the fore in her nightmares and conscious fantasies following the cessation of the petit mal and the headaches. While the dynamic role of oedipal conflicts and of the castration complex and penis envy were obvious in these fantasies and in her behavior, analysis revealed that on a deeper level these fantasies expressed her concepts of birth and her attempts to deal with this first and irreparable separation.

Analysis by exposing and linking her fantasies to traumatic events in her life did not change their content but released the affects connected with them. Of particular importance was the feeling of panic in frustrating situations which unconsciously were associated with traumatic situations of early childhood. By modifying her ego and superego structure, analysis enabled her to adopt more appropriate defenses and to tolerate some of her impulses, feelings, fears, and fantasies, consciously.

Interestingly, the analytic relationship enabled her to give up her spells before the underlying fantasies had been analyzed. In my experience this kind of transference response is an important factor in facilitating the flow of repressed material and is a favorable prognostic sign because it indicates that the patient has accepted the analyst as an ally and as an ego and superego support in the struggle against dangerous impulses. The technical aspects of her analysis cannot be dealt with here. However, one factor needs to be emphasized, and that is the importance of analyzing from the very beginning and consistently throughout the analysis, the transference in all its manifestations in order to forestall or to invalidate the patient's attempt to turn the analyst into a parent substitue. In this way, the patient was helped to form a new relationship and to resolve her separation conflict sufficiently to attain a degree of independence sufficient for autonomous functioning.

PART 9

PSYCHOSOMATIC SKIN DISORDERS

22

The Object Under the Skin

by Otto E. Sperling, M.D.

It has always been known that the skin is an organ of expression; people blush with shame or anger, turn pale with fright or rage, perspire with anxiety, etc. But psychological factors in skin diseases were not suspected before the middle of the nineteenth century. Wood (1856) described a case of chronic eczema which was relieved when the cause of anxiety ceased. In the last two decades of the nineteenth century different skin lesions were produced experimentally by suggestion in hypnosis. Most convincing were the experiments by Heller and Schultz (1909). They suggested to a subject that a coin placed on his hand would cause a blister at 5:00 p.m. In order to exclude fraud the subject was placed in the hospital, a bandage was applied and sealed. At 5 o'clock, when the bandage was unsealed, a blister was noted. Klauder (1936) cites reports by Doswald, Kreibich, Sack, and Kronfeld on cutaneous lesions— such as erythema, vesicles, bullae, and bloody exudates— produced by hypnotic suggestion.

During an analytic session, Needles (1943) observed in a Jewish man spontaneous bleeding through the normal skin of the palm of his right hand. Though it appeared to be a

stigmatization, it had no religious meaning. Rather, it represented punishment for masturbation, menstruation in identification with his mother, but the most important motivation was
punishment and defense against aggressive tendencies against
the father and other father figures.

Extreme guilt for aggression against family figures was also
found by Saul and Bernstein (1941) in a case of urticaria. Miller
(1942) also found that his patients suffered from guilt which
they expiated in the form of eczema and neurodermatitis.
Scarborough (1948), Klein (1949), and Graham and Wolfe
(1950) found that scratching in skin lesions represented
hostility turned inward. Wittkower and Russel (1953) noted
that not only eczema patients, but also those with pruritus
vaginae and ani and those with seborrheic dermatitis showed
powerful sadistic impulses turned upon themselves.

Analytic investigations of skin disorders in children emphasize the importance of the mother. Woodhead (1946), in a study
of thirteen cases of various skin disorders, considers the
presence of psychological problems in the parents as most
significant among etiological factors. In her opinion, treatment
of child and parents is necessary. She reports that in some cases
the improvement of the condition of the child resulted in an
aggravation of the mother's neurosis. Carpentieri and Jenson
(1949) report the case of a four-and-a-half-year-old girl with
dermatitis factitia in which the parents' attitude was found to be
an important factor. The mother especially showed a morbid
concern about the lesions. When this was brought to the
attention of the parent, the skin lesions gradually and
spontaneously cleared up and did not return.

Mittelmann (1947a) in the psychoanalytic investigation of an
eight-year-old boy with eczema, learning difficulties, and
hypermotility, found that the eczema first appeared on his
penis; to prevent him from scratching his mother had tied his
hands. Spitz (1951) studied twenty-eight children who developed skin affections during the first year of life. He found that
these children often had an anxiety-ridden mother who avoided
touching her baby because of her repressed aggression. In this
way the child was deprived of tactile experiences. "The infant's
libidinal and aggressive drives, which normally would be

discharged in the course of the handling of the mother and converted into identifications, remain undischarged. It seems that they are discharged in the form of a skin reaction."

Melitta Sperling felt that the interplay of unconscious fantasies between the mother and the child was the most important factor in eczema and neurodermatitis. Mutual unconscious needs were projected upon the skin. Seitz (1949), using brief psychotherapy, encountered acting out, temporary therapeutically induced aggravation, and relapse within a year following the treatment and early termination of treatment by the patient. Negative reactions to therapy can occur also in psychoanalysis, but in psychoanalysis these reactions can be analyzed, and they can in this way contribute to the understanding of the case. The following is an example of the difficulties and vicissitudes which may be encountered in the treatment of psychosomatic skin diseases.

Ayn (13½)

Ayn, a girl of thirteen and a half, was referred to me by her minister. Her fingers, face, neck, and the insides of her elbows were covered with itching sores, which had existed in different degrees of intensity since the age of two. (While she was in kindergarten it had been better, but when children began to tease her, it grew worse.) Several reliable dermatologists had made a diagnosis of dry neurodermatitis. Although all tests for allergy had proven negative, she called it her allergy.

Ayn told me that at age three and a half, she had had a tetanus infection, and the allergy had grown worse. At age eight it was infected and covered with pus. During summers, in camp, it got better: "Perhaps because I like swimming and volleyball." The itch was more pronounced when in bed and in school. When she talked to people, the itch was so strong that she could not control herself, but must scratch until she "draws blood." She had hoped that the onset of menses would cure her, but two years previous, when she had her menarche, the itch got worse, rather than better.

Since the age of one and a half, Ayn had had the habit of pulling out her hair and dropping it on the floor. Her hair became thin and short, but she was never bald. She did not like her hair because it was kinky, but later, even though it had straightened, she still pulled it out.

Since her childhood she had had a phobia of dogs and cats. At one time it was so bad that she recalled screaming and refusing to enter if there were a dog in the elevator. She still could not touch a dog for fear of being licked or bitten. Her parents were also somewhat afraid of dogs. She was saving money to buy herself a dog, hoping in this way to overcome her fear.

In the past year Ayn had developed a fear of burglars, especially while taking a bath or in bed. She left all the lights on if she was at home alone. She wished her mother would adopt another sister for her.

Ayn suffered from car sickness and tried to sleep in the back seat.

She described to me her agonies of shyness. When a teacher asked her something, her face became red, her eyes watery, and she blushed all over her body. During examinations she had chills and perspired. Once, when an English teacher wanted to read her composition to the class, she cried and left the room. At parties, when they sang "Happy Birthday," either to her or her sister, she suffered embarrassment. She could not read aloud in school. If someone gave her a compliment, she felt like crying. At camp reunions she infuriated her mother because she could not even say hello to the children she knew. She could recognize from the voices or faces of people whether they were bored or interested in what she was saying. She was more comfortable with older or younger children, but not with her peer group. When she tried to talk to boys, she became tongue-tied. Ayn preferred to stay in her own room. She liked "to have peace."

Ayn confessed to a "bad habit." Although it made her feel guilty, she told lies. Once she had spilled ink on the bed and pretended not to know about it. She told her cousin that she read a book when in reality she did not do any reading. She said that she went to a Halloween party to which she had not been invited. Her mother used to ask questions about other children, but Ayn told only lies until her mother stopped asking. "Once I told my mother the truth, but she did not believe me, so I decided I might as well lie."

Two years previous Ayn had begun to take dimes from the washing machine, a practice she continued for three months. Finally, her mother accused her, point blank, and then she did not do it any more. At present she asked her mother for money. "It was simpler before."

When Ayn was angry she talked to herself in the bathroom or in her bedroom.

Examinations by internists and neurologists had shown normal results. She had no tics, did not bite her nails, and had not been a bed wetter. A complete psychological report had recently been made with the diagnosis—schizophrenia. To the question "How many people in the United States?" she answered, "900." To "Where is London?" "Not in Paris."

Ayn had innumerable complaints. Her father always wanted everything to be perfect. Recently he had threatened that if she didn't stop scratching he would have her committed to an insane asylum. She had controlled her desire to cry, but was convinced that she would be taken away that very day, be placed in solitary confinement, and be denied the privilege of seeing her family. (This is one of the many examples of exaggerated obedience in fending off outside influences.) For a while she stopped scratching, but the next day the itch became so strong that she could no longer control herself.

Ayn felt that her mother had rejected her because she had been an ugly baby. She treated her sister Bea, four years her senior, quite differently. At the age of two, when she had refused to swallow her food, her mother had frightened her by threatening that she and her sister would walk out on her. Ayn had screamed, but remained a poor eater. She had stopped playing the piano because she had felt her mother's disappointment at her. She felt that she could never tell her mother she was wrong. On the other hand, when her mother flew to Florida, Ayn was afraid the plane would crash.

Her sister, Bea, was very popular. She was beautiful and elegant, like their parents. The telephone was always ringing for *her*. Bea often teased her and would not tell her what was going on until she cried. Bea was "rotten" because she awakened Ayn when she came in late. She often had fist fights with Bea, but always lost. Ayn could not hit back. "I'm supposed to love my sister, but I've no pattern for love."

What made Ayn most unhappy was the behavior of other children. Every year, on the first day of school, Ayn would be sent home to bring a certificate from her doctor as to whether her dermatitis was infectious. Some children would shun her because they were afraid of infection. When she invited girls to her home after school they were busy and did not want to have anything to do with her. She had never been invited to a party, and never had the courage to invite children to a party of her own. Children teased her, boys more than girls. She was not able to tease them in return. If they hit her, she was not able to hit back. She was afraid they would kill her. The boys said she was a "goody-goody." In the sixth grade some girls had frightened her with a dog. She ran away so violently that she ran into a pane of glass and cut herself on both arms and under her nose. Her mother wrote a protesting note to the teacher who tried to curb the teasing, but it did not help.

Ayn entered treatment with many resistances. She suggested that she go to a hospital to find out why she had "the allergy." She professed a preference to talk to her mother and father, rather than see a psychiatrist. She was disgusted and discouraged if something did not go easily: "Analysis is like an operation; there is always a chance things will go wrong, and in principle I don't like other people handling my insides."

When I asked her about her dreams, she said she hoped that she would never dream because "that is not real." Instead, she disclosed some of her fantasies. For instance: she would go to the police and cause them to lock up her mother because she had annoyed her, or she would escape from an insane asylum and when the men from this asylum pursued her, for fear of being killed, she would run to her cousin Eve, where her aunt and uncle would keep her.

I first intervened when she related that a teacher had once told her that she should look up unfamiliar words whenever reading a book. Since that time it would take her hours to read half a page, and then she would not know what she read. On this occasion I explained to her that she had tried to make a fool of the teacher by her exaggerated obedience. I permitted her to read easy fiction and to read fast. The reading inhibition was the first symptom to give way and she soon enjoyed reading. This encouraged her to establish a working alliance, so that she began to tell her dreams and to bring in associations.

For a while she tried to convince me that she was a good girl. She dreamed that when her sister was not accepted in college, she went before the committee and pleaded for her. (In reality, her sister had often defended Ayn when children attacked her and had frequently played the part of mother when their mother was absent.) At this time, she told her mother that she wanted to become a physician because she had had experience with bandages. (In reality, she had been treated with bandages for her dermatitis, and often enough she had torn them off claiming they had come undone.) Meanwhile, she told me repeatedly how much she would like to have a dog, but because her parents were afraid of them, she was making the "sacrifice" not to have one. (I was able to show her that she talked abut dogs whenever she was bored with people. In the dog phobia, she used heredity; in the case of dermatitis, she used organicity as an excuse to avoid responsibility. I did not interpret for her the counterphobic nature of her dream of helping her sister, the wish for a career as a physician, or the wish for the dog.)

Ayn cried frequently in treatment, and complained how difficult her homework was. She wanted me to help her with it. "My mother always helps me with my schoolwork." When I explained to her what psychoanalysis is about, and that I was neither her tutor nor her mother, she had a temper tantrum. "You don't understand me. You are like other doctors. No one understands me. These skin doctors don't know how to treat my skin, so they try to treat my personality. Instead of relieving my itch, they want to relieve my social inhibitions. Everybody wants to change me. I can't change. This is how I am." (Intellectually, she could understand the difference between her basic personality and a pathological character trait, but emotionally, she experienced a rejection.) This was an occasion to show her how she had provoked other people to do "injustice" to her. In her dreams she had experienced rejections where she had met with success in reality. I reminded her of a dream in which she had failed a Spanish test with a mark of 50. Her mother had screamed at her, and she had hated her for it. Actually, her mark on the real test had been 85. I told her she was looking for a justification to hate everybody. I reminded her that the girls in her class had voted her "The Best Dressed Girl." I was able to convince her that her mother loved her, and that she, in spite of her frequent assertations to the contrary, loved her mother, and that this was also the case with her father, sister, and cousin. Confirming this interpretation, she dreamed that somebody had asked her for a favor. When she had said no, a gang of girls threw rocks at her.

At this time she was making a greater effort to communicate with her classmates. She was better able to defend herself. Her newfound trust in me led her to confide that two years ago she had changed the spelling of her name to Ayn because Anne was so common. She wanted to be sophisticated and popular, but admitted, "it goes slow."

She reported frequent daydreams of flirting with her minister but then realizing that since he was a married man with three children, it wasn't right to seduce him. In another fantasy, she would take her sister's boyfriends. (This was the beginning of the period of a very demanding positive transference which led to an analysis of her Oedipus complex.) Later her interest turned to delivery boys, especially if they were handsome. She started telling her classmates that she had dates. Another time she made up the story that she had gone to a movie and been thrown out. "One can only have a good time when one does something that is forbidden."

In another dream Ayn kissed her sister all over. In her associations she remembered that Bea once said, "Whatever Ayn says is stupid." (In the dream she denied the hatred of her sister and exaggerated the command to love her.) In speaking about her sexuality, it turned out that she refused to acknolwedge the existence of a vagina, had an anal concept of childbirth, had no concept of ovaries, and regarded menstruation as a punishment for masturbation. Once her father had told her that she masturbated during her sleep and she shouldn't do it. He didn't threaten her but since then she had refrained. She was afraid that she might hurt herself. In the course of analysis it became clear that some of her masturbation fantasies were of a homosexual nature.

At this time, Ayn was frightened by a dream that she was cutting off her arms. In new associations she said, "I hate myself because of this scratching. My sister could overcome her nail biting. Why can't I overcome the scratching?" She had asked her mother to hit her if she caught her doing it.

Some dreams dealt with terrible things happening to her parents, others with her running away from home. She realized she was in a conflict about her mother. She hated her, but at the same time she wanted to protect her. She realized that she couldn't separate herself from her mother. Let me cite several dreams. In one she ran away from home, but when she heard her mother was ill, she ran back to rescue her. In another, there were four treasure hunters digging secretly for a treasure. When they saw they were observed, they stopped. (The four treasure hunters are the four fingers used for scratching; the treasure is her mother.)

In another dream, body snatchers were trying to exhume a body from the cemetery but were caught by the police. In her associations, she talked about the ticks which dogs can have. She heard that if one has ticks and scratches, the head remains under the skin. "How does one get the head from under the skin?" In still another dream, she and her cousin Eve were weeding in the backyard. She said to Eve, "You have to dig deeper to get the whole root out."

On the basis of this and similar material, she realized that her mother was like a foreign body under the skin. She had been trying to separate herself from the mother by scratching her out of her skin.

Secondarily, the disease involving bandages and salves had given her an opportunity to have something in common with her mother: that is, it kept her mother busy with her and gained her attention and sympathy. Furthermore, dealing with dirty matters such as soiled bandages, pus, and blood had given her an opportunity for anal activities. (These interpretations helped to stop the scratching.)

Playing with her hair had become a fetish because she had felt neglected by her mother. The hair was always there when her mother wasn't. The more the resentments against her mother accumulated, the more playing with the hair became a pulling-out of the hair. Aggression against her mother would be punished but not against her own hair. At the age of two, she had had a period of hyperactivity which her mother had resented very much. By having dermatitis she had regained the love of her mother. The hyperactivity had remained in her fingers especially when she was bored or in the state of anxiety. Besides her hair pulling, she would squeeze blackheads for hours. In the course of psychoanalysis, this hyperactivity in her fingers was rechanneled to crocheting and knitting.

Her associations in connection with her hair pulling dealt with the bad insides which had to come out. When she had a cold, she had to take aspirin and be covered with a heavy blanket in order to sweat out the poison of the disease. Wax had to come out of the ear. She had the concept that breasts were first inside and then penetrated the chest. When she went fishing with her father he had shown her how to open a fish and take out the inside." All kinds of animals are shedding their hair. Every hair has to fall out anyhow at one time or another. I just can't wait until it falls out by itself. I have to help it out." When she had a bowel movement, it wasn't enough to wait until it came, she had to press hard. "Perhaps I am impatient. But obstetricians are also impatient. They don't wait until the baby comes out by itself, they pull it out." Finally, she realized that her hair represented her mother. She had been pulling it out in order to get rid of her.

In connection with a dream of playing with a dog and then the dog's running after her, it turned out that the dog had wanted to bite her because she had pulled its ear. As a child she had plucked hair from fur and also from dogs. The dog phobia was a defense against her cruelty to dogs. She also had the fear that terrible things could happen to her mother, a defense against her murderous and cruel impulses. In this connection, she realized that her car sickness was motivated by the fear that her father would kill somebody while driving.

The hair pulling as well as the dermatitis were also expressions of the tendency to make herself ugly. It is true that she tried to please people by dressing well and by giving compliments, but otherwise in her behavior there was a distinct awkwardness. The compliments given under the direct command of her mother sounded insincere. Her approaches to friendship by means of invitation were abrupt and almost explosive. They did not come about naturally. It was obvious that she issued them under pressure without expectations of success as a form of exaggerated obedience to her mother. I was able to show her that such self-defeating actions had the purpose of saving face. If she had done her best to gain a friendship and had still been rejected, it would have been more painful. By bringing out the rejection herself she avoided a narcissistic mortification. In this connection we discussed the obtuse answers she had given in her psychological test. She had felt offended by the testing of her intelligence and fought back by giving a stupid answer to a stupid question and an intelligent answer to an intelligent one. I was able to show her that she had intentionally tried to make a fool of the psychologist and failed her test in order to preserve the illusion that she was of "superior intelligence."

Very soon, a new symptom appeared; she wet her bed while asleep. This had not happened since she was about one and a half years old. In her associations, it evolved that she had reacted negatively to every kind of treatment that she had gotten from her dermatologists. The prescribed bandages had cut off circulation, making her hands feel dead; the different salves and creams had only increased the itching; the Florida climate change had only increased her dermatitis. Furthermore, after working with a tutor, her marks in school had become lower. The bed wetting was not repeated.

An approaching graduation speech made her wish heartily to be sick because she was afraid she would make herself look ridiculous. She could not produce any symptoms. Her dermatitis was healing and her hair was growing longer. She delivered her speech without any parapraxis. She went to the class dance, but danced only with girls. It was now nine months since she had begun her analysis.

This year in camp she had good relationships with girls, but none with boys. In the fall, in association to a dream in which her aunt committed a murder, her hatred for boys came to the fore. Because she was not popular with boys she would have liked to kill them all. She recognized that she could not defend herself because she might really murder them. She hated high school, particularly social studies and mathematics, but discovered something she enjoyed, baby-sitting. She liked children.

In her associations to a dream in which her mother gave her one of her dresses, she talked about her wish to be a boy. Then she would chase girls and fight with boys. On the other hand, as a boy, she couldn't go to tap dancing classes.

While she told me in analysis of her plan to become one of the Rockettes, she hid from me a new symptom which surprised her parents in spite of my having warned them of this possibility. One night when she had acute anxiety and was afraid to go to sleep, she admitted to her parents that she had a new girlfriend, Ronnie, and had joined her truancy. That day Ronnie had accused her of squealing and had threatened her with a knife. For ten minutes Ayn could neither speak nor think and her left arm had become paralyzed. The next day her foot was caught in the subway door. After a man helped free her, she had fainted, and her lips had gone cold and numb. The analysis of these incidents revealed that in truancy, she was trying to show me that I was wrong when I said she didn't have to be afraid of criminal impulses. Her phobias were necessary; otherwise, she would become a criminal. She punished herself for her truancy by the accident in the subway, by fainting, and by the paralysis. The anxiety in the night when she couldn't sleep was a return to the technique of using anxiety for the control of murderous impulses. In her temper tantrum she had shown how much she resented anybody's attempt to change her personality. In the episode of stealing, she had shown her mother "You are not satisfied with my personality, so I'll change it, but you will not be happy about the change." She had done the same with her truancy. Later in the analysis she produced new symptoms of restlessness and pain in the heart, but these were the last symptoms and were easily overcome.

In the spring her mother called me. A boy had called Ayn and she didn't want to talk to him. The mother wept and Ayn wept and, finally, Ayn came to the telephone. Ayn explained she thinks the boy is ugly. Boys had rejected her because she is ugly, so she has a right to reject the boy because he is ugly.

Another time, she had to call a girl who was supposed to get her into a sorority. She cried and cried because she was so sure she would be rejected. She doesn't want to ask anybody for a favor because she doesn't want to experience the pain of rejection. At the same time, she was doing crossword puzzles in her sessions. I was able to show her that doing crossword puzzles in the classrooms and in the analytic hour is a provocation and that is why she gets rejected. Then she could feel sorry for herself and this numbed the conscience. In turn she did something which was forbidden—that is, provoking people. This was a vicious cycle. In this way, she could always feel that an injustice was being done to her.

I was able to show her that her "sensitivity" provided her with an excuse for being sadistic. By going through the long list of complaints which had prevailed at the beginning of the analysis, I pointed out how she was responsible, if not for the traumata, then for her reaction to these traumata. In this way, a basis could be established for a real reconciliation with her mother and with the world. She had always wanted to run away from her mother, but she couldn't. That is why she had to scratch. In the transference, she had wanted to run away from me. There was a temptation to make me an object under the skin and to scratch during the session.

After the analysis of her transference neurosis, when her sister came home she was happy. "Last year when my sister came home I was unhappy because she got all the attention." It was different now. In general, she didn't hate people. She had more friends than ever before. Her skin was normal, her hair had grown, she had gotten a dog, and there were no monologues anymore. She talked to her dog. After two years, the analysis was terminated.

The Mother

Before and during the analysis of Ayn, I saw her mother several times. She suffered from a mild compulsion neurosis. She confessed that she was disappointed when Ayn was born. She had wished for a boy because she already had a daughter. Moreover, Ayn was an ugly baby. She was not affectionate. She turned her head away and did not want to be kissed. There was no difficulty in bowel training, which was completed at fourteen months, but when Ayn began to walk, she needed continuous, exhausting supervision because she was a very active child. Ayn also carried on terribly if she and her husband wanted to go out in the evening. This remained a sore point. Ayn had to know where her parents could be reached "in case of an emergency."

When her child was covered with sores, she felt she had a leper in the house. She would use gloves because she didn't want to be in contact with dirty bandages, with pus and salves. Ayn was also supposed to wear gloves all the time, especially during her sleep. But Ayn either refused or said yes and took them off when nobody was around. The whole house was centered around Ayn's dermatitis. She felt it was God's punishment for her sins. She compared herself to Job.

In the beginning the mother felt that Ayn hated her, but later I was able to convince her that Ayn really loved her. At the end of Ayn's treatment a reconciliation between the mother and daughter was effected.

Discussion

Ayn's difficulties started at the age of two when her mother could not tolerate her hyperactivity and Ayn could not tolerate separation from her mother. Ayn found two solutions: (1) developing a skin disease, which would bind her mother to her, and (2) playing with her hair as a fetish. Instead of passively suffering the going away of the mother, she symbolically expelled her by pulling out her hair and digging her out from under her skin. It could be argued that the interpretation that the mother was the object under the skin which she tried to dig out in her neurodermatitis was a secondary meaning; that is, whatever the causation of her dermatitis might have been, it had additionally acquired the meaning of separation from her mother because this was the conflict which was going on while she was suffering from this disease. I have given serious consideration to this possibility but I convinced myself that the object under the skin was really the most important factor. First, because in the analysis it was therapeutically most important; second, it was repeated in the transference neurosis. We also have to consider that the symptom occurred first at the age of two when the separation from the mother was indeed the most important problem. As defense against sadistic impulses toward animals, she established a dog phobia and as a defense against murderous impulses toward people, she avoided them. She also feared that her father would kill people with the car and therefore she developed a car sickness. Her treatment was aided by counterphobic tendencies. In her superego was firmly established a demand not to be afraid and to do the things which she feared. This helped to establish a therapeutic alliance.

When she went to kindergarten, her libido turned from her mother to her father and her dermatitis got better. At the same time, she also established good relations with her cousin Eve and with other children. But when she had to give up her oedipal wishes toward her father, she turned again to her mother, and fighting against this dependence, started again to dig her out from under the skin. The massive rejections by boys and girls her age resulted in her withdrawal of her libido to her own person in the form of a pathological narcissism. She cherished the solitude in her room and talked to herself. She defended herself against further injuries by bringing about these rejections herself; she refused to greet the children she knew and scratched herself whenever she talked with people. Another form of defense was a defiant denial: "It isn't true that I am ugly. The opposite is true, I am more beautiful than my mother or sister. How did I get into this ugly family? . . . I will be a Rockette. I will be a physician." These were fleeting fantasies, not real ideas of grandeur. Another narcissistic defense was her stubborn rejection of advice or criticism of her personality. "You are not satisfied with the way I am so I'll be worse. I can be a thief or I can also be a truant." When her mother didn't believe her, she punished her by lying. When a teacher advised her to look up words in the dictionary, she stopped reading altogether. When a physician prescribed for her, she got worse. When she had the psychological test and the psychologist tested her with what she considered to be a stupid question, she mocked him. This manifested itself also in the psychoanalysis in the form of a resistance which has been best formulated by Shakespeare in Hamlet "Do you think I am easier to be played on than a pipe? Call me what instrument you will, though you can fret me, you can not play upon me."

In the psychoanalysis she reexperienced her Oedipus complex. With the development from the preoedipal to the phallic phase her symptoms changed from the psychosomatic disease to those characteristic of conversion hysteria (paralysis, fainting, etc.) and finally subsided. The underlying schizophrenia, which had been established in the psychological test beyond a doubt, remained latent and might remain so for the rest of her life. In the following four years she had no recurrence of her symptoms, nor a manifestation of schizophrenia. This confirmed my repeated experience that the diagnosis of schizophrenia should not deter us from treating psychosomatic diseases with psychoanalysis. This case is in some way similar to the case of neurodermatitis in an adult by Schur (1955). In his case, the skin disease was cured in spite of its long duration and accessibility to all kinds of physical treatment.

23

A Case of
Angioneurotic Edema
by Otto E. Sperling, M.D.

Angioneurotic edema is a sudden eruption of one of several edematous areas. It involves not only the skin, but also the underlying structures, and lasts but a few days. It can affect the back of the hands of feet, eyelids, lips, and genitalia. If it involves the throat, it can be life threatening (Socarides, 1954). If it is recurring and not a reaction to insect stings, drugs, certain foods, or chronic infection, a psychological causation should be suspected (Rose, 1954).

Nancy (16)
   Nancy, at age sixteen, was referred by a dentist. The diagnosis was angioneurotic edema. She had consulted him several times because of a swelling of the left cheek and some pain in the left jaw. Careful examination revealed no pathology. After a day or two, the swelling and the pain would disappear.
   Nancy felt offended by the referral to a psychiatrist; there was nothing psychologically wrong with her. She was a good student and had many friends. Her mother complained that Nancy was having an affair with Fred, a married man, and she suspected that the symptom had something to do with it. There had been no history of angioneurotic edema in the family.

In the course of the treatment (psychoanalytically oriented psychotherapy) it was observed that she had had hypochondriasis concerning her skin for the past several years. Every pimple was a catastrophe for her. She had to concede that the symptom occurred after every sexual intercourse with Fred. She had met Fred after a lecture he had given in a meeting hall. She had approached him after the lecture and started a discussion which he suggested continuing in a coffee house. Later he had met her regularly in a private dining room in a French restaurant. She attributed the "toothache" to the food, which was fancy and strange to her. At home she had always eaten simple food.

Her father had died when she was nine years old, and her mother had then started a boarding house which kept her very busy. After some positive transference had been established, she remembered the circumstances under which the first "toothache" had appeared. Approximately two years previous, she had discovered that her mother was having an affair with Carl, one of the roomers. She was appalled because her mother had presented a front of strict adherence to Catholic principles. She and her mother shared a bedroom and her mother had always been affectionate and oversolicitous with her. She did not confront her mother with her discovery, but she became interested in Carl and started to flirt with him. A year ago she had had her first sexual intercourse with him. When she left his room, thinking she had kept it a secret from her mother, to her surprise she found her mother standing in front of the door. Her mother was enraged and slapped her face. It hurt and the left cheek was swollen. Nancy was angry and said, "If you can do it, I can do it also." She felt that her mother was a hypocrite. She had pretended to love only her father and declared that she would never remarry. She decided to defy her mother and to repeat the experience. Again she was caught by her mother and again she was slapped in the face. This time, however, her mother talked to her woman to woman. Nancy felt pity for her and promised to stay away from Carl—a promise which she kept faithfully.

The relationship with her mother was a very close one. As a child, when she was sick (and she was sick frequently) her mother had nursed her lovingly, but under normal circumstances her mother was strict. Besides her love for her mother there were resentments. Among other things she remembered that as a child when she had a toothache her mother would bring her to a clinic where monks pulled teeth free of charge. They were not dentists. They did not use any anesthesia nor modern instruments, just hooks. Her mother said they were experienced and fast, but Nancy thought that her mother did not want to spend the money for a real dentist. Another resentment went back to the age of four, when her father had insisted that she should sleep in another room. She resented that he had displaced her from her mother's bed, and she hated her mother because she had permitted this. Later in the treatment she remembered that she had been removed from her mother's bed because she had observed the sexual intercourse of her parents and had complained about it. She had not been shocked by it, but her mother's consequent discussion with her father made her think that she should not have seen it. I was able to show her that she had unconsciously arranged the scene at the door where her mother had slapped her face. Because she had been a witness to her mother's intimacy with her father as a child, she was now making her mother a witness to her own sexual intercourse with Carl.

After the death of her father she moved into the bed next to her mother. This prevented her from masturbation. Occasionally she had the fantasy of substituting for her father; she would earn a lot of money so that her mother wouldn't have to work. At that time she had envied boys, but was not much of a tomboy.

Among other things in the transference, she repeated the situation of jealousy. She accused the therapist of spending more time with other patients and felt guilty about her possessive tendencies. Finally she brought about a reconciliation with her mother. Her "toothache" disappeared and did not recur. Nancy lost interest in Fred and started a relationship with a medical student.

The treatment lasted only four months. When I saw the patient nine years later she was still free of symptoms. She had married the medical student, now a physician, and had two children.

On the basis of analytical material, it could be understood that the swelling of the cheek represented a pregnancy. The analysis did not go deep enough to substantiate the phallic meaning of this symptom, which is probably related to tumescence and detumescence in the cheek and to the fact that in her unconscious she played the role of husband (a jealous husband at that) to her mother. The symptom formation was facilitated by the real somatic reaction when her mother slapped her face. A further predisposition had been established by her experiences in the monks' clinic. At that time the extraction of teeth left not only a physical, but also a narcissistic wound. The psychosomatic object relationship also was important (see chapter 2). Her mother had affection and love for her when she was sick but was strict when she was in good health. Her positive relationship with her mother prevented her from making an open break by running away. The disfigurement in the face was a confession to her mother that she had had sex. In this way she succeeded in making her a witness and punishing her for her affair with Carl. At the same time the pain and the disfigurement appeased her mother and her own superego.

Angioneurotic edema was first described by Sydenham (1642-1689) when he wrote on the hysterical diseases. Crowder and Crowder (1917) were the first to state that sometimes "physic influences seem to call forth an attack. The great emotions of fear and anger or prolonged and arduous mental application have been observed to precede the first attack." Menninger (1926) innumerated sixteen different drugs which were used during his time for the treatment of angioneurotic edema. He himself observed a "case in which the patient made close mental association between onanism, which he practiced, and the attacks of edema, which curiously enough nearly always affected the genitals." In the psychoanalytic literature I could find only a few references to this disease. (Menninger, 1926; Oberndorf, 1912; Woodhead, 1955; Freedman and Redlich, 1956; Musaph and Prakken and Bastains, 1964; Selesnick and Sperber, 1965).

One case was reported by Lorand, in 1936. For two years he treated a fifteen-year-old girl who, after an automobile accident, suffered from angioneurotic edema of the face, hands, and ankles. Her father had abandoned the family. Two older brothers and an older sister were very critical of her, and she could not defend herself. She also had a sister two years younger, whom she felt was more beautiful and preferred by the mother. Furthermore, she suffered from the tyranny of the mother, who demanded that she come home early from every date. She bathed twice daily and was very worried about acne and about her skin in general. The patient used the symptom to get more love and attention from her mother. Lorand was able to deal with the fixation as well as with the present conflict. As a result of the treatment the symptom disappeared and the patient established an alliance with her younger sister and learned to defend herself against her old siblings.

Angioneurotic edema also played a role in the symptomatology of Michael's mother (see chapter 17).

24

A Case of
Giant Hives

Allergies in children are not limited to the upper respiratory system, although this is a preferred area. Certain alimentary and skin reactions, such as infantile eczema, are attributed to allergic factors. A startling discovery I made in the psychoanalytic treatment of allergic children and their mothers was the fact that these allergic reactions were in many cases responses of the child to neurotic needs of the mother and, also, that they disappeared once the mother became aware of her needs and was able to control them. This psychological sensitization and desensitization of allergic reactions in children which can, in some cases, be treated through the mother alone without direct treatment of the child, is a remarkable phenomenon.

The following is an episode which occurred during the treatment of an adolescent girl who since the age of five had suffered from dermatitis, with excessive itching and hives without proven specific allergy. In the fifth month of her treatment, she developed an acute allergic reaction with hives, swelling of her eyelids, and itching of the entire body while horseback riding. Before starting treatment she had been in a bad condition. Her dermatitis had flared up and she was in a depressed mood. She went to a ranch for two weeks as a sort of therapy and she actually improved. She had been horseback riding since she went to camp when she was seven years old without having shown any allergic reaction.

The setting in which the attack of hives occurred was as follows: she had expected to ride a certain horse but could not get it. This was her horse, so to speak. She was always riding this particular horse. That afternoon she had to ride a horse which she did not like and which she considered wild. Yet she did not say anything and accepted it although she felt uncomfortable. She had never been anxious on a horse before. Shortly after she got on the horse, she broke out in a sweat. She felt faint and discovered that she was full of giant hives. She received an adrenalin injection which cleared up her hives.

At this time, we had found in her treatment that she suffered from an intense castration complex and penis envy which she had completely denied to herself and which manifested itself in her symptoms and her behavior. There was a marked exhibitionistic quality in her dermatitis and itching. The dermatitis was mainly on her neck, arms, and hands. At times she would scratch until she was bleeding. The repressed penis envy manifested itself also in her horse hobby. The horse unconsciously represented the penis to her, actually her father. She could show that she was very good at it and in full control. The fact that she could not get the horse she wanted had the effect of mobilizing the repressed disappointments that she had not gotten what she wanted as a child, that is, a penis and her father. This represented an acute threat to the maintenance of her denial. The outbreak of hives occurred in this situation and was her way of magically creating what she missed. In this way, she established omnipotent control over an uncontrollable situation. After this, she remembered that she had had a similar reaction, though less severe, once before. That reaction, too, occurred on an occasion when she was given a strange horse. "I've never thought of it in this connection," she said in a rather surprised tone and then began to tell me that her immediate reaction to being given a new horse was to decline. So it was not the horse but the fact that she could not get the horse she wanted and what this represented to her unconsciously which precipitated the allergic reaction.

The analysis of her dermatitis and itching showed that this had become her way of reacting to frustration and anger in general and to her mother in particular. She once said, "Isn't it funny, as soon as I get out of the subway and walk toward my house, I begin to itch terribly, as if I were allergic just to the sight of my horse." We decided to test whether it was the horse or her feeling about it that had produced the allergic reaction. The next day she asked for this very horse and was able to ride it without any reaction. But here we must put the emphasis on the fact that she asked for it and not that it was given to her against her wishes.

25

Analysis of a Recurrent Case of Ulcer of the Skin

Barbara, at seven and a half years, became ill of ulcerative colitis. She had been under psychoanalytic treatment for one year during which period the analysis brought to light Barbara's jealousy of her brother Jim (four years younger than she), her hostility toward him, resentment and anger toward the mother, the mother's ambivalent attitude, and the unconscious rapport between Barbara and her mother. The symptom of ulcerative colitis disappeared under treatment, but Barbara then produced a new symptom—an ulcer of the leg. The subsequent material covers two years of treatment, begun when Barbara was eight and a half.

Barbara (8½)

The ulcer of the leg began with a purplish red swelling of the ankle, which opened after a few days, secreting a bloody fluid and then becoming necrotic. The patient ran a fever which was treated with penicillin. Wet compresses were applied locally. The attending physician advised hospitalization because Barbara's lack of cooperation (she had to be forced to allow him to examine her leg) made it impossible for him to treat her. He could not establish a diagnosis of the ulcer.

Barbara was not hospitalized; at this point, her conflict was presented to her as one in which she would either get well and go to school, thereby relinquishing her mother, or remain sick and maintain her hold on her mother like a helpless, dependent baby. In this way she would be taking the mother away from the brother. The ulcer cleared in a very short time without hospitalization or medical treatment and Barbara was able to return to school and participate in all activities.

The mother, however, was constantly worried, anticipating some disaster. She observed that Barbara would run freely on the street with her friends, but in the mother's presence she would limp and drag her foot. The mother suspected that Barbara was making use of her leg as a worrying device. One such episode impressed her dramatically.

During this period, Barbara was under pressure at school where she had to make up two terms of work which she had missed. There was mounting tension between Barbara and her mother; when the mother insisted one day that Barbara stay home because of a cold, she flew into a rage, accused her mother of wanting her to be sick and threatened to "get even" with her. She refused to eat and instead forced her mother to look on while she would take one bite and crumble the rest. If her mother attempted to leave the room, Barbara held on to her or ran after her. She threatened an ulcerative colitis attack and screamed that she would make her mother empty the bedpan for her. Although Barbara was up all that night with the bedpan at her side, she was able to produce neither bloody diarrhea nor any of the other colitis symptoms. But she did produce a new ulcer on the same leg.

The consulting surgeon suspected an underlying osteomyelitis and hospitalized her. In the hospital she ran a high fever for which she got penicillin injections regularly but with no apparent effect on temperature or ulcer. The bacteriological findings were negative. X-rays did not reveal any bone pathology. No diagnosis could be established and therefore no specific treatment could be given. The ulcers were treated locally with boric acid. At the onset of the leg ulcer, the full meaning of the symptom was obviously not apparent to me, and I had interpreted only one of its causative factors to Barbara.

I saw her regularly in the ward during the six weeks of hospitalization, and in this period interpreted to her that this leg ulcer, like the colitis before it, was a new way of destroying her brother Jim, and consequently herself. Barbara became disturbed at this and pleaded, "Don't let me do it."

Barbara was much more rational in behavior than she had been formerly when hospitalized for the ulcerative colitis, but she was still fearful about showing her leg to the doctors. Her attitude toward me may well be described by her remark, "Little Barbara doesn't have much to do with this now—she only started it." (During our sessions, we spoke of her unconscious impulses as "little Barbara.") The ulcer was clearing, but because of its size, grafting was suggested, which Barbara accepted when she was told it would shorten her stay in the hospital. The skin for grafting was taken from her abdomen.

When Barbara had been home for a week, her mother, greatly agitated, came to see me, accusing herself of having made Barbara sick again. On entering the child's room she had found her masturbating. Seeing that Barbara was flushed and perspiring and was moving about restlessly under her covers as she had been on other such occasions, the mother cautioned Barbara against masturbating. She warned her that the excitement and perspiration, especially in her present condition, would retard the healing of the wound on her abdomen and that her leg would be made worse. The next day Barbara's leg began to swell and her temperature rose.

Barbara was again hospitalized on advice of the surgeon. This time she was placed on the Surgical Service and upon direction from the Chief Surgeon, who was antagonistic to psychiatric treatment, Barbara was put through the entire series of examinations for ulcerative colitis, which had been performed several times during earlier phases of her illness on the pediatric service. X-ray and rectoscopic examination revealed the typical findings of residues of a chronic ulcerative colitis. All bacteriological findings again proved negative. No diagnosis of the condition of her leg could be established. The dermatological description of the ulcer was, "Not typical for any specific type of infection. This type or similar ulcers not infrequently seen in association with colitis in adults." This apparently prompted the chief surgeon to put Barbara on a "colitis diet," to urge an ileostomy, and to declare psychiatric treatment contraindicated. This was opposed by the chief pediatrician, who knew Barbara from her previous hospitalizations for ulcerative colitis, and felt that she had responded remarkably to psychiatric treatment. She again received penicillin injections without any apparent effect on temperature or ulcer. She also had some x-ray radiations.

Barbara resented intensely her stay on the Surgical Service and feared that if she were not left alone she would "get sick all over again." Her resentment was also directed toward me because she felt that I should have protected her from all this. I finally succeeded in convincing the surgeon in charge that the ulcerations of her leg were psychosomatic in nature. The diet and all the treatment, except the penicillin injections, were now discontinued and Barbara was left to my care.

Analysis of her negative transference had to be carried on in the ward. I had to show her that she was now ready to destroy herself out of frustration, fury, and disappointment in me. She told me that she had felt that I, too, no longer cared—had deserted her—and that, being all alone, she hadn't felt like fighting "little Barbara" (her own sadistic, destructive impulses). We made a deal. I would take her out of the hospital regardless of the surgeon's opinion or permission if she were willing to help both herself and me by fighting "little Barbara" rather than me and the doctors. I also pointed out to her that if I took her out of the hospital she would have to accept the responsibility for her symptoms herself. Barbara was very optimistic saying, "You'll see for yourself soon."

The effect of this discussion with Barbara was striking. When I had spoken to the treating surgeon, he thought it unwise to take her out of the hospital for several weeks. When I saw him two days later, after my discussion with Barbara, he was amazed by the visible improvement in her leg and the change in her entire condition although nothing had changed in the treatment. Her temperature had dropped almost immediately after my talk with her, and the ulcer was healing rapidly.

I now took Barbara out of the hospital with the consent of the surgeon, who, nevertheless, did not seem convinced that Barbara would be able to stay out of the hospital for any length of time. Since she still had a temperature of about 101° to 102°, he advised that penicillin injections be continued.

This suggestion could not be carried out since it was difficult to find a physician who was willing to take charge of the case. One doctor, who was willing to treat her, first wanted to acquaint himself with her hospital record. However, within several days Barbara's temperature dropped without the use of medication. Her ulcer also was practically healed, and there was apparently no further need for any medical treatment.

Occasionally Barbara would have a sudden rise in temperature for no obvious reason. The mother reported she had observed that on several occasions there was a marked rise in Barbara's temperature after they had quarreled. I had also been aware that the rise in Barbara's temperature seemed to coincide with the emotional upheavals between mother and child. I encountered a similar condition in the case of Robert (see chapter 7). I advised the mother to adopt a more casual attitude toward it than she generally had, and I interpreted to Barbara that her rise in temperature was an expression of anger toward her mother. Elevated temperatures soon disappeared.

An episode illustrating the mother's sober handling of Barbara's tendency to produce an elevated temperature follows: the day her father returned to work after a two-week vactaion during which he had devoted a great deal of time to Barbara, she complained of chills, fatigue and moodiness. She requested her mother to take her temperature and although it was found to be rather high (103°) the mother in a reassuring way made light of it. The next day the spell was over and Barbara was well again.

Barbara took care of her leg herself and insisted on walking after she bandaged it. She had good bowel control, but when she was very angry she would run to the bathroom, expecting her mother to come in and wipe her. Although she and her mother were more agreeable, there were still numerous quarrels, especially about Jim, of whom Barbara was openly resentful.

Barbara now began to show signs of anxiety. Often she was afraid of falling asleep. In speaking of it to me, she was able to analyze this fear herself. "Little Barbara" she said, "really wants Jim to die during the night and is then afraid it will be her."

One day after a quarrel with her mother, she fell while playing ball. She was very upset and implored her mother not to scold. Barbara's interpretation of the accident was that it was really not an accident but that "Little Barbara did not want her to be well, play ball, and do what other children do. Little Barbara is around again," she said, "because Mother nags and scolds me all the time and I had a quarrel with her just before I fell."

Barbara was still wearing a big bandage over her abdomen where she had a scar with a few scabs from the grafting. When I suggested that she take this bandage off, she said, "You don't know little Barbara. She'll want to scratch." So I suggested that she leave the bandage off during the day and put it on at night. A few days later Barbara's mother very much disturbed, called to inform me that Barbara had developed a sore on her abdomen. When I saw Barbara she showed me the sore, which had evidently resulted from scratching and pulling off scabs. It was not very extended but rather deep and it exuded a secretion. She said, "You see what she can do." She had achieved her purpose: to prove to me again how dangerous "little Barbara" was and that it was therefore safer to have this sore covered. She did this by applying some powder and gauze and the sore heeled up very quickly.

Several days later the mother reported that Barbara had awakened in the night crying and asked to be taken to the bathroom. She feared something would happen to her stomach (meaning abdomen). The mother felt that that child's disturbance was related to the bandage on her abdomen. Whereas, formerly she would coerce Barbara to take it off, she said nothing to her about it but merely listened to her complaints in the bathroom until Barbara said, "Now I feel better," and permitted her mother to go to bed.

Barbara spontaneously told me about the bad night. She told me she could not fall asleep because she was afraid of what "little Barbara" would do to her stomach and that it was "not the scratching but something else." When she fell asleep that night she had a nightmare in which she found herself at the hospital. We discussed why she should be so scared of little Barbara at this point. We knew that whenever this was the case it was because she was angry at somebody—usually her mother or her brother, or both. Barbara said, "I have to tell you something. You know, it's about the dog; not that my mother wants to give it away, but she doesn't let me take it out in the yard. And what good is a dog if you don't feel it's yours and can't do whatever you want with it?

Several weeks before, Barbara got a sudden urge to have a dog and persuaded her mother to get her one the very same day. (It may be interesting to note that one of Barbara's severe attacks of ulcerative colitis more than a year ago had occurred after her mother, who disliked dogs, had disposed of her dog.)

In discussing the urgency of her wish for a dog, we came to understand that the dog represented a penis symbol to her. In one of the preceding sessions Barbara had brought out her belief that she (like all girls) was really born with a penis and that her mother, punishing her in anger for her masturbation, had taken her penis away. She also related to me her feelings about the threats her mother had made about masturbation. Mother had told her that "it would get rotten and foul, and fall off." What would fall off she didn't know. We also came to understand that the leg represented both Jim's penis and at the same time Jim himself. Thus her fear of the surgeon revealed itself as a castration fear, namely, that he, as executor of her mother's castration threats, would cut off her leg-penis. This was something she dreaded and wished for at the same time, the idea being "to get it over with." As she later remarked, "It seems little Barbara won't rest until I have my leg cut off."

At the end of this session Barbara was resentful and angry with me. She blamed me for insisting upon bringing up such material and said, "Little Barbara is angry at you because you found out about her secrets." As a reaction to this session Barbara suddenly wanted a dog badly and insisted that her mother give it to her immediately. To Barbara, obtaining the dog meant getting her mother to return the penis she had taken away from her. When this was interpreted to her, she asked, "Is it bad if I think of my dog as my penis?" Significantly enough, her interest in the dog diminished so markedly after this interpretation that her mother one day remarked: "It seems that Barbara doesn't care for this dog at all any more. I can't understand that; she wanted it so badly."

Another of my patients, suffering from a severe depression with psychosomatic manifestations, recalled how, as a little girl of five, she used to hold her dog close to her body, pretending it was her penis. Whenever she did that she was afraid of being caught by her mother, who she feared would punish her severely. This patient had two brothers. She was extremely jealous of the one three years her junior. During her analysis she developed pain and swelling in her ankle, and she wore a bandage. Whenever her penis envy and her jealousy of her younger brother, which she had unconsciously displaced onto her younger son, were discussed, she registered her feelings in her ankle. At such times she would have the sensation that her leg was expanding and was throbbing (erection). After this had been analyzed, her leg symptom disappeared and she discarded the bandage.

Another incident Barbara's mother mentioned is also illustrative of her castration fear. One night, in her sleep, Barbara called out, "Nurse!" (She did this occasionally when her sleep was disturbed.) When her mother came to the bed, she observed Barbara, half asleep, touching and moving her leg. She then smiled, as if reassured that it was still there.

In discussing her nightmare, she realized she had feared she would have to tear open the healing wound on her abdomen. Barbara had not believed her mother when, upon my suggestion, the mother had retracted the masturbation threats. "This," Barbara said, "she only told me so that I shouldn't be upset, but she didn't mean it." The grafting apparently had supported Barbara's belief that the penis could be taken away, and the operation had been conceived of as a punishment for her sadistic impulses, namely, ripping off the penis and also her mother's belly (the baby inside). This was also expressed in her remark, "Little Barbara was glad that I was cut on my stomach."

When we discussed why she distrusted her mother so, she asked, "Do you think this was so even before Jim was born?"

"Perhaps," I said, "but I am sure that Jim's birth had a lot to do with it."

"Yes," she said, "she took my penis away and gave it to Jim."

I was startled by this remark, made very casually. I collected myself quickly and said, "I see. And so this is why you are trying to get it back from him at all costs."

After a while, she asked, "Why should little Barbara insist upon being a baby?" I suggested, "Maybe that's how she thinks she's forcing mother to attend to her, and in that way she takes Jim's place."

Speaking about Jim and the consideration her mother expected her to show to him, she remembered an incident. When Jim was very little, he had got caught between two dressers while she was watching over him. She got frightened and had to call her father to rescue him because she could not pull him out. She remembered the beating she received for it from her mother. "You know," Barbara said, "I think maybe it's not even the penis little Barbara wants and thinks mother took away from her and gave to Jim. Maybe it's the breast or love, or something she took away from me and gave to him." She recalled that during her last hospitalization, when I was present at meal time, she had refused to eat and had taken only ice cream and milk; and that she whispered to me, "You know, babies drink only milk."

I cannot resist relating a little episode that reflects Barbara's fine analytic understanding. One day on entering the playroom she noticed a piece of art that another little patient had left. It showed two clay figures, one larger and one smaller, tied together on a clay boat. Barbara asked me what it was. "Well," I said, "You know we can't discuss what other patients do here." "Let me guess," she said, "This is a man and a little boy." "How can you tell?" I asked her. "Don't you see what a big penis he has?" and she pointed to the tall hat with a feather on the larger figure." And he had one, too," she said, pointing to the smaller figure that was also wearing a similar hat. After a moment of thought, she said, "I was much worse off than he, because little Barbara was mad at both of them [mother and father]. This little boy at least has his father with him."

Material brought out by the mother indicated that, although Barbara's feelings about her were exaggerated, there was some basis in the disturbed relationship of the parents. The mother revealed that her marriage was unhappy and sexually frustrating. She had married her husband, for whom she did not really care, only because her mother thought that he would be the right man for her. The husband was a rather sadistic fellow, she claimed, who showed little concern for her. He made sexual overtures to her in the most unpredictable way. While visiting at her mother's or at her friend's, he would pull her away and force her to have sexual intercourse. As a matter of fact, she was frigid and never submitted to intercourse unless she was coerced. Barbara's concept of sexual intercourse as a struggle between man and wife can more readily be understood since we know that she had been a witness to such scenes. Some of her remarks bear this out: "She doesn't want to sleep with him," and "She kicks him."

The mother never slept in the same room with her husband. Before Jim's birth she had slept with Barbara, who resented it greatly when her mother began to sleep with Jim and put her into a room with her father. The mother recalled how infuriated she had been with this behavior; Barbara was then four.

The mother related the following episode which illustrates Barbara's awareness of the relationship between her parents. One day when she was out shopping with Barbara, the butcher jokingly asked: "Do your mother and father fight?" And Barbara said, "Oh, yes, and my mother spits in his face," for which the mother gave her a terrific beating.

According to the mother, Barbara had always avoided any physical contact with her and antagonized her by preferring the grandmother, and even strangers, to her. At that time (age four) she developed a facial tic that persisted until she became ill with ulcerative colitis; it reappeared as an intermediate symptom during the analysis and the dissolution of her ulcerative colitis. Her knuckle-cracking as well as picking and pulling at her skin also originated at that time. These were all manifestations of strongly repressed anger. Barbara could not afford to go into fits of temper, because her mother would not tolerate them. She therefore had to repress and convert her sadistic impulses into symptoms. "I wouldn't let her grow up to be like one of my husband's family," her mother once said to me.

After the father's induction into the navy, Barbara, who was then seven and one half, was left alone in her room, while her mother continued to sleep with Jim. It was then that Barbara became ill with ulcerative colitis. Only after the mother caught herself becoming sexually excited on many occasions while sleeping with Jim did she sense the nature of her strong attachment for him. Preceding her husband's discharge from the navy, she decided to move Jim out of her bed and have him share Barbara's bedroom.

In relating this, she expressed anxiety at losing Jim's affection due to the necessity of devoting so much attention to Barbara. At least she had possessed Jim, had been sure of his love. But could she be sure of receiving Barbara's love? It seemed very important to her to feel that there was somebody who loved her and was completely dependent on her. She questioned her ability to experience deep feeling. She had become anxious about it when her father was seriously ill. She told me that she felt like a heel when everyone, even strangers, cried at the thought of his death while she could neither shed a tear nor feel anything at all. When others told her not to take it too hard, she felt like a monster. Also, when Barbara was so ill and it was feared she might die, she stayed at her post "like a soldier" but apparently without feeling. When I interpreted that she was thereby overreacting to her intense feeling, and fear of being swept away by these feelings should they come to consciousness, she opened up and told me she had been called "a cry baby" as a child. Now, she can cry only when alone, and usually for no tangible reason. It was possible to show her that she had projected onto Barbara her own fear of loss of control and that Barbara, through her display of uncontrolled behavior and masturbation, represented a threat to the mother's own balance. She also spoke of a fear of insanity, again projected onto Barbara. To rationalize her fear about Barbara, she gave the case of a girl she knew who had displayed peculiar behavior, and no one but she had suspected the girl insane. Now this girl is in a mental institution.

As the mother brought out this material, there was considerable improvement in her relationship with Barbara. Barbara, in turn, began to speak of things which, she explained, she had hitherto hesitated to reveal because she thought I might laugh at her, as her mother was prone to do. In her daydreams she saw herself as a dancer or an actress admired by others. Actually, she felt she would never be able to expose her abdomen and leg because of the scars, which were horrible to her. Her feeling changed markedly, however, when she recognized the association with masturbation.

She thought she would never be able to achieve any of her wishes in reality. I told her that it was "little Barbara" who did not want her to achieve anything, but that by exercising her foot, she would be able to do anything she wished—dance or jump. She understood me. Soon her mother reported that Barbara was very persistent in training her foot. One day Barbara came in beaming, "You know, I won a contest in jumping rope today. I can jump rope and skate now just as well as any other girl on the block."

She also began to talk about her concrete difficulties. The prospect of school worried her. My suggestion that she get a tutor to help her with math and spelling before returning to school was accepted by her and carried out by the mother.

When the time for my vacation approached, both Barbara and her mother seemed worried about it. It was possible to help the mother understand that her feelings of insecurity, her fear that everything would go wrong, were a reaction to my leaving and that she, like Barbara, felt that I was deserting. Barbara's reaction expressed itself in physical symptoms. A few days before my departure she lost her appetite and felt tired and worried. The extent of her dependence on me was expressed by her need to see me the day I was leaving, as if to halt my departure. Barbara declared that not only was I leaving her but that she would have to put up with a tutor whom she did not like. She was apprehensive about going back to school before I returned. It was now exactly two months since Barbara had left the hospital.

Barbara did not write to me as she had promised. The mother, however, wrote to inform me that Barbara had been quite sick but that the insight she had gained from me enabled her to handle the child. On my return, I learned that Barbara had complained of pain in the wrists and shoulders so severe as to make her cry. She was not put to bed in spite of pain, fatigue, and listlessness. In a sympathetic way, the mother made light of it all and even took Barbara out, thus avoiding any acknowledgment of illness. For several days Barbara had a series of aches—a severe pain in the knee, swelling of the ankle (where the ulcer had formerly appeared), and swelling and pain in the knuckles. These symptoms had appeared once before, during one of her attacks of ulcerative colitis. At that time a tentative diagnosis of rheumatic fever had been made. However, as all examinations for rheumatic fever had been negative (Barbara was then in the hospital), this diagnosis was dropped.

Although the mother was upset, she managed to carry out the technique of reassurance without treating Barbara as sick. She was able to dissuade Barbara from using the bandage or wintergreen when her leg swelled, pointing out that there was apparently no value in it since the other pains and swellings had disappeared without treatment.

Two startling episodes of this period illustrate the degree of insight which the mother had achieved and the security which she felt in taking responsibility. When Barbara was still feeling so weak and tired that she could hardly walk, the mother took her to a movie, against the advice of relatives. On coming out of the movie, Barbara appeared energetic and completely well. Another day she had the swelling on her ankle and ran a high temperature (105°). At Barbara's request her mother took her out on the bicycle she had received as compensation for the dog which had been stolen. At a clinical conference at our hospital where I presented both the child and the mother to our pediatric staff, the mother explained to the staff that she had been able to handle these situations in the way described because she had convinced herself that I had put her on the right track and because she had been determined to prove to me that she was able to pull Barbara through without breaking down herself.

That Barbara was aware of the use she had made of her symptoms may be seen in her reaction to an accident in which her brother Jim fell and hurt his eye so that it became blackened and swollen. The mother was very worried about it, at which Barbara remarked: "You're too upset about it. He isn't going to die. You wouldn't worry about me like that." The mother, realizing that Barbara was jealous of the attention her brother was getting, explained that she was only doing for him what she would do for Barbara—taking him to the doctor to make sure that nothing serious had happened. Barbara's reply to this was, "So it wouldn't pay for me to have a black eye."

Barbara kept herself and her mother in suspense about going back to school. She decided, of her own accord, to return at the beginning of the term. The mother reported a very interesting incident which showed her understanding of Barbara and her ability to handle the situation successfully. On the first day of school, the mother expected that Barbara would refuse to eat her lunch because of excitement. However, contrary to her expectation, Barbara came home quite cheerfully asking for lunch. When the mother put the meal on the table Barbara asked to be fed. This the mother did not refuse. She started to feed her with a spoon, remarking pleasantly, "So you think that now you are going to school you are not my little girl anymore and that I won't care for you." Barbara began to laugh and said, "I can eat by myself."

When I saw Barbara she did not speak very much about having been sick while I was away. She was very casual about it, saying, "You know little Barbara. You did leave her, didn't you? But," she added, "I showed her that I am big Barbara after all, and she really doesn't bother me much."

She looked very well and told me how active she had been and that she could now roller-skate as well as any child on her street. School still presented a difficult situation but Barbara seemed to feel confident that she would be able to cope with it since she had a tutor to help with her work. "It helps that Jim is going to school too," she said, implying he was not left at home with her mother anymore.

Barbara spoke about the stolen dog and expressed the feeling that he had "left" her—that he had run away from her. Apparently the dog's disappearance had upset her, and she had therefore sustained a double loss, the analyst and the dog; this may have contributed in bringing on the symptoms previously described.

Barbara's readiness to react with specific physical symptoms to specific emotional stimuli may be further illustrated. For some time the mother had noted a change in Barbara's attitude toward her. In general, the relationship between them had again become tense. The mother herself told me she could not look straight at Barbara because she felt like "bashing her head in." She understood how Barbara felt and why she, in turn, could not look at her mother. The mother thought that Barbara was angry with her because she was giving more attention to Jim, who was then ill with mumps.

One day, when the mother had scolded Jim and given him a

spanking, Barbara said, "You wouldn't dare to beat me up." The mother said, "If you deserved it, I certainly would." Although she realized that Barbara was challenging her, she fell for Barbara's provocation and spanked her on the buttocks. Several days later Barbara complained that she could not sit, and upon examination the mother found that Barbara had a lump about the size of a fist on her buttock and that it was sensitive to touch. I advised the mother to apply a wet compress to the swelling and to minimize the importance of it to the child.

Barbara was very pleased to have the compress applied, and the next day the lump had gone down considerably to about the size of a walnut.

When I saw Barbara, she showed me the bump in a casual manner, telling me that it had been much bigger but had gone down. She did not attribute the improvement to the epsom salt compress but said, "It's because I caught little Barbara in time." In discussing what was upsetting her she referred to her brother's mumps and also to the fact that she was not getting along too well with her mother. She expressed a fear that "little Barbara" wanted to get her back to the hospital. In this connection we began to discuss masturbation. Barbara said that she had not been masturbating, adding, "When you speak about these things to me, you look like a witch."

The mother, however, told me that some time before, on entering Barbara's bedroom she had found her masturbating. Barbara seemed very frightened when caught and looked very guilty. The mother had made no threats on this occasion. But she remembered that when Barbara had complained of Jim's thumb-sucking, she had told Barbara she would rather see him do that than "something else." Barbara had apparently understood what she meant. The mother added that she watched Barbara a great deal to observe whether she was masturbating. She apparently did not realize that Barbara sensed this and that by her provocative behavior she was trying to find out whether her mother wanted to punish (castrate) her or whether Barbara could trust her. The following is significant in this connection: one day, Barbara asked her mother, "Who are you really?" Once before, Barbara had said to her mother, "You are like two people; only one is my mother." That night her mother overheard her saying, in her sleep (Barbara frequently talked in her sleep) again and again, in a pleading voice, "Please, mother, don't!"

This change in the quality of the relationship between Barbara and her mother, we came to understand as an expression of intense accumulated resentment in both. When Barbara's maternal grandfather died, she was permitted to sleep at her grandmother's house, assuming the role of guardian. She felt very important and enjoyed the experience. After a few days, however, her mother felt that Barbara was being indulged and would not allow her to sleep there. Barbara apparently felt this was a demotion from a position of responsibility. Although denying to me and to herself that she had been hurt, she told her mother that I had pointed out this was really the cause for her anger.

The mother complained she was overwhelmed by Barbara and that both were slipping. At this point, I interpreted to her that in this incident of Barbara and her grandmother, she had been acting out her jealousy of her own mother as well as of Barbara. It was difficult at first for her to accept this. However, on reflection, she confirmed this interpretation by telling me that on entering her mother's bedroom and seeing her mother and Barbara in bed together, she "saw red." She expressed strong resentment toward her mother for having rejected and neglected her. She was able to recognize how frustrated she felt by Barbara, who instead of rewarding her mother (who had done so much for her), gave her love to the grandmother. She also realized that this was the very same feeling she had had when Barbara, as a very young child, showed preference for her grandmother. She suddenly understood Barbara's reacting with rage to a telephone conversation she had with a niece of whom she was very fond but of whom Barbara had always been very jealous.

For years, Barbara had not gone to a dentist. She had a great number of cavities that needed treatment but was terrified of the dentist. We were able to analyze her fears as a projection of her own sadistic impulses, colored by sexual fears. This helped Barbara to accept dental treatment, even to the extent of going to the dentist's office by herself. She had an abscessed tooth which had to be extracted. Her reaction to this was traumatic and revived intense resentment of her imagined castration, as well as her own sadistic castrative wishes. After analysis of this material, Barbara asked me to show her the "baby book" (a book with pictures of pregnant women, the birth process, and the fetus), thus confirming that castration and giving birth, penis and baby, were interchangeable concepts to her. This material seems to be so revealing that I should like to report it in even greater detail:

Barbara had been disturbed for a few days after the extraction; she got up at night, asked to have the lights put on, and went to the bathroom. She spoke of her annoyance with her brother Jim, whose thumb-sucking upset her and disturbed her sleep. Although Jim had always been a severe thumb-sucker, significantly enough it was only at this point that it had begun to disturb Barbara. While she was talking to me about it, her own finger went into her mouth. When I drew her attention to this, she laughed and said, "I have one, too." She had immediately made the association between finger and penis.

I said, "It seems that little Barbara would also like to suck." She looked at me and answered, "But not the thumb. I have a funny idea. I think . . ." and she hesitated. "I think she would really like to suck a penis. You know," she went on, "the other day my father got very angry when I walked into the bathroom and he was just making. Since Sunday I have a stomachache and have been running to the bathroom very often. I'm getting a stomachache right now."

While discussing what had happened recently to make "little Barbara" want to have a penis so badly again, she thought for a while and then said, "Do you know that I went to the dentist and had a tooth pulled out?" And she asked, "Can little Barbara bring on an abscess of a tooth?"

In explaining her question, she told me of her surprise at the sudden disappearance of the swelling, almost as soon as the tooth had been pulled. As mentioned before, we had discussed her fear of the dentist and understood it to be castration fear, closely related to her own sadistic castrative impulses toward Jim. Now she remembered a nightmare she had had the night before: "I, Mother, Father, and Jim were walking on the street. I wanted to get on the trolley and broke my ankle (the one that had the ulcer). I had to go to the hospital and my leg had to be cut off. I had crutches and I couldn't walk. Jim was teasing me. I spit out all the food that I took in."

"Do you remember that little Barbara thought the doctors would cut off my leg?" she asked me. "She didn't even want me to show it to you. She didn't trust you. She was glad that I was cut on my stomach" (the grafting).

"Why should she have felt like that?" I asked. "Are you still afraid of the things that will happen to you when you play with yourself?"

"Since you told me that nothing could happen to me," she said, "I'm not even doing it anymore."

She went on to tell me that when Jim was very little, two or three years of age, she would masturbate in his presence and ask him to do it too. "But he couldn't see anything in it." She used to think of what married people do. The thought of kissing was very exciting to her.

She summed up her dream with the following remark: "It seems little Barbara won't rest until I have my leg cut off. Do I just want Jim's penis," she asked, "or any old boy's?" She answered herself, "Mother didn't give my penis to any old boy, but to Jim."

Several weeks later Barbara herself was able to interpret the connection between her disturbance and the dentist. She told me that she had received a note from him informing her that he was back from his vacation and could resume treatment. In a very dramatic session that day, Barbara revealed her most secret masturbation fantasy. (It was dramatically brought out to me by Barbara, how essential it is to analyze the oedipal conflict in a patient as deeply as possible, whether the patient is a child or an adult.) She was actually trembling with excitement and at one point, in fixing the collar of my blouse, she got panicky and could not speak for a while. She then told me she had had an impulse to choke me when her hand was close to my neck. But now she was not afraid of little Barbara any more and could tell me everything. And she really poured forth. She traveled all through her analysis and reminded me of a dream she had told me in the very beginning of our association. In this dream she had asked first me, and then her mother, to explain something about soldiers and sailors. (Her father had been a sailor at that time.) But neither her mother nor I would help her. She vomited and had to go to the hospital.

She indicated that had we understood this dream, it might not have been necessary for her to be so sick. We could understand now that this dream, as well as the nightmare in which she had her leg amputated and spit out all the food, dealt with her oedipal wishes orally expressed. (Vomiting with severe anorexia and abdominal pain had been an outstanding symptom of her colitis.)

Her masturbation fantasy was also an oral one: There are two boys and each shows her his penis, which she kisses. She asked me again whether it was possible to have a baby in that way, saying, "But a little boy can't do it anyway." Her question, "Whose penis do I really want?", she could now understand to mean not only Jim's penis, which she thought her mother had taken away from her and given to him, but also her father's penis (baby), which he gave to her mother and not to her. Barbara understood that spitting and vomiting meant that undoing of the incestuous impregnation and that it also meant childbirth. At the end of this session, Barbara said, "We did some cleaning today."

The effect of this catharsis was amazing. When Barbara came out of my office after this session, she hugged her mother, telling her that she loved her and that she was so happy she did not know what to do. This demonstrative behavior was unusual for Barbara. That night she ate ravenously.

The striking change that took place in Barbara's personality with the working through of this material can best be evaluated in the light of Barbara's remark to her mother: "I will not go to the hospital this winter and not next winter. I won't go at all. You know when I will go to the hospital again—when I have a baby." This was the first time that Barbara openly expressed her willingness to be a girl, a woman, a mother. She had always said, "I will never get married or have any children." In school, too, she was able to establish a very good relationship with the children and the teacher and was chosen president of the class. This pleased her greatly.

The mother's feeling for Barbara may be seen from her own statement: "She is openly affectionate to me. It is remarkable how well she is able to analyze her sudden changes of mood and to overcome them just as quickly. I should never have believed that such a change was possible, or have I changed, too? I couldn't wish for Barbara to be any better physically and in every other respect. The other day, when I got excited, Barbara said, 'All right, take it easy; we don't have to fight.'"

One day, Barbara, who had become quite friendly with boys and enjoyed the attention they were giving her, told her mother a dirty joke. When Barbara's little friend came in and learned that Barbara had told this joke to her mother, the friend blushed. At this, Barbara said, "Oh, I can say these things to my mother. You can trust her; she understands."

Summary and Conclusions

In examining the causative factors in Barbara's illness, I feel that the relationship with her mother was of primary importance. In her case, there existed an unconscious rapport between Barbara and her mother. Barbara reacted to her mother's unconscious hostility, characterized by ambivalence and, at times, open sadistic attitudes, with an increase of sadism and narcissism, accompanied by an unconscious obedience, almost as though she *had to do* what her mother unconsciously wanted her to do. "All right, you want me to be sick; I'll be sick but you'll be sorry," Barbara once actually said to her mother preceding the onset of the leg ulcer. One day when her mother admonished her to be careful and not to fall on crossing the slippery street, Barbara's reaction was, "Please don't tell me this or I'll have to fall." Her mother's mention of the possibility of falling was to Barbara a suggestion or, rather, a command to fall. She was reacting to her mother's unconscious wish that she fall and not to the countercathexis in the form of a concern about her falling.

Thus, in unconscious obedience, she also fulfilled her mother's castration threats, namely, that "It would get rotten, foul, and fall off," or as Barbara expressed it, "Little Barbara won't rest until I have my leg cut off." When the mother found Barbara masturbating, following the recurrence of the leg ulcer, the mother had not only repeated the masturbation threats but specifically said, "It will make your leg worse; it won't let it heal." To Barbara this meant that her leg would have to come off; thus the threat precipitated the last recurrence of the ulcer.

The choice of the leg as a representation of the penis in the unconscious is a rather common phenomenon in neurotic women, expecially those with exhibitionistic tendencies. This was true of Barbara, who had very strong exhibitionistic feelings about her legs, manifested in her desire to be admired as a dancer and in her extreme feelings of frustration that she would not be able to exhibit her leg because of the scars.

Other unconscious forces motivating Barbara may be seen in her resentment toward her mother and her jealousy and envy of her brother. Barbara's emotional development had been severely affected by the mother's neurotic need to fight her own undesirable impulses (including her hatred of her husband and his family), by projecting them onto Barbara. According to the mother, Barbara "never smiled and always used to shy away" from her. This very unsatisfactory relationship was shattered almost beyond repair by the birth of Barbara's brother Jim when Barbara was about four years of age. Barbara reacted to this with manifestly neurotic symptoms, such as facial tics, knuckle-cracking, picking at her nails and skin. However, she still had her father, with whom she now shared the bedroom while her mother took Jim into her room. The fact that this happened at the height of the oedipal conflict only increased Barbara's difficulties, namely, through an overexposure to her father, which evoked wishes and expectations that could not be fulfilled. After her father's induction into the navy, she felt completely deserted and soon after developed the first signs of ulcerative colitis.

In the organic symptoms, the extraordinary degree of repressed sadism was turned masochistically toward her own self. The pronounced narcissism made it difficult for her to tolerate any psychic tension for any length of time. Since to feel an impulse meant to act it out immediately, Barbara could not afford to be conscious of her sadistic impulses but had to release them in physical symptoms.

When, through analysis, the sadism contained in the symptoms of ulcerative colitis was released, Barbara for the first time in her life experienced and exhibited signs of severe anxiety. This anxiety is in proportion to the severer sadism of such a patient and is quantitatively different from similar occurrences in conversion hysteria. It was at this phase of her analysis that she changed from the symptom of ulcerative colitis to the symptom of ulcer of the leg. This was a definite indication that Barbara, at this point, was not yet able to tolerate her sadistic impulses, but had to act them out immediately in physical symptoms. "If I feel like doing something terrible to Jim or my mother, isn't it better I do it to myself?" she once asked me in a state of severe anxiety preceding the onset of the ulcer of her leg.

The guilt feeling and anxiety of the mother provided Barbara with sadistic satisfaction, "I am sick but it is your fault," and with the justification for releasing sadism toward her mother. It was, therefore, essential to treat the mother simultaneously in order to deprive Barbara of this gain which made her illness worthwhile.

Barbara's wish for a penis and her reactive castrative tendencies would appear to be the manifestations of the phallic phase. Closer analysis, however, revealed them to be of a pregenital nature both in regard to the object and to the mechanism applied in securing this object. To Barbara, in her own words, the penis stood for the "breast," "love," or "something" that mother took away from her and gave to the brother. It was something essential to life, as is the breast or mother's love to an infant. The means for regaining it were also infantile, namely biting, scratching, and clawing. These are expressions of oral sadism and perhaps of an even earlier sadistic phase preceding the development of teeth and characterized by scratching as the first sadistic activity of the child.

In the ulcerative colitis, the orally incorporated object (breast, baby; Jim, penis) had been eliminated through hemorrhagic transudation and ulceration of the mucous membrane of the colon. After this had been made conscious to her, she changed the locus of elimination from the colon to the leg, while the mode remained the same, namely, hemorrhagic transudation and ulceration of the skin. The minor ulcerations that Barbara had on her thigh and her abdomen (where the skin for the graft had been taken) were of a completely different nature. They were the result of scratching and represented means of acquiring the object by ripping it off or clawing it. The hemorrhagic transudation and ulceration of both the mucous membrane of the colon and of the skin on the leg, however, were expressions of restitution and elimination of the sadistically incorporated object, which, on different levels, was either the breasts, the baby (Jim), or the penis.

The element of somatic compliance that is always present in conversion, whether hysterical or pregenital, showed itself in Barbara's case in the readiness to form a serous-hemorrhagic transudate into the mucous membrane and skin with necrosis. Psychogenic skin ulcers beginning with inflammation and ending with necrosis have been observed by Werther (1911, 1929), Stern (1922), Bunnemann (1922), and others. The psychogenic nature was established beyond a doubt. They could be produced and cured by suggestion. The association of ulcerative colitis with swelling of the joints has been observed by Cullinan (1938), Sullivan (1932), and others. Skin lesions in association with ulcerative colitis have been observed by Bargen (1935). Barbara, however, ist he first child in whom it was possible to study these phenomena psychoanalytically for almost three years.

References

Aarons, Z. 1958. Notes on a case of maladie des tics. *Psychoanalytic Quarterly* 27:194-204.

Abraham, K. 1927a. Contributions to a discussion of the tic. In *Selected Papers*. London: Hogarth.

———. 1927b. The first pregenital stage of the libido. In *Selected Papers*. London: Hogarth.

———. 1927c. The Influence of oral erotism on character formation. In *Selected Papers*. London: Hogarth.

———. 1927d. The narcissistic evaluation of excretory processes in dream and neurosis. In *Selected Papers*. London: Hogarth.

———. 1927e. A short study of the development of the libido. In *Selected Papers*. London: Hogarth.

Abramson, R.A. 1961a. Intractable asthma: conflict of period of toilet training. *Journal of Psychology* 53:223-234.

———. 1961b. Psychodynamics of the intractably asthmatic state. *Journal of Children's Asthma Research Institute and Hospital* 1:18-27.

———. 1963. Some aspects of the psychodynamics of intractable asthma in children. In *The Asthmatic Child*, ed. H. I. Schneer, pp. 27-38. New York: Harper.

Alexander, F. 1931. The influences of psychological factors upon gastrointestinal disturbances. *Psychoanalytic Quarterly.* 3:501-539.

———. 1935. The logic of emotions and its dynamic background. *International Journal of Psycho-Analysis* 16:399-413.

———. 1942. *Proceedings of the Brief Psychotherapy Council,* Institute for Psychoanalysis, Chicago. October 1942.

———. 1943. Fundamental concepts of psychosomatic research: psychogenesis, conversion, specificity. *Psychosomatic Medicine.* 5:205-210. Also in *Psychosomatic Medicine,* ed. F. Alexander and T. French, New York: Norton, 1950.

Arlow, J.A. 1959. The structure of the déjà vu experience. *Journal of the American Psychoanalytic Association* 7:611-630.

Ascher, E. 1948. Psychodynamic considerations in Gilles de la Tourette's disease (maladie des tics). *American Journal of Psychiatry* 105:267-276.

Bacon, C. 1934. Typical personality trends and conflicts in cases of gastric disturbance. *Psychoanalytic Quarterly* 3:540-557.

———. 1956. The role of aggression in the asthmatic attack. *Psychoanalytic Quarterly* 25:309-324.

Bandler, B.; Kaufman, I C.; Dykens, J. W.; Schleifer, M.; Shapiro, L. N.; and Arico, J. F., 1958. Role of sexuality in epilepsy. *Psychosomatic Medicine* 20:227-234.

Baraff, A. A., and Cunningham, A. P. 1965. Asthmatic and normal children. *Journal of the American Medical Association* 192:13-15.

Bargen, J. A. 1935. *The Management of Colitis.* Chicago: Natural Medical Book.

Barinbaum, M. 1932. Eine vorlaufige Mitteilung uber die Bedeutung der Freudschen Psychoanalyse fur die Dermatologie. *Dermatologische Wochensohrift* 95:1060-1067.

Barker, W. 1948. Studies on epilepsy: the petit mal attack as a response within the central nervous system to distress in organism-environment integration. *Psychosomatic Medicine* 10:73-94.

Bartemeier, L. H. 1932. Some observations of convulsive disorders in children. *American Journal of Orthopsychiatry* 11:260-267.

———. 1943. Concerning the psychogenesis of convulsive disorders. *Psychoanalytic Quarterly* 12:330-337.

Benedek, T. 1938. Adaptation of reality in early infancy. *Psychoanalytic Quarterly* 7:200-214.

Berg, C. 1941. Clinical notes on a case diagnosed as epilepsy. *British Journal of Medical Psychology* 19:9-18.

Berlin, I. N. 1951. Adolescent alternation of anorexia and obesity. *American Journal of Orthopsychiatry* 21:387-419.

Blitzer, J. R.; Rollins, N., and Blackwell, A. Anorexia nervosa. *Psychosomatic Medicine* 23:368-383.

Bloomfield, A. L. 1932. Diseases of the gastrointestinal tract. In *Internal Medicine*, ed. J. H. Musser. Philadelphia: Lea and Febiger.

Bolton, G. C. 1922. Vom 'hysterischen Oedem'. Deutsche Zeitschrift Fur Nervenheilkund 73:319-328.

Bridger, W., and Reiser, M. F. 1959. Psychophysiologic studies of the neonate. *Psychosomatic Medicine* 21:265-276.

Brody, S. 1952. Psychiatric observations in patients treated with cortisone and ACTH. *Psychosomatic Medicine* 14:94-103.

―――. 1956. *Patterns of Mothering: Maternal Influences During Infancy*. New York: International Universities Press.

Brown, W. T.; Preu, P. W.; and Sullivan, A. J. 1938. Ulcerative colitis and the personality. *American Journal of Psychiatry* 95:407-420.

Bruch, H. 1945. Psychosomatic approach to childhood disorders. In *Modern Trends in Child Psychiatry*, ed. Lewis and Pacella, pp. 57-58. New York: International Universities Press.

―――. 1962. Perceptual and conceptual disturbances in anorexia nervosa. *Psychosomatic Medicine* 24:187-194.

―――. 1971. Anorexia nervosa in the male. *Psychosomatic Medicine* 33.

―――. 1973. *Eating Disorders: Obesity, Anorexia Nervosa and the Person Within*. New York: Basic Books.

Bruch, H., and Thum, L. C. 1970. Maladie des tics and maternal psychosis. *Journal of Nervous and Mental Diseases* 146:436-456.

Brush, A. L. 1939. Recent literature relative to the psychiatric aspects of gastrointestinal disorders. *Psychosomatic Medicine* 1:423-428.

Bruun, R. D., and Shapiro, A. K. 1972. Differential diagnosis of Gilles de la Tourette syndrome. *Journal of Nervous and Mental Diseases* 155:328-334.

Bunnemann, O. 1922. Uber psychogene Dermatosen. Eine biologische Studie, Zugleich ein Beitrag zur Symptomatologie der Hysterie. *Zeitschrift fur die Gesamte Neurologie und Psychiatrie* 78:115-152.

Cannon, W. B. 1920. *Bodily Changes in Pain, Hunger, Fear and Rage*. New York: Appleton and Company.

Carpentieri, J., and Jensen, R. A. 1949. Psychosomatic medicine and pediatrics. *Quarterly Journal of Child Behavior* 1:72.

Cesio, F. R. 1954. Psychoanalysis of headache in three patients (Spanish). *Revista de Psicoanalisis* 11. Abstract *Annual Survey of Psychoanalysis* 5:149.

Charlton, M. H. 1965. Borderland of petit mal. *American Journal of Psychiatry* 122:669-672.

Clark, L. P. 1917. *Clinical Studies in Epilepsy*. Utica, N.Y.: State Hospitals Press.

————. 1931. The psychobiologic concept of epilepsy. *Association for Research in Nervous Mental Disease* 7:65-79.

Coolidge, J. C. 1956. Asthma in mother and child as a special type of intercommunication. *American Journal of Orthopsychiatry* 26:165-178.

Corbett, J. A. 1971. The nature of tics and Gilles de la Tourette syndrome. *Journal of Psychosomatic Research* 15:403-409.

Cremerius, J. 1965. Discussion. In *Anorexia Nervosa*, ed. Meyer and Feldman, pp. 67-69. Stuttgart: Georg Thieme.

Crisp, A. H. 1969. Psychological aspects of breast-feeding with particular reference to anorexia nervosa. *British Journal of Medical Psychology* 42:119-132.

Crohn, B. B. 1963. Psychosomatic factors in ulcerative colitis in children. *New York State Journal of Medicine* 63:1456-1457.

Crowder, J. R., and Crowder, T. R. 1917. Five generations of angioneurotic edema. *Archives of Internal Medicine* 20:840-852.

Cullinan, E. R. 1938. Ulcerative colitis: clinic aspects. *British Medical Journal* 2:1351.

Dally, P. J. 1969. *Anorexia Nervosa*. New York: Grune and Stratton.

Daniels, G. E. 1940. Treatment of a case of ulcerative colitis associated with hysterical depression. *Psychosomatic Medicine* 2:276-285.

————. 1940. Psychiatric aspects of ulcerative colitis. *New England Journal of Medicine* 226:178-184.

Deutsch, F. 1923. Uber die Ursachen der Kreislaufstorungen bei den Herzneurosen. *Zeitschrift fur die gesamte experimentelle Medizin* 34:1, 2.

————. 1933. Studies in Pathogenesis: biological and psychological aspects. *Psychoanalytic Quarterly* 2:225-243.

————. 1939. The choice of organ in organ neuroses. *International Journal of Psycho-Analysis* 20:252-262.

Deutsch, H. 1925. Zur Psychogenese eines Tic Falles. *Internationale Zeitschrift für Psychoanalyse* 11:325-332.

————. 1929. The genesis of agoraphobia. *International Journal of Psycho-Analysis* 10:51-69.

Diethelm, O. 1930. Disturbances of vision and consciousness in petit mal attacks. *Human Biology* 2:547-554.

————. 1934. Epileptic convulsions and the personality setting. *Archives of Neurology and Psychiatry* 31:755-767.

————. 1947. Brief psychotherapeutic interviews in the treatment of epilepsy. *American Journal of Psychiatry* 103:806-810.

Doswald, D. D., and Kreibich, K. 1906. Zur Frage der posthypnotischen Hautphanomene. *Monatshefte f. prakt. Dermat.* 43:634-640.

Dunbar, H. F. 1938a. *Emotions and Bodily Changes*. New York: Columbia University Press.

――――. 1938b. Psychoanalytic notes relating to syndromes of asthma and hay fever. *Psychoanalytic Quarterly* 7:25-68.

――――. 1947. *Mind and Body: Psychosomatic Medicine.* New York: Random House.

Dunlap, J. R., 1960. A case of Gilles de la Tourette's disease (maladie des tics): a study of the intrafamily dynamics. *Journal of Nervous and Mental Diseases* 130:340-344.

Eisenberg, L.; Ascher, E.; and Kanner, L. 1959. A clinical study of Gilles de la Tourette's disease (maladie des tics) in children. *American Journal of Psychiatry* 115:715-723.

Elkish, P. 1947. A case of child tiqueur. *American Journal of Psychotherapy* 1:279-312.

Engel, G. L. 1955. Studies of ulcerative colitis: III. The nature of the psychobiologic processes. *American Journal of Medicine* 19:231.

――――. 1962. *Psychological Development in Health and Disease.* Philadelphia: Saunders.

Engel, G. L.; Hamburger, W. W.; Reiser, M.; and Plankett, J. 1953. Electroencephalographic and psychological studies of a case of migraine with severe pre-headache phenomena. *Psychosomatic Medicine* 15:337-348.

Engels, W. D., and Wittkower, E. 1970. Psychophysiological, allergic, and skin diseases. In *Comprehensive Textbook of Psychiatry*, ed. Freedman, Kaplan, and Sadok, pp. 1655-1693.

Escalona, S. K. 1954. Emotional development during the first year of life. In *Problems of Infancy and Childhood*, ed. M. J. E. Senn. New York: Josiah Macy Foundation.

Falstein, E. I. 1956. Anorexia nervosa in the male child. *American Journal of Orthopsychiatry* 26:751-772.

Federn, P. 1934. Personal communication.

Feldman, H. 1965. Zur Frage der Psychodynamischen Faktoren bei der Pubertamagersucht. In *Anorexia Nervosa*, ed. Meyer and Feldmann, pp. 103-107. Stuttgart: Georg Thieme.

Fenichel, O. 1931. Respiratory introjection. In *Collected Papers* 1:221-240. New York: Norton, 1953.

――――. 1943. The psychopathology of coughing. *Psychosomatic Medicine* 5:181-184.

――――. 1945a. Anorexia. In *Collected Papers* 2:228-295. New York: Norton, 1954.

――――. 1945b. Nature and classification of the so-called psychosomatic phenomena. *Psychoanalytic Quarterly* 14:287-312.

――――. 1945c. *The Psychoanalytic Theory of Neurosis.* New York: Norton.

Ferenczi, S. 1916. *Contributions of Psycho-Analysis.* Boston: Richard C. Badger.

—————. 1921. Psychoanalytic observations on tics. In *Further Contributions to the Theory and Technique of Psychoanalysis.* London: Hogarth, 1926.

—————. 1926. *Further Contributions to the Theory and Technique of Psycho-Analysis.* London: Hogarth.

—————. 1955. Ein Fall von déjà vu. *Final Contributions.* New York: Basic Books.

Finch, S. M. 1952. Psychosomatic problems in children. *Nervous Child* 9:261-269.

Finch, S. M., and Hess, J. H. 1962. Ulcerative colitis in children. *American Journal of Psychiatry* 118:819-826.

Frahm, H., 1965. Results of somatic treatment in anorexia nervosa. In *Anorexia Nervosa,* ed. Meyer and Feldmann, pp. 64-66. Stuttgart: Georg Thieme.

Freedman, D. A., and Adatto, C.P. 1968. On the precipitation of seizures in an adolescent boy. *Psychosomatic Medicine* 30:437-447.

Freedman, D. X.; Redlich, F. C.; and Igersheimer, W. W. 1956. Psychosis and allergy: experimental approach. 112:873-877.

French, T. M., and Alexander, F. 1941. Psychogenic factors in bronchial asthma. *American Journal of Psychiatry Monographs,* vol. 2 and 4. Washington: National Research Council.

Freud, A. 1928. Introduction to technique of child analysis. New York: Nervous and Mental Disease Publication Company.

—————. 1946. The psychoanalytic study of infantile feeding disturbances. *Psychoanalytic Study of the Child* 2:119-132.

Freud, A., and Burlingham, D. T. 1943. *War and Children.* New York: International Universities Press.

Freud, S. 1905a. Fragment of an analysis of a case of hysteria. *Standard Edition* 7:40 (1953).

—————. 1905b. Three essays on the theory of sexuality. *Standard Edition* 7:163-248 (1953).

—————. 1909. Analysis of a phobia in a five-year-old boy. *Standard Edition* 10:3-147.

—————. 1914. Fausse reconnaissance (déjà raconte) in psychoanalytic treatment. *Standard Edition* 14:201-209 (1957).

—————. 1915. The unconscious. *Standard Edition* 14:159-204 (1957).

—————. 1917. Mourning and melancholia. *Standard Edition* 14:237-260 (1957).

—————. 1928. Dostoevsky and parricide. *Standard Edition* 21:175-194 (1961).

Friedman, A. P.; Katz, J.; and Gisolfi, A. 1950. Psychologic factors of migraine in children. *New York State Journal of Medicine* 50:19, 2269-2270.

Fries, M. E. 1944. Psychosomatic relationship between mother and infant. *Psychosomatic Medicine* 6:159-162.

———. 1946. The child's ego development and the training of adults in his environment. *Psychoanalytic Study of the Child* 2:85-112.

Fromm-Reichmann, F. 1937. Contribution to the psychogenesis of migraine. *Psychoanalytic Review* 24:26-33.

Garma, A. 1959. Observations on the visual symptomatology in migraine. *Psychoanalytic Quarterly* 28:242-246.

Gerard, M. W. 1946a. Bronchial asthma in children. *Nervous Child* 5:327-331.

———. 1946b. The psychogenic tic in ego development. *Psychoanalytic Study of the Child* 2:133-162.

Gero, G. 1953. An equivalent of depression: anorexia. In *Affective Disorders*, ed. P. Greenacre, pp. 117-189. New York: International Universities Press.

Giovacchini, P. L. 1959. The ego and the psychosomatic state. *Psychosomatic Medicine* 21:218-227.

Giovacchini, P. L., and Muslin, H. 1965. Ego equilibrium and cancer of the breast. *Psychosomatic Medicine* 27:524-532.

Goitein, P. L. 1942. Potential prostitute: role of anorexia nervosa in defense against prostitution desires. *Journal of Criminal Psychopathology* 3:359-367.

Gottschalk, L. A. 1956. The relation of psychologic states and epileptic activity. *Psychoanalytic Study of the Child* 10: 352-380.

Graham, D. T., and Wolfe, S. 1950. Pathogenesis of urticaria. *Psychosomatic Medicine* 13:122.

Graven, P. S. 1924. Die aktive analytische Behandlung der Epilepsie. *Fortschr. Sexualwiss. Psychoanal.* 1:58-69.

Greenacre, P. 1941. The predisposition to anxiety. *Psychoanalytic Quarterly* 10:66-95.

———. 1944. Infant reactions to restraint: problems in the face of infantile aggression. *American Journal of Orthopsychiatry* 14:204-218.

Groddeck, G. W. 1923. *Das Buch vom Es: psychoanalytische Briefe an eine Freundin*. Vienna: Internationaler Psychoanalytischer Verlag.

Groen, J. J., and Feldman-Toledano, Z. 1966. Educative treatment of patients and parents in anorexia nervosa. *British Journal of Psychiatry* 112:671-681.

Groethuysen, H. C.; Robinson, D.; Haylett, C.; Estes, H. R.; and Johnson, A. M. 1957. Depth electrographic recording of a seizure during a structured interview. *Psychosomatic Medicine* 19:353.

Gull, W. W. 1874. Anorexia nervosa (apepsia hysterica, anorexia hysterica). *Transactions of the Clinical Society of London* 7:22-28.

————. 1888. Anorexia nervosa. *Lancet* 1:516-517.

Halliday, J. L. 1943. Principles of aetiology. *British Journal of Medical Psychology* 19:367-380.

Hallowitz, D. 1954. Residential treatment of chronic asthmatic children. j2American Journal of Orthopsychiatry 24:567-587.

Hamill, R. C. 1936. Petit mal in children. *American Journal of Psychiatry* 93:303-312.

Heilig, R., and Hoff, H. 1928. Uber psychogene Entstehung des Herpes Labialis. *Med. Klin.* 24:1472.

Heller, F., and Schultz, J. H. 1909. Uber einen Fall von Hypnotisch erzeugter Blasenbildung. *Munchen. Med. Wchnschr.* 56:2112.

Hendrick, I. 1940. Psychoanalytic observations on the aurae of two cases with convulsions. *Psychosomatic Medicine* 2:43-52.

Hug-Helmuth, H. von. 1919. *A Study of the Mental Life of the Child.* Washington: Nervous and Mental Diseases.

Hulse, W., and Rapoport, J. 1952. What can pediatrics expect from psychoanalysis? *Nervous Child* 9:270-277.

Jelliffe, S. E. 1933. Migraines. In *Encyclopedia of Medicine*, vol. 81. Philadelphia: David.

————. 1935. Dynamic concepts and the epileptic attack. *American Journal of Psychiatry* 92:565-574.

Jelliffe, S. E., and Evans, E. 1916. Psoriasis as an hysterical conversion symptom. *New York Medical Journal* 104:1077-1086.

Jelliffe, S. E., and White, W. A. 1915. *Diseases of the Nervous System.* Philadelphia and New York: Lea and Febiger.

Jessner, L. 1955. Emotional impact of nearness and separation for the asthmatic child and his mother. *Psychoanalytic Study of the Child* 10:353-375.

Jessner, L., and Abse, D. W. 1960. Regressive forces in anorexia nervosa. *British Journal of Medical Psychology* 33:301-311.

Johnson, A. M. 1946. A case of migraine. *The Proceedings of the Third Psychotherapy Council*, pp. 69-118, Chicago: Institute for Psychoanalysis.

Kardiner, A. 1932. *The Bio-Analysis of the Epileptic Reaction.* Albany, New York: Psychoanalytic Quarterly Press.

Kaufman, M. R., and Heiman, M., eds. 1964. *Evolution of Psychosomatic Concepts. Anorexia Nervosa: A Paradigm.* New York: International Universities Press.

Kay, D. W., and Shapiro, K. 1965. Prognosis in anorexia nervosa. In *Anorexia Nervosa*, ed. Meyer and Feldmann, pp. 113-117. Stuttgart: Georg Thieme.

Kerman, E. F. 1946. Bronchial asthma and affective psychoses: two cases treated with electric shock. *Psychosomatic Medicine* 8:53-57.

Klauder, J. V. 1936. Psychogenic aspects of skin diseases. *Journal of Nervous and Mental Diseases* 84:249-273.

Klein, H. S. 1949. Psychogenic factors in dermatitis and their treatment in group therapy. *British Journal of Medical Psychology* 22:32-52.

Kleitman, N. 1939. *Sleep and Wakefulness.* Chicago: University of Chicago Press.

Knapp, P. H. 1960. Acute bronchial asthma: II. Psychoanalytic observations of fantasy, emotional arousal and partial discharge. *Psychosomatic Medicine* 22:88-105.

————. 1963. The asthmatic child and the psychosomatic problem of asthma: toward a general theory. In *The Asthmatic Child,* ed. H. I. Schneer, pp. 234-255. New York: Harper and Row.

Knapp, P. H., and Nemetz, S. J. 1957. Sources of tension in bronchial asthma. *Psychosomatic Medicine* 19:466-485.

Knapp, P. H.; Nemetz, S. J.; Gilbert, R. R.; Lowell, F. C.; and Michelson, A. L. 1957. Personality variations in bronchial asthma. *Psychosomatic Medicine* 19:442-465.

Knopf, O. 1935. Preliminary report on personality studies in thirty migraine patients. *Journal of Nervous and Mental Diseases* 82:270-285.

Korelitz, B. I. 1964. Ulcerative colitis in children. *New York State Journal of Medicine* 64:1851-1856.

Korelitz, B. I., and Gribetz, D. 1962. The prognosis of ulcerative colitis with onset in childhood: II. The steroid era. *Annals of Internal Medicine* 57:592-597.

Kovacs, V. 1925. Analyse eines Falles von Tic convulsif. *Internationale Zeitschrift fur Psychoanalyse* 2:318-327.

Krug, O.; Hayward, H.; and Crumpacker, B. 1952. Intensive residential treatment of a 9-year old girl with an aggressive behavior disorder, petit mal and enuresis. *American Journal of Orthopsychiatry* 22:405-427.

Kulovesi, Y. 1929. Zur Enstehung des Tics. *Internationale Zeitschrift fur Psychoanalyse* 15:82-85.

Lamont, J. H. 1963. Which children outgrow asthma and which do not? In *The Asthmatic Child,* ed. H. I. Schneer, pp. 16-26. New York: Harper and Row.

Leonard, C. E. 1944. An analysis of a case of functional vomiting and bulimia. *Psychoanalytic Review* 31:1-18.

Levy, D. M. 1944. On the problem of movement restraint: Tics, stereotyped movements, hyperactivity. *American Journal of Orthopsychiatry* 14:644-671.

Lidz, T.; Carter, M.D.; Lewis, B. I.; and Suratt, C. 1952. Effects of ACTH and cortisone on mood and mentation. *Psychosomatic Medicine* 14:366-377.

Lieberman, M., and Lipton, E. 1963. Asthma in identical twins. In *The Asthmatic Child*, ed. H. I. Schneer, pp. 58-74. New York: Harper and Row.

Long, R. T.; Lamont, J. H.; Whipple, B.; Baudler, H.; Blom, J. E.; Burgin, L.; and Jessner, L. 1958. A psychosomatic study of allergic and emotional factors in children with asthma. *American Journal of Psychiatry* 114:890-899.

Lorand, S. 1936. Psychogenic factors in a case of angioneurotic edema. *Journal of Mount Sinai Hospital* 2:231-236.

———. 1943. Anorexia nervosa: case. *Psychosomatic Medicine* 5:282-292.

Lynn, H. B. 1965. Early surgery urged in childhood colitis. *Medical Tribune*, March 3, p. 1.

McDermott, J. F., and Finch, S. M. 1967. Ulcerative colitis in children: reassessment of a dilemma. *Journal of the American Academy of Child Psychiatry* 6:512-525.

MacDonald, I. J. 1963. A case of Gilles de la Tourette syndrome with some etiological observations. *British Journal of Psychiatry* 109:206-210.

MacKay, M. C., and Heimlich, E. P. 1972. Case report: psychotherapy with paraverbal therapy in a case of Gilles de la Tourette syndrome. *American Journal of Psychotherapy* 26:571-577.

MacKenzie, J. N. 1886. The production of "rose asthma" by an artificial rose. *American Journal of Medical Science* 91:45-57.

Maeder, A. 1909. Sexualitat und Epilepsie. *Jahrb. fur Psychoanalysche Psychopath. Forsch.* 1:119-154.

Mahler, M. S. 1949. A psychoanalytic evaluation of tic in psychopathology of children: symptomatic and tic syndrome. *Psychoanalytic Study of the Child* 3/4:285-300.

Mahler, M. S., and Gross, I. 1945. Psychotherapeutic study of a typical case with tic syndrome. *Nervous Child* 4:358-373.

Mahler, M. S., and Rangell, L. 1943. A psychosomatic study of maladie des tics. *Psychoanalytic Quarterly* 17:579-603.

Margolis, P. M., and Jenberg, A. 1960. Analytic therapy in a case of extreme anorexia. *British Journal of Medical Psychology* 33:291-300.

Marsh, C. A. 1920. A psychological theory of the cause of epilepsy. *American Journal of Medical Science* 159:450-458.

Maslow, A. H., and Mittelmann, B. 1951. *Principles of Abnormal Psychology*. New York: Harper and Brothers.

Mason, J. W.; Walle, J. H.; Nauta; Brady, J.V.; Robinson, J. A.; and Thache, J. S. 1960. Limbic system influences on the pituitary adrenal cortical system, abstr. *Psychosomatic Medicine* 22:322.

―――. 1963. Psychoendocrine differentiation of emotional responses in the monkey. *Proceedings of Research in Nervous Mental Diseases.*

―――. 1963. Comments on the psychoendocrine approach to psychosomatic research. Discussion in *Proceedings 44th Conference on Pediatric Research.* Columbus, Ohio.

Masserman, J. H. 1941. Psychodynamisms in anorexia nervosa and neurotic vomiting. *Psychoanalytic Quarterly* 10:211-242.

Mayr, J. K. 1927. Psychogenese von Hautkrankheiten. *Zentrabl. f. Haut-u. Geschlechtskr* 23:1-22.

Meige, H., and Feindel, E. 1907. *Tics and Their Treatment.* London: Appelton.

Menninger, K. A. 1926. Psychoanalytic study of a case of organic epilepsy. *Psychoanalytic Review* 13:187-199.

―――. 1934. Some unconscious psychological factors associated with the common cold. *Psychoanalytic Review* 2:201-207.

Menninger, W. C. 1926. the treatment of angioneurotic edema. *Journal of the Medical Society of New Jersey* 23:68-71.

Miller, H., and Baruch, D. 1948. Psychosomatic studies of children with allergic manifestations. *Psychosomatic Medicine* 10:275-278.

Miller, M. L. 1942. A psychological study of a case of eczema and a case of neurodermatitis. *Psychosomatic Medicine* 4:82-93.

―――. 1948. Psychodynamic mechanisms in a case of neurodermatitis. *Psychosomatic Medicine* 10:310-316.

Millman, D. H. 1960. Multiple tics. *American Journal of Psychiatry* 116:955-956.

Mittelmann, B. 1947a. Psychoanalytic observations on skin disorders. *Bulletin of the Menninger Clinic* 11:169-176.

―――. 1947b. Psychopathology of epilepsy. In *Epilepsy,* ed. P. H. Hoch and R. P. Knight, pp. 136-148. New York: Grune and Stratton.

Mirsky, I. A. 1958. Physiologic, psychologic, and social determinants in the etiology of duodenal ulcer. *American Journal Digest* 3:285-314.

Moersch, F. P. 1924. Psychic manifestations in migraine. *American Journal of Psychology* 3:697-715.

Mohr, G. J.; Tausend, H.; Selesnick, S.; and Augenbrand, B. 1963. Studies of eczema and asthma in the preschool child. *Journal of Child Psychiatry* 2:271-291.

Mohr, G. J.; Josselyn, I. M.; Spurlock, J.; and Barron, S. H. 1958. Studies in ulcerative colitis in children. *American Journal of Psychiatry* 114:1067-107

396 References

Monsour, K. 1960. Ulcerative colitis, migraine, and abortion. Read at Meeting of the American Psychoanalytic Association in Atlantic City, N. J.

Moos, R. H., and Solomon, G. F. 1965. Psychologic comparisons between women with rheumatoid arthritis and their nonarthritic sisters: I & II. *Psychosomatic Medicine* 27:135-149.

Mueller, H. L. 1961. The dangers and consequences of steroid therapy in children. *New York State Journal of Medicine* 61:2743-2749.

Muralt, L. 1902. Zur frage der epileptischen Amnesien. *Zeitschrift fur Hypnotismus* 10:75-90.

Murray, C. D. 1930a. A brief psychological analysis of a patient with ulcerative colitis. *Journal of Nervous and Mental Diseases* 72:617-627.

———. 1930b. Psychogenic factors in the etiology of ulcerative colitis and bloody diarrhea. *American Journal of Medical Science* 180:239-248.

Musaph, H.; Prakken, J. R.; and Bastians, J. 1964. *Itching and Scratching: Psychodynamics in Dermatology.* New York: S. Karger, Bassel.

Needles, W. 1943. Stigmata occurring in the course of psychoanalysis. *Psychoanalytic Quarterly* 12:23-39.

Neuhaus, E. C. 1958. A personality study of asthmatic and cardiac children. *Psychosomatic Medicine* 20:181-186.

Niederland, W. 1959. Schreber: father and son. *Psychoanalytic Quarterly* 28:151-169.

Noyes, A. P., and Kolb, L. 1958. *Modern Clinical Psychiatry.* Philadelphia: W. B. Saunders.

Oberholzer, E. 1914. The role of the unpleasure motive in epileptic amnesia and its cure. *Psych.-Neur. Wochenschrift* 16:128-131.

Obendorf, C. P. 1912. Disappearance of angio-neurotic edema after appendectomy. *Journal of the American Medical Association.* 59:623.

O'Donovan, W. J. 1927. *Dermatological Neuroses.* Kegan Paul, Trench Trubner.

Pacella, B. L. 1944-1945. Physiologic and differential diagnostic considerations of tic manifestations in children. *Nervous Child* 4:313-317.

Palmer, H. A. 1939. Beriberi complicating anorexia nervosa. *Lancet* 1:269.

Patterson, M., 1945. Spasmodic torticollis. *Lancet* 249:556-559.

Peshkin, M. M. 1963. Diagnosis of asthma in children: past and present. In *The Asthmatic Child,* ed. H. I. Schneer, pp. 1-15. New York: Harper and Row.

Portis, S. A. 1949. Idiopathic ulcerative colitis: newer concepts concerning its cause and management. *Journal of American Medical Association* 139:208-214.

Prugh, D. G. 1959. Variations in attitudes, behavior and feeling states as exhibited in the play of children during modifications in the course of ulcerative colitis. *Proceedings of the Association for Research in Nervous and Mental Disease* 29:692-705.

———. 1951a. The role of emotional factors in idiopathic celiac disease. *Psychosomatic Medicine* 13:220-241.

———. 1951b. The influence of emotional factors on the clinical course of ulcerative colitis in children. *Gastroenterology* 18:339-354.

Purcell, K.; Bernstein, L.; and Bukantz, S. 1961. A preliminary comparison of rapidly remitting and persistently steroid-dependent asthmatic children. *Psychosomatic Medicine* 23:305-314.

Rank, B. 1948. Significance of "emotional climate" in early feeding difficulties. *Psychosomatic Medicine* 10:279-283.

Rapoport, J. 1959. Maladie des tics in children. *American Journal of Psychiatry* 116:177-178.

Reich, W. 1925. Der Psychogene Tic als Onanie Aequivalent. *Internationale Zeitschrift fur Psychoanalyse* 17:263-275.

———. 1931. Uber den epileptischen Anfall. *Internationale Zeitschrift fur Psychoanalyse* 17:263-275.

Ribble, M. 1936. Ego dangers and epilepsy. *Psychoanalytic Quarterly* 5:263-275.

———. 1944. *The Rights of Infants.* New York: Columbia University Press.

Richmond, J. B.; Lipton, E. I.; and Steinschneider, A. 1962. Autonomic functions in the neonate. V. *Psychosomatic Medicine* 24:66-74.

Richter, H. E. 1965. Die dialogische Function der Magersucht. In *Anorexia Nervosa*, ed. Meyer and Feldmann, pp. 108-112. Stuttgart: Georg Thieme.

Ricklin, F. 1903. Zur Anwendund der Hypnose bei epileptische Anfallen. *Journal fur Psychoanalyse und Neurologie* 2:28-30.

Ritvo, S. 1944-1945. Survey of the recent literature on tics in children. *Nervous Child* 4:308-312.

Riviere, J. 1936. On the genesis of psychical conflict in earliest infancy. *International Journal of Psycho-Analysis* 17:395-422.

Rogerson, C. H.; Hardcastle, D. H.; and Duguid, K. 1935. A psychological approach to the problem of asthma and the asthma-eczema-prurigo syndrome. *Guy's Hosp. Rep. 85:289-308.*

Rose, A. G. 1954. Angio-neurosis and hypnosis. *British Journal of Medical Hypnotism* 6:43-50.

Sack, W. T. 1925. Die Haut als Ausdrucksorgan. *Arch. f. Dermat. u. Syph.* 151:200-206. 14.

Sadger, J. 1911a. Is bronchial asthma a sexual neurosis? *Zentralbl. fur psychoanlyse und Psychotherapy* 1:200-213.

Sargent, W. 1951. Leucotomy in psychosomatic disorders. *Lancet* 261:87-91.

Saul, L. J. 1935. A note on the psychogenesis of organic symptoms. *Psychoanalytic Quarterly* 4:476-483.

———. 1938. Psycho-genic factors in the etiology of the common cold. *International Journal of Psycho-Analysis* 19:451-470.

Saul, L. J., and Bernstein, C. 1941. The emotional settings of some attacks of urticaria. *Psychosomatic Medicine* 3:349-369.

Saul, L. J., and Lyons, J. W. 1955. Motivation and respiratory disorders. In *Recent Developments in Psychosomatic Medicine*, ed. E. D. Wittkower and R. A. Cleghorn, pp. 267-280. Philadelphia: Lippincott.

Scarborough, L. F. 1948. Neurodermatitis from the psychosomatic viewpoint. *Diseases of the Nervous System* 9:90-93.

Schick, A. 1949. A contribution to the psychopathology of genuine epilepsy. *Psychoanalytic Review* 36:217-239.

Schilder, P. 1928. *Introduction to a Psychoanalytic Psychiatry*. Nervous and Mental Diseases Monograph Series, No. 50. New York: Nervous and Mental Disease Publishing.

———. 1936. Remarks on the psychophysiology of the skin. *Psychoanalytic Review* 23:274-285.

Schindler, R. 1927. *Nervensystem und Spontane Blutungen*. Abh. aus d. Neur., Psychiatrie, Psychologie und ihren Grenzgebieten, Monograph No. 42. Berlin: S. Karger.

Schmale, A. H., Jr. 1958. Relationship of separation and depression to disease: I. *Psychosomatic Medicine* 20:259-277.

Schneck, J. M. 1960. Gilles de la Tourette's disease. *American Journal of Psychiatry* 117:70.

Schneer, H. I. 1963. The death of an asthmatic child. In *The Asthmatic Child*, ed. H. I. Schneer, pp. 166-181. New York: Harper and Row.

Schur, M. 1955. Comments on the metapsychology of somatization. *Psychoanalytic Study of the Child* 10:119-164.

Scott, D. 1969. *About Epilepsy*. New York: International Universities Press.

Scott, M. J. 1960. *Hypnosis in Skin and Allergic Disease*. Springfield, Illinois: Charles C Thomas.

Seitz, P. F. D. 1949. An experimental approach to psychocutaneous problems. *Journal of Investigative Dermatology* 13:199-205.

———. 1953. Experiments in the substitution of symptoms by hypnosis. *Psychosomatic Medicine* 15:405-424.

Selesnick, S. T., and Sperber, Z. 1965. The problem of the eczema-asthma complex: a developmental approach. In *Psychoanalysis and Current Biological Thought*, ed. N. S. Greenfield and W. C. Lewis. Madison: University of Wisconsin Press.

Selinsky, H. 1939. Psychological study of the migrainous syndrome. *Bulletin, New York Academy of Medicine* 15:757-763.

Selvini, M. 1965. Interpretation of mental anorexia. In *Anorexia Nervosa,* ed. Meyer and Feldmann, pp. 96-103. Stuttgart: Georg Theime.

Shanahan, W. T. 1928. Convulsions in infancy and their relationship, if any, to a subsequent epilepsy. *American Journal of Psychiatry* 7:591-606.

Shirley, H. 1948. *Psychiatry for the Pediatrician.* New York: Commonwealth Fund.

Simmel, E. 1932. The psychogenesis of organic disturbances and their psychoanalytic treatment. *Psychoanalytic Quarterly* 1:166-170.

———. 1933. Pregenital primacy and intestinal stage of the libido organization. *Internationale Zeitschrift fur psychoanalyse* 19:245-246.

———. 1944. Self-preservation and the death instinct. *Psychoanalytic Quarterly* 13:160-185.

Singer, K. 1963. Gilles de la Tourette's disease. *American Journal of Psychiatry* 120:80-81.

Socarides, C. W. 1954. Psychologic factors in angioneurotic edema of the pharynx. *U.S. Armed Forces Medical Journal* 5:6.

Solomon, G. F., and Moos, R. H. 1965. The relationship of personality to the presence of rheumatoid factors in asymptomatic relatives of patients with rheumatoid arthritis. *Psychosomatic Medicine* 27:350-360.

Sontag, L. 1944. Differences in modifiability of fetal behavior and physiology. *Psychosomatic Medicine* 65:151-154.

Sours, J. 1969. Anorexia nervosa: nosology, diagnosis, developmental patterns and power control dynamics. In *Adolescence,* ed. G. Caplan and S. Lebovici, pp. 185-212. New York: Basic Books.

Sperling, E. 1965. The magersucht Familie und Ihre Behandlung. In *Anorexia Nervosa,* ed. Meyer and Feldmann, pp. 156-160. Stuttgart: Georg Thieme.

Sperling, M. 1948. Diarrhea: a specific somatic equivalent of an unconscious emotional conflict. *Psychosomatic Medicine* 10:331-334.

———. 1949. Neurotic sleep disturbances in children. *Nervous Child* 8:28-46.

———. 1950a. Children's interpretation and reaction to the unconscious of their mothers. *International Journal of Psycho-Analysis* 31:1-6. (*See also* M. Sperling, 1974, chapter 3.)

———. 1950b. A contribution to the psychodynamics of depression in women. *Samiksa* 4:86-101.

———. 1950b. Enuresis: In a seminar on psychiatric problems in the practice of medicine. *Jewish Hospital of Brooklyn* 8-17.

———. 1950d. Indirect treatment of psychoneurotic and psychosomatic disorders in children. *Quarterly Journal of Child Behavior* 2:250-

266. (*See also* M. Sperling, 1974, chapter 2.)

———. 1950e. Psychosomatic diseases in children: In a seminar on psychiatric problems in the practice of medicine. *Jewish Hospital of Brooklyn* 1-8.

———. 1950f. The structure of envy in depressions of women. In *Feminine Psychology*, pp. 17-23. New York Medical College, Symposium Proceedings.

———. 1951. The neurotic child and his mother. *American Journal of Orthopsychiatry* 21: 351-364.

———. 1952a. Animal phobias in a two-year-old child. *Psychoanalytic Study of the Child* 7:115-125. (*See also* M. Sperling, 1974, chapter 9.)

———. 1952b. Psychotherapeutic techniques in psychosomatic medicine. *Specialized Techniques in Psychotherapy*, ed. G. Bychowski and J. Despert, pp. 279-301. New York: Basic Books.

———. 1953. Food allergies and conversion hysteria. *Psychoanalytic Quarterly* 22:525-538.

———. 1954. The use of the hair as a bi-sexual symbol. *Psychoanalytic Review* 41:363-365.

———. 1955a. Etiology and treatment of sleep disturbances in children. *Psychoanalytic Quarterly* 24:358-368.

———. 1955b. Observations from the treatment of children suffering from non-bloody diarrhea or mucous colitis. *Journal of Hillside Hospital* 4:25-31.

———. 1955c. Psychosis and psychosomatic illness. *International Journal of Psycho-Analysis* 36:320-327.

———. 1957. The psychoanalytic treatment of ulcerative colitis. *International Journal of Psycho-Analysis* 38:341-349.

———. 1958. Pavor nocturnus. *Journal of the American Psychoanalytic Association* 6:79-94.

———. 1959a. Current concepts of ulcerative disease of the gastrointestinal tract. *New York State Journal of Medicine* 59:3800-3806.

———. 1959b. Equivalents of depression in children. *Journal of Hillside Hospital* 8:138-148. (*See also* M. Sperling, 1974, chapter 23.)

———. 1959c. Psychiatric aspects of ulcerative colitis. *New York State Journal of Medicine* 59:3801-3806.

———. 1959d. A study of deviate sexual behavior in children by the method of simultaneous analysis of mother and child. *Dynamic Psychopathology in Childhood*, ed. L. Jessner and E. Pavenstedt, pp. 221-242. New York: Grune and Stratton. (*See also* M. Sperling, 1974, chapter 13.)

———. 1960a. The psychoanalytic treatment of a case of chronic regional ileitis. *International Journal of Psycho-Analysis* 41:612-618.

————. 1960b. Symposium on disturbances of the digestive tract II: Unconscious phantasy life and object-relationships in ulcerative colitis. *International Journal of Psycho-Analysis* 41:450-455.

————. 1961a. Analytic first aid in school phobia. *Psychoanalytic Quarterly* 30:504-518. (*See also* M. Sperling, 1974, chapter 8.)

————. 1961b. A note on some dream symbols and the significance of their changes during analysis. *Journal of Hillside Hospital* 10:161-266. (*See also* M. Sperling, 1974, chapter 6.)

————. 1964a. The analysis of a boy with transvestite tendencies. *Psychoanalytic Study of the Child* 19:470-493. (*See also* M. Sperling, 1974, chapter 14.)

————. 1964b. A case of ophidiophilia: a clinical contribution to snake symbolism, and a supplement to a "psychoanalytic study of ulcerative colitis in children." *International Journal of Psycho-Analysis* 45:227-233.

————. 1964c. Dynamic considerations and treatment of enuresis. *Journal of American Academy of Child Psychiatry* 4:19-31. (*See also* M. Sperling, 1974, chapter 17.)

————. 1965a. Psychosomatic disorders. *Tokyo Journal of Psychoanalysis* 23:202-216.

————. 1965b. Ulcerative colitis in adolescent girls. Paper read in part at the Symposium on Adolescence, Georgetown University, Washington, D.C.

————. 1967a. Pregenital fixations and somatic symptomatology in phobias. Paper read at the Fall Meeting of the American Psychoanalytic Association, New York.

————. 1967b. School phobias: classification, dynamics and treatment. *Psychoanalytic Study of the Child* 22:375-401. (*See also* M. Sperling, 1974, chapter 7.)

————. 1967c. Transference neurosis in patients with psychosomatic disorders. *Psychoanalytic Quarterly* 36:342-355.

————. 1968a. Acting-out behavior and psychosomatic symptoms: clinical and theoretical aspects. *International Journal of Psycho-Analysis* 49:250-253.

————. 1968b. Psychologic desensitization of allergy. *Bulletin of the New York Academy of Medicine* 44:587-591.

————. 1968c. Trichotillomania, trichophagy and cyclic vomiting: a contribution to the psychopathology of female sexuality. *International Journal of Psycho-Analysis* 49:250-253.

————. 1969a. Migraine headaches, altered states of consciousness and accident proneness: a clinical contribution to the death instinct theory. In *Psychoanalytic Forum*, ed. J. Lindon, pp. 69-100. New York: Jason Aronson.

————. 1969b. Sleep disturbances in children. In *Modern Perspectives in International Child Psychiatry*, ed. J. Howells, pp. 418-454. Edinburgh: Oliver and Boyde. (*See also* M. Sperling, 1974, chapter 4.)

————. 1970. The clinical effects of parental neurosis on the child. In *Parenthood*, ed. E. Anthony and T. Benedek, pp. 539-569. New York: Little, Brown. (*See also* M. Sperling, 1974, chapter 1.)

————. 1973. Conversion hysteria and conversion symptoms: a revision of classification and concepts. *Journal of the American Psychoanalytic Association* 21:772-787.

————. 1974. *The Major Neuroses and Behavior Disorders in Children*. New York: Jason Aronson.

Sperling, O. 1944. On appersonation. *International Journal of Psycho-Analysis* 25:128-132.

————. 1950. Interpretation of the trauma as command. *Psychoanalytic Quarterly* 19:352-370.

Spitz, R. 1945. Hospitalism: an inquiry. *Psychoanalytic Study of the Child* 1:53-74.

————. 1946. Anaclitic depression. *Psychoanalytic Study of the Child* 2:313-342.

————. 1951. The psychogenic diseases in infancy, an attempt at their etiologic classification. *Psychoanalytic Study of the Child* 6:255-278.

Stahl, G. E. 1702. De medicina medicinae necessaria. Quoted from G. Zilboorg, *A History of Medical Psychology*. New York: W. W. Norton, 1941.

Stekel, W. 1924. Der epileptische Symptomenkomplex und seine Behandlung. *Fortschr. Sexualwiss. Psychoanal.* 1:17-57.

Sterba, E. 1949. Analysis of a psychogenic constipation in a two-year old. *Psychoanalytic Study of the Child* 3/4:227-252.

Stern, F. 1922. Zur Frage der psychogenen Dermatosen. *Zeitschrift fur die gesamte Neurologie und Psychiatrie* 79:218-253.

Sullivan, A. J. 1932. Ulcerative colitis of psychogenic origin. A report of six cases. *Yale Journal of Biology and Medicine* 4:779-796.

Swanton, C. 1947. Asthma and other psycho-physical interrelations. *Medical Journal of Australia* 1:138-145.

Sydenham, A. 1946. Amenorrhea at Stanley Camp, Hong Kong, during internment. *British Medical Journal* 2:159.

Sylvester, E. 1945. Analysis of psychogenic anorexia in a four-year-old child. *Psychoanalytic Study of the Child* 1:167-188.

Szollosy, L. von. 1907. Ein Fall von multipler neurotischer Hautgangran in ihrer Beziehung zur Hypnose. *Munchener Medizinische Wochenschrift* 54:34-35.

Taipale, V.; et al. 1971. Anorexia nervosa: an illness of two generations. *Acta Paedopsyca* 38:1, 21-25.

———. 1972. Anorexia nervosa in boys. *Psychosomatics* 13:236-240.

Thoma, H. 1967. *Anoerxia Nervosa*. Trans. G. Brydme. New York: International Universities Press.

Tolstrup, K. 1965. Die Charakteristika der juengen faelle von Anorexia Nervosa. In *Anorexia Nervosa*, ed. Meyer and Feldmann, pp. 51-59. Stuttgart: Georg Thieme.

Touraine, G. A., and Draper, G. 1934. The migrainous patient. *Journal of Nervous and Mental Disease* 80:183-201.

Trowbridge, L. S.; Cushman, D.; Gray, M. G.; and Moore, M. 1943. Notes on the personality of patients with migraine. *Journal of Nervous and Mental Diseases* 97:509-517.

Tucker, W. L. 1952. Lobotomy case histories: ulcerative colitis and anorexia nervosa. *Lahey Clinic Bulletin* 7:239-243.

Waller, J. V. 1942. Anorexia nervosa: psychosomatic entity. *Psychosomatic Medicine* 2:3-16.

Walsh, P. J. 1962. Compulsive shouting and Gilles de la Tourette's disease. *British Journal of Clinical Practice* 16:651-655.

Weber, H. 1932. The psychological factor in migraine. *British Journal of Medical Psychology* 12:151-173.

Weiss, E. 1923. Psychoanalysis of a case of nervous asthma. *International Journal of Psycho-Analysis* 4:3-66.

Weiss, E., and English, O. 1949. *Psychosomatic Medicine*. Philadelphia: Saunders.

Werther, J. 1911. Uber hysterische Hautnekrose mit erythematosem und exsudativem Vorstadium. *Dermat. Ztschr.* 18:341-348.

———. 1929. Die psychogenen Dermatosen. *Ztschr. f. arztl. Fortbild.* 26:341-346.

White, B. V.; Cobb, S.; and Jones, C. M. 1939. *Mucous Colitis, A Psychological Medical Study of Sixty Cases*. Psychosomatic Medicine Monograph No. 1. Washington, D.C.: National Research Council.

Wilder, J. 1946. Tic convulsif as a psychosomatic problem. *Nervous Child* 5:365-371.

Wilson, G. 1934. Typical personality trends and conflicts in cases of spastic colitis. *Psychoanalytic Quarterly* 3:558-573.

Winnicott, D. W. 1966. Psycho-somatic illness in its positive and negative aspects. *International Journal of Psycho-Analysis* 47:510-516.

Wittels, F. 1924. Eine Epilepsie-Analyse. *Fortschr. Sexualwiss. Psychoanal.* 1:178-199.

———. 1940. Phantom formation in a case of epilsepsy. *Psychoanalytic Quarterly* 9:98-107.

Wittkower, E. 1938. Ulcerative colitis: personality studies. *British Medical Journal* 2:1356-1360.

Wittkower, E., and Russel, B. 1953. Emotional factors in skin disease. New York: Hoeber.

Wolff, E. W., and Bayer, L. M. 1952. Psychosomatic disorders of childhood and adolescence. *American Journal of Orthopsychiatry* 22:510-521.

Wolff, H. G. 1937. Personality features and reactions of subjects with migraine. *Archives of Neurology and Psychiatry* 36:895-921.

Wood, A. 1856. On the nervous element in inflammation and its influence on treatment. *Edinburgh Medical Journal* 1:586-605.

Woodhead, B. 1946. The psychological aspect of allergic skin reactions in childhood. *Arch. Dis. Childhood* 21:98-105.

———. 1955. The eczema-asthma syndrome: psychiatric considerations. *British Journal of Dermatology* 67:50-52.

Wulff, M. 1932. An interesting oral symptom complex and its relation to addiction. *Internationale Zeitschrift fur Psychoanalyse* 18:281-301.

Acknowledgments

The authors wish to thank the publishers of the books and periodicals enumerated below for permission to reprint the following articles:

Chapter 2: Problems in the analysis of children with psychosomatic disorders. *Quarterly Journal of Child Behavior* 1(1949): 12-17.

Chapter 3: The role of the mother in psychosomatic disorders in children. *Psychosomatic Medicine* 11(1949): 377-385. Published by Paul B. Hoeber, Inc.

Chapter 4: Psychosomatic medicine and pediatrics. In *Recent Developments in Psychosomatic Medicine*, ed. Eric D. Wittkower and R.A. Cleghorn, pp. 381-396. London: Pitman, 1954.

Chapter 5: Psychosomatic disorders in adolescents. In *Adolescents: Psychoanalytic Approach to Problems and Therapy*, ed. S. Lorand and H. Schneer, pp. 202-216. New York: Hoeber, 1961.

Chapter 6: Ulcerative colitis in children: current views and therapies. *Journal of the American Academy of Child Psychiatry* 8(1969): 336-352.

Chapter 7: Psychoanalytic study of ulcerative colitis in children. *Psychoanalytic Quarterly* 15(1949): 302-329.

Chapter 8: Observations from the treatment of children suffering from non-bloody diarrhea or mucous colitis. *Journal of the Hillside Hospital* 4(1955): 25-31.

Chapter 9: Psychogenic diarrhea and phobia in a six-and-a-half-year-old girl. In *Case Studies in Childhood Emotional Disabilities*, ed. George E. Gardner. New York: American Orthopsychiatric Association, 1953.

Chapter 10: Mucous colitis associated with phobias. *Psychoanalytic Quarterly* 19(1950): 318-326.

Chapter 14: Asthma in children: an evaluation of concepts and therapies. *Journal of the American Academy of Child Psychiatry* 7(1968): 44-58.

Chapter 15: A psychoanalytic study of bronchial asthma in children. In *The Asthmatic Child*, ed. H. Schneer, pp. 138-165. New York: Harper, 1963.

Chapter 18: Contains excerpts from A psychoanalytic study of migraine and psychogenic headache (*The Psychoanalytic Review* 39: 152-163, 1952) and A further contribution to the psychoanalytic study of migraine and psychogenic headaches (*The International Journal of Psycho-Analysis* 45: 549-557, 1964).

Chapter 20: Psychodynamics and treatment of petit mal in children. *International Journal of Psycho-Analysis* 34(1953): 248-252.

Chapter 25: Analysis of a case of recurrent ulcer of the leg. *Psychoanalytic Study of the Child* 3/4(1949): 391-407.

The preface and chapters 1, 22 and 23 were written by Otto E. Sperling. The introduction and chapters 11, 12, 13, 17, 18, 19, 21, and 24 were written by Melitta Sperling specifically for this book.

Index